CONTEMPORARY ENDOCRINOLOGY

Series Editor
P. Michael Conn, PhD
Oregon Health & Science University
Beaverton, OR

For other titles published in this series, go to
www.springer.com/series/7680

Nanette F. Santoro · Genevieve Neal-Perry
Editors

Amenorrhea

A Case-Based, Clinical Guide

Humana Press

Editors
Nanette F. Santoro
Department of Obstetrics and Gynecology
University of Colorado Denver School
of Medicine
Aurora, CO, USA
Nanette.Santoro@ucdenver.edu

Genevieve Neal-Perry
Department of Obstetrics and Gynecology
Division of Reproductive Endocrinology
and Infertility
Albert Einstein College of Medicine
Bronx, NY, USA
Sienna3598@aol.com

ISBN 978-1-60327-863-8 e-ISBN 978-1-60327-864-5
DOI 10.1007/978-1-60327-864-5
Springer New York Dordrecht Heidelberg London

Library of Congress Control Number: 2010936295

Printed on acid-free paper

Springer is part of Springer Science+Business Media (www.springer.com)

Preface

Female reproductive success relies upon coordinated interactions among the hypothalamus, the pituitary, and the ovaries and the subsequent hormonal priming of the endometrium for implantation. The absence of oocyte fertilization or the failure of embryo implantation results in ovarian hormone withdrawal, the onset of menses, and the beginning of the next reproductive cycle. Failure of any single organ in the quartet to play its part can result in amenorrhea.

Although amenorrhea is a common problem that affects up to 10% of reproductive aged women, there has not been a major textbook solely dedicated to this clinical problem for more than 20 years. The main purpose of this first edition of *Amenorrhea: A Case-Based Clinical Guide* was to organize a comprehensive review that updates clinicians on our current knowledge regarding normal female reproductive physiology and to discuss the pathophysiology, diagnostic algorithms, and therapeutic intervention for amenorrhea. With this principal goal, we have invited several world experts on female reproductive physiology to provide clinicians with highly practical information regarding the epidemiology and management of amenorrhea. To that end, the content of this textbook has been divided into three sections; the first section is composed of two chapters that provide a comprehensive updated review on our basic science and clinical knowledge about the organ systems responsible for normal physiology of the menstrual cycle. This section focuses on the roles of the endometrium and the hypothalamic–pituitary–ovarian axis in the menstrual cycle. The second section includes discussions about menstrual cycle disruption as it relates to hypothalamic–pituitary dysfunction, surgical and natural menopause, genetic defects, premature ovarian failure/insufficiency, and the effects of caloric excess and restriction. The third section of this book provides an update on the physiological effects of prolonged amenorrhea induced surgically or by hypothalamic dysfunction. The third section also includes an original chapter that focuses solely on the impact of race and ethnicity on the prevalence and diagnosis of amenorrhea. When appropriate, we have also created clinical scenarios and management plans that readers may be confronted with in their daily practice.

We would like to express our deep gratitude to our incredibly supportive administrative staff, Karen Knickens and Elizabeth Abbate, without whose determined efforts this project could not have been completed. We would also like to thank all of the contributors to this book for their diligence and outstanding efforts to update clinicians on the physiology of the menstrual cycle and pathophysiology and the clinical consequences of amenorrhea. We hope that the readers will find this book to be a complete resource for information regarding amenorrhea and that this book will be a well-used reference for doctors and other health professionals who care for women.

Nanette F. Santoro and Genevieve Neal-Perry

Contents

Contributors

Jonathan S. Berek MD, MMS
Department of Obstetrics & Gynecology, Stanford University Hospital and Clinics, 300 Pasteur Drive Room HH333, Stanford, CA 94305-5317, USA

Sarah L. Berga MD
Department of Gynecology and Obstetrics, Emory University, 1639 Pierce Drive, Suite 4208-WMB, Atlanta, GA 30322, USA

Enrico Carmina MD
Department of Medical and Biological Sciences, University of Palermo, Via delle Croci 47, 90139 Palermo, Italy

Amber R. Cooper MD
Department of Obstetrics and Gynecology Division of Reproductive Endocrinology and Infertility, Washington University School of Medicine, St. Louis, MO, USA

Sharon N. Covington MSW
Integrative Reproductive Medicine Unit, Intramural Research Program on Reproductive and Adult Endocrinology, Eunice Kennedy Shriver National Institute of Child, Health and Development, Bethesda, MD, USA

M.J. De Souza PhD
Women's Health and Exercise Laboratory, Noll Laboratory, Department of Kinesiology, Penn State University, University Park, PA 16802, USA

Cary Dicken MD
Department of Gynecology and Obstetrics and Women's Health and, The Dominic Pupura Department of Neuroscience, Albert Einstein College of Medicine, Bronx NY, USA

Pouneh Fazeli MD
Neuroendocrine Unit, Massachusetts General Hospital and Harvard Medical School, Boston, MA, USA

Benjamin M. Lannon MD
Division of Reproductive Endocrinology and Infertility, Department of Obstetrics and Gynecology and Reproductive Biology, Beth Israel Deaconess Medical Center, Harvard Medical School, Boston, MA 02215, USA

Lawrence Layman MD
Section of Reproductive Endocrinology, Infertility, and Genetics, Department of Obstetrics and Gynecology, Developmental Neurobiology Program, Institute of Molecular Medicine and Genetics, Medical College of Georgia, Augusta, GA 30912-3360, USA

Tammy L. Loucks MPH
Department of Gynecology and Obstetrics, Emory University, Atlanta, GA, USA

Marie Menke MD
Department of Gynecology and Obstetrics and Women's Health and The Dominic Pupura Department of Neuroscience, Albert Einstein College of Medicine, Bronx, NY, USA

Sara Morelli MD
Department of Obstetrics, Gynecology and Women's Health, University of Medicine and Dentistry of New Jersey, Newark, NJ, USA

Lisa B. Nachtigall MD
Neuroendocrine Clinical Center unit, Massachusetts General Hospital and Harvard Medical School, Boston, MA 02114, USA

Anjana R. Nair MD
Department of Obstetrics and Gynecology, New York Downtown Hospital, New York, NY, USA

Genevieve Neal-Perry MD, PhD
Department of Gynecology and Obstetrics and Women's Health and Domnick Purpura Department of Neuroscience, Albert Einstein College of Medicine of Yeshiva University, Jack and Pearl Resnick Campus, 1211 Ullmann Building, 1300 Morris Park Avenue, Bronx, NY 10461, USA

Lawrence M. Nelson MD
Integrative Reproductive Medicine Unit, Intramural Research Program on Reproductive and Adult, Endocrinology, Eunice Kennedy Shriver National Institute of Child, Health and Development, Bethesda, MD, USA

Alex J. Polotsky MD, MS
Department of Obstetrics and Gynecology, University of Colorado Denver School of Medicine, Aurora, CO, USA

Nanette Santoro MD
Department of Obstetrics and Gynecology, University of Colorado Denver School of Medicine, Aurora, CO, USA

Donna Shoupe MD, MBA
Division of Reproductive Endocrinology, Department of Obstetrics and Gynecology after Division of Reproductive Endocrinology Keck School of Medicine, University of Southern California School of Medicine, Los Angeles, California

Hugh S. Taylor MD
Division of Reproductive Endocrinology and Infertility, Department of Obstetrics and Gynecology Yale University School of Medicine, 333 Cedar Street, New Haven, CT 06510, USA

Kimberley Thornton MD
Division of Reproductive Endocrinology and Infertility, Department of Obstetrics and Gynecology and Reproductive Biology, Beth Israel Deaconess Medical Center, Harvard Medical School, Boston MA, USA

R.J. Toombs BSc
Women's Health and Exercise Laboratory, Noll Laboratory, Department of Kinesiology, Penn State University, University Park, PA, USA

Gerson Weiss MD
Department of Obstetrics, Gynecology and Women's Health, University of Medicine and Dentistry of New Jersey, Newark, NJ, USA

Chapter 1
The Hypothalamic-Pituitary-Ovarian Axis

Cary Dicken, Marie Menke, and Genevieve Neal-Perry

Introduction

The hypothalamic-pituitary unit is the most evolutionarily conserved brain structure. It is responsible for integrating incoming information from the external (e.g., light, pain, temperature, smell) and internal environment (e.g., blood pressure, blood glucose, blood osmolality) and maintaining physiological homeostasis by coordinating endocrine, autonomic, and behavioral responses. In addition to preserving physiological homeostasis, the hypothalamic-pituitary axis synchronizes neuroendocrine physiology essential for ovarian physiology and reproduction. Key hormones responsible for hypothalamic-pituitary-gonadal (HPG) axis competency and reproductive success include gonadotropin releasing hormone (GnRH), follicle stimulating hormone (FSH), luteinizing hormone (LH), estradiol, progesterone, inhibin, activin, and follistatin. While the hypothalamic-pituitary axis is important for homeostasis, this chapter will primarily describe the role of HPG axis in the regulation of the menstrual cycle.

The Neuroendocrine Axis

Hypothalamus

Anatomy

The hypothalamus forms the floor of the third ventricle and is located beneath the thalamus at the base of the brain. Although the hypothalamus is small, occupying

G. Neal-Perry (✉)
Department of Gynecology and Obstetrics and Women's Health and Domnick Purpura Department of Neuroscience, Albert Einstein College of Medicine of Yeshiva University, Jack and Pearl Resnick Campus, 1211 Ullmann Building, 1300 Morris Park Avenue, Bronx, NY 10461, USA
e-mail: Sienna3598@aol.com

N.F. Santoro and G. Neal-Perry (eds.), *Amenorrhea: A Case-Based, Clinical Guide*, Contemporary Endocrinology, DOI 10.1007/978-1-60327-864-5_1,

about 10 of the total 1,400 g of adult human brain, it is composed of a complex group of highly specialized cells that are responsible for homeostasis and reproduction, and exhibit physiological characteristics consistent with neurons and endocrine gland cells [1].

The hypothalamus can be grossly divided in the medial–lateral plane into the medial, lateral, and periventricular regions. It can also be divided in the anterior–posterior plane to yield the anterior, posterior, and middle regions. It has several specific nuclei including the arcuate, supraoptic, suprachiamatic, paraventricular, dorsal medial, ventromedial, posterior hypothalamic, premammillary, lateral mammillary, and the medial mammillary. The periventricular region consists of the regions bordering the third ventricle and houses neurons important for the preservation of the circadian rhythm and autonomic neuroendocrine responses to stress. The periventricular fiber system conveys the axons of the parvocellular neuroendocrine neurons in the paraventricular and arcuate nuclei to the median eminence for control of the anterior pituitary. They are met in the median eminence by the axons from the magnocellular neurons, which continue down to the posterior pituitary. The medial region of the hypothalamus participates in the control of reproduction, osmoregulation, and thermoregulation. The lateral region of the hypothalamus is involved in behavior and arousal. The most anterior aspect of the hypothalamus overlies the optic chiasm and is called the preoptic area. The preoptic area houses the preoptic nuclei which contain neurons responsible for the regulation of blood pressure and body temperature. The middle region of the hypothalamus, located just above the pituitary stalk, contains the dorsomedial, ventromedial, paraventricular, supraoptic, and arcuate nuclei. The paraventricular, arcuate, and supraoptic nuclei all contain neuroendocrine neurons that regulate pituitary physiology. The dorsomedial and ventromedial nuclei project mainly within the hypothalamus and to the periaqueductal gray matter. These nuclei regulate growth, feeding, maturation, and reproduction. Finally, the posterior third of the hypothalamus includes the mammillary body and the overlying posterior hypothalamic area. The function of the mammillary bodies is unknown. The posterior portion of the hypothalamus contains the tuberomammillary nucleus, a histaminergic cell group that regulates arousal and wakefulness. From a reproductive perspective, the arcuate nucleus and the preoptic area are the most critical regions because they house GnRH neurons, the primary controllers of pituitary reproductive function.

Maintenance of the human menstrual cycle is directly dependent upon coordinated complex changes in patterns of neurotransmitter and neuropeptide released from the hypothalamus from the median eminence into portal system. These hypothalamic neuropeptides and neurotransmitters communicate with the anterior pituitary and affect anterior pituitary peptide secretion. Retrograde flow will bring pituitary hormones from the pituitary to the hypothalamus for feedback control. Conversely, the axons of the magnocellular neurons in the paraventricular and supraoptic nuclei project directly to the posterior pituitary to release oxytocin and vasopressin.

Physiology

Once the menstrual cycle is established, an event which on average is achieved within 5 years postmenarche, women enter into their reproductive prime. This period is most often coincident with maximal reproductive potential and characterized by the existence of a mature and functional hypothalamic-pituitary axis. The mature hypothalamic-pituitary axis subsequently functions to regulate ovarian physiology and menstrual cyclicity.

GnRH Neurons

Hypothalamic GnRH neurons, the maestros of reproductive success, originate from epithelial cells located in the olfactory placode. GnRH neurons, like olfactory neurons, have cilia and migrate along the cranial nerves until they reach the forebrain and their final residence within the medio-basal hypothalamus of the preoptic area and the arcuate nucleus. Critical to this migration is a neuronal cell surface glycoprotein that mediate cell-to-cell adhesion. Several genes and their related proteins are involved in cell adhesion and are important for GnRH neuronal migration. An example is anosmin-1, a protein encoded by the KAL1 gene, which is responsible for X-linked Kallmann syndrome [2]. Mutations of genes that encode adhesion molecules are often associated with anosmia, GnRH deficiency, and hypogonadotropic hypogonadism. Fibroblast growth factor receptor one also plays a role in GnRH neuronal migration, and mutations in this receptor generate a Kallmann syndrome phenotype [3].

About 1,000–3,000 GnRH neurons can be found in the arcuate nucleus. GnRH neurons exist in a complex network that involves interconnections between GnRH neurons and several other neurotransmitter systems that modulate GnRH release and GnRH neuronal activation. This complex arrangement allows GnRH neurons to communicate with each other and to integrate and transmit input received from multiple estradiol-responsive neurotransmitter systems and growth factors that affect gonadotropin release. Delivery of GnRH to the portal circulation occurs via an axonal pathway – the GnRH tubero-infundibular tract. Axons from GnRH neurons project to the median eminence and terminate in the capillaries that drain into the portal vessels. The portal vein is a low-flow transport system that descends along the pituitary stalk and connects the hypothalamus to the anterior pituitary. The direction of the blood flow in this hypophyseal portal circulation is generally from the hypothalamus to the pituitary. The peak concentration of GnRH in human portal blood is about 2 ng/mL.

GnRH is a 10 amino acid neuropeptide derived from the posttranslational processing of a large 92 amino acid precursor molecule (pre-pro-GnRH) that contains 4 parts: a 23 amino acid signal domain, the GnRH decapeptide, a 3 amino acid proteolytic processing site, and a 56 amino acid GnRH-associated peptide (GAP) [1]. GnRH and GAP are transported to the nerve terminals before secretion into the portal circulation. Pre-pro-GnRH is the product of the short arm of chromosome 8. The physiologic role of GAP has not yet been established. GnRH peptide has a half-life of 2–4 min. The short half-life of GnRH reflects rapid cleavage of the bonds between several amino acids (5 and 6, 6 and 7, and 9 and 10).

The short half-life and the large peripheral dilution effect of the vascular system prohibit the measurement of GnRH outside the central nervous system. LH has a half-life that is approximately 10–15 times longer than that of GnRH and each pulse of LH measured in the peripheral blood corresponds to a hypothalamic pulse of GnRH in the portal system in a one-to-one relationship [4]. Therefore, LH pulsing is often used as a surrogate marker for GnRH pulsatile secretion.

GnRH neurons release GnRH in a pulsatile fashion. The periodicity and amplitude of the pulsatile rhythm of GnRH are critical to reproduction because it ultimately drives gonadotropin and gonadal steroid secretion, gamete maturation, and ovulation. GnRH peptide regulates GnRH receptor expression on gonadotropin-producing cells by a process also known as self-priming. GnRH self-priming is maximized when GnRH release occurs every 60–90 min. Less frequent GnRH pulse frequency results in anovulatory amenorrhea. Slow pulse frequency also decreases gonadotropin secretion due to inadequate stimulation. In contrast, prolonged exposure or increased GnRH frequency results in gonadotroph receptor downregulation and decreased gonadotropin secretion.

During puberty, hypothalamic reproductive activity begins with a low frequency of GnRH–LH release and proceeds with cycles of accelerated frequency characterized by passage from relative inactivity, to nocturnal activation, and finally to the full adult pattern. In adult females, LH pulse amplitude increases throughout the menstrual cycle, peaking in the early luteal phase. Pulsatile frequency of LH in the early follicular phase is every 90 min. The frequency increases to every 60 min in the late follicular phase and decreases to 100 min during the early luteal phase and 200 min in the late luteal phase. Normal menstrual cycles depend on maintaining the pulsatile release of GnRH within this critical range of amplitude and frequency. In general, more rapid pulse frequency favors LH secretion, whereas a slower pulse frequency favors that of FSH.

Control of the reproductive system by GnRH is governed by gonadal steroid feedback effects. Negative feedback prevents the growth of multiple large follicles and positive feedback is necessary for the LH surge and ovulation. Multiple neurotransmitters and neurohormones have been implicated as having roles in the control of GnRH secretion. An example of some of these neuroendocrine modulators includes catecholamines, opiates, neuropeptide Y (NPY), corticotrophin-releasing hormone, prolactin, and gonadal steroids. Sex steroids have both positive and negative feedback effects on GnRH pulse frequency. Estrogen alpha receptors (ERα), the mediators of estradiol positive feedback, have not been localized in hypothalamic GnRH-secreting neurons [5]. Adjacent neurons have been found to have ERα and are therefore likely to be critical in transmitting sex steroid feedback to GnRH neurons [6].

Estradiol increases GnRH pulse frequency, whereas elevated progesterone levels decrease GnRH pulsatility. Although GnRH neurons only express ERβ, studies with transgenic ERα and ERβ knockout mice demonstrate that ERα is necessary for estradiol positive feedback control of the hypothalamic-pituitary axis. This suggests that gonadal steroids do not directly regulate GnRH activity. Instead, estradiol mediates its effects on GnRH neurons through indirect mechanisms that most likely involve regulation of other hormone-responsive neurotransmitter systems like glutamate, GABA, norepinephrine, endorphins, and others.

Hypothalamic Neuropeptides and GnRH Neurons

Neuropeptide Y

NPY is a 36 amino acid peptide neurotransmitter whose main role is the regulation of energy balance. The majority of NPY expressing hypothalamic neurons are located in the arcuate nucleus [7]. The regulation of NPY secretion stems from nutritional status. States of negative energy balance in which circulating leptin is reduced are associated with the stimulation of NPY [8]. It is hypothesized that NPY increases food intake by modulating corticotropin releasing hormone (CRH) and decreases physical activity, thereby increasing the proportion of energy stored as fat [9, 10].

In addition to its stimulatory effect on food intake, NPY is hypothesized to affect reproduction positively through regulation of GnRH pulsitility. GnRH neurons expressing one or more of the six NPY receptor subtypes receive direct synaptic input from NPY-containing neurons [11]. The effect of NPY on GnRH depends on the presence or absence of gonadal steroids. In the presence of gonadal steroids, NPY stimulates the pulsatile release of GnRH and potentiates gonadotropin response to GnRH neurons by increasing the number of GnRH receptors on the pituitary gonadotrophs. However, in the absence of gonadal steroids, NPY inhibits gonadotropin secretion.

Proopiomelanocortin

Proopiomelanocortin (POMC) is a precursor polypeptide composed of 241 amino acids and part of the endogenous opiod peptide family. It undergoes extensive posttranslational processing via cleavage enzymes and has eight potential cleavage sites. Depending on the type of cleavage enzyme present within the tissue, POMC has the potential to yield ten biologically active peptides.

POMC is split into two fragments – an ACTH intermediate fragment and β-lipotropin. β-Lipotropin has no opioid activity, but is broken down in a series of steps to α, β, and γ melanocyte stimulating hormone (MSH); enkephalin; and the ṕ-, β-, and γ-endorphins. MCH interacts with one of five distinct receptor subtypes (MCR). αMSH is important for the regulation of skin pigmentation and, through interactions with NPY, food intake and energy homeostasis. Enkephalin and the ṕ-, β-, and γ-endorphins act at opioid receptors. β-Endorphin and other opioids affect reproduction by suppressing GnRH release [12].

Kisspeptin

Kisspeptin, a 54 amino acid peptide, is the product of the Kiss1 gene and binds to an endogenous receptor G-protein coupled receptor 54 (GPR54). Kisspeptin neurons are found in both the arcuate and anteroventral periventricular nucleus, and send their projections to GnRH cell bodies. Kisspeptin and its cognate receptor GPR54 directly and indirectly contribute to regulation of GnRH secretion and have an important role in the pubertal transition [13]. Mutations in GPR54 are responsible for some cases of hypogonadotropic hypogonadism and a failed pubertal transition [14].

Kisspeptin may have a role in mediating feedback control on GnRH secretion. Studies in rodents suggest kisspeptin neurons located in the anteroventral periventricular nucleus are proposed to be important for positive feedback effects of estradiol on the LH surge [15] and kisspeptin neurons located in the arcuate nucleus are proposed to be important for negative feedback [16].

Hypothalamic Neurotransmitters and GnRH Neurons

In addition to peptidergic input, GnRH neurons receive afferent input from a variety of neurotransmitter pathways. Changes in the release of amino acid neurotransmitters glutamate and GABA in response to gonadal steroids are critical for the pubertal transition, the LH surge, and reproductive senescence [17–22]. Similarly, the neurotransmitters norepinephrine and dopamine are thought to be important modulators of GnRH neuron activity and gonadotropin release [23–26]. Dopaminergic neurotransmission also regulates prolactin secretion.

Pituitary

Embryology and Anatomy

Fetal pituitary is derived from the fusion of the neuroectoderm that gives rise to Rathke's pouch and the diencephalon, and begins to develop approximately between the fourth and fifth weeks of gestation. By the ninth week of gestation, a rudimentary anterior pituitary can be recognized and between the 12th and 17th week of gestation, a functional hypothalamic-pituitary axis is established.

Several transcription factors have been linked to embryologic pituitary development, including HESX1, LHX3, LHX4, PIT1 (PROP1), POU1f1, PITX2, T-PIT (TBX19), SOX2, and SOX3 [27]. Mutations in these genes have been associated with syndromes that include pituitary abnormalities ranging from combined pituitary hormone deficiency to isolated hormonal deficiencies [28]. Although genetic variants include phenotypes with primary amenorrhea, the deficiency is more often identified in childhood as part of a wider clinical syndrome such as septo-optic dysplasia [29]. When hormone deficiencies do occur, abnormalities in growth hormone production and its consequences are usually the earliest sign.

With an average weight between 0.4 and 0.8 g in human adults, the pituitary can be found in the sella turcica where it is covered by dura. The sella turcica is located at the base of the brain and inferior to the hypothalamus. The optic chiasma lies just above the sellar diaphragm, with visual symptoms presenting as an early clinical sign of gross pituitary enlargement.

The arterial vascular supply to the pituitary consists primarily of the superior and inferior hypophysial arteries; branches of the internal carotid arteries. Venous blood return occurs through the internal jugular veins [30]. Blood supply to the median eminence and infundibular stalk arises from the superior hypophysial arteries. From these sites, a dense capillary network coalesces to allow blood flow directly to the anterior pituitary through a portal system that traverses the pituitary stalk. This capillary network supplies approximately 80–90% of blood pituitary flow [12].

The Anterior Pituitary

The anterior pituitary is derived from Rathke's pouch and the posterior pituitary is derived from the diencephalon. The anterior hypothalamus, also known as the adenohypophysis, is composed of the pars distalis, pars intermedia, and pars tuberalis, all of which account for 80% of the pituitary gland. Of these structures, the pars distalis and pars tuberalis represent the sites of hormonal synthesis. The pars intermedia has no known function in humans. The anterior pituitary lacks direct innervation; regulation is solely through hypothalamic hormonal control via the portal system. Retrograde flow allows feedback loops between the hypothalamus and anterior pituitary.

Six major cell types reside in the anterior pituitary: 40–50% somatotrophs (growth hormone), 14–25% lactotrophs (prolactin), 10–20% corticotrophs (adenocorticotrophic hormone), 5% thyrotrophs (thyroid-stimulating hormone), 10% gonadotrophs (FSH and LH), and folliculostellate cells. The anterior pituitary's intimate role in reproduction results from the secretion of the glycoproteins FSH and LH. Until recently, histologic classification of anterior pituitary cells rested entirely on immunohistochemical findings of acidophilic, basophilic, or chromophobic cells. This classification system has largely been replaced with descriptive terms determined by cellular peptide production. Acidophilic cells are now classified as somatotropes or lactotropes, and basophilic cells are classified as corticotropes, thyrotropes, or gonadotropes. Cells previously classified as chromophobic generally fall into one of the above hormone-producing cell types.

The Posterior Pituitary

The posterior pituitary, also called the neurohypophysis, is composed of the infundibular stalk and the pars nervosa. The infundibular stalk is surrounded by the pars tuberalis, and together they constitute the hyopophyseal stalk. The posterior pituitary has a collection of nerve terminals that arise from magnocellular secretory neurons located within the paraventricular and supraoptic nuclei of the hypothalamus. Upon stimulation, the nerve terminals secrete vasopressin and oxytocin into the pituitary capillary plexus in close proximity to the axons. Alteration in concentrations of these neuropeptides within the peripheral vasculature results in changes in blood osmolality, blood pressure, and fluid balance.

The pituitary gland is regulated by three interacting elements: hypothalamic inputs, steroid feedback, and pituitary paracrine and autocrine actions. Hypothalamic input to the pituitary varies according to local hormonal and physiological cues that modulate neuropeptide and neurotransmitter secretion into the median eminence and the pituitary capillary plexus. Thus steroid feedback directly and indirectly affects pituitary reproductive physiology.

Pituitary Gonadotropins

FSH and LH belong to a superfamily of heterodimeric glycoprotein hormones. They are formed by noncovalent linkage of the α- and β-subunits. Like other members of this superfamily, FSH and LH share a common 92 amino acid α polypeptide stabilized by five disulfide bonds on ten cysteine residues and composed of asparagine-linked glycosylation sites. The human α-subunit gene is located on the short arm of chromosome 6 (p21.1-23). Although encoded from different chromosomes, a high degree of sequence homology exists among the β-subunits. FSH and LH bind to different transmembrane G protein-coupled receptors with unique ligand recognition domains. Mutations in the β-subunit of FSH or LH or their cognate receptors have been described and are generally equated with precocious puberty, primary amenorrhea, and/or infertility [31, 32].

By 16 weeks of gestation, portal circulation is developed and fetal secretion of all pituitary hormones is detectable with peak levels achieved by 28 weeks of gestation. Postnatally, gonadotropins rise briefly during the first year of life. A wide range of values are observed in neonates, with FSH ranges of 12–26 IU/L and less marked elevations of LH (0.5–3.5 IU/L) [33]. In premature infants born between 24 and 29 weeks of gestation, these variations are even more pronounced. FSH levels have been reported to range between 1.2 and 167.0 IU/L and LH levels to range between 0.2 and 54.4 IU/L. The progressive decline of FSH levels with fetal maturity suggests ongoing maturation of the hypothalamic-pituitary-ovarian axis, which subsequently continues postnally [34]. After the first year of life, childhood levels of gonadotropins are nearly undetectable, with little additional change occurring before the onset of puberty [35].

FSH

FSH has a molecular weight of approximately 29,000 Da. The human β-subunit gene for FSH is located on the short arm of chromosome 11 (p13). The FSH β-subunit contains 111 amino acids, 5 sialic acid residues, and 2 asparagine-linked glycosylation sites. Circulating estradiol (E2) affects FSH isoforms by modulating carbohydrate moieties. Elevated serum E2 levels increase an FSH isoform with decreased sialic acid residue sites. Reduced numbers of sialic acid residue sites shorten the half-life of FSH and increase receptor affinity [36]. In contrast, FSH isoforms with increased numbers of sialic acid residues have reduced receptor affinity and lengthened half-lives [37].

LH

LH is composed of the shared α-subunit and a 121 amino acid β-subunit. As with FSH, the oligosaccharide component of the β-subunit specifies the half-life of LH. The Gal-N-Ac sulfate located on LH allows rapid recognition and metabolism by hepatic cells and results in its 20–30 min half-life [37]. Mutations of the LH β-subunit gene have been associated with primary infertility [38] and precocious puberty in males [39, 40]. Although LH β-subunit variants have been identified in subgroups of PCOS women, they do not demonstrate differences in prevalence between normal and polycystic ovarian syndrome populations [41].

Prolactin

Lactotropes secrete prolactin. Transcription of the prolactin gene is regulated by Pit-1, which also plays a role in secretion of growth hormone and thyroid stimulating hormone. As previously described, mutations in Pit-1 have been implicated in defects of the anterior pituitary, including combined pituitary hormone deficiency. Although prolactin's primary function is thought to be regulation of lactogenesis, prolactin is also synthesized in the uterus where it is believed to play a role in implantation.

Roles for prolactin outside of pregnancy and lactation are not known. However, transgenic prolactin receptor knockout mice have disordered estrous cycles [42, 43]. Additionally, prolactin receptor knockout mice have fewer primary follicles, fewer ovulatory events, poor progression of fertilized oocytes to the blastocyst stage, and decreased estradiol and progesterone levels. These studies strongly suggest that prolactin may also be important for gonadotropin secretion.

Hyperprolactinemia inhibits GnRH secretion [44]. In conditions of hyperprolactinemia, LH pulse amplitude and frequency are decreased [45, 46]. LH secretion normalizes when prolactin levels are normalized [47]. Short-term treatment with opioid antagonists suggests that prolactin inhibition is mediated by opioid activity [48]. However, long-term opioid antagonist treatment does not restore menstrual cycles resulting from hyperprolactinemic states [49].

The Ovary

Ovarian Embryology

Embryonic gonadal development follows a pre-programmed transition from the indifferent gonad stage to sex-specific female or male germ cells. In the indifferent gonad stage, primordial germ cells first appear in the endoderm of the yolk sac, allantois, and hindgut. By way of ameboid movement, primordial germ cells migrate to the genital ridge by 5–6 weeks of gestation. The mechanism for this migration is not fully understood; however, electron microscopic studies demonstrate formation of pseudopod-like cytoplasmic processes that allow movement through the mesenchyme [50].

Upon arrival to the genital ridge, replication of germ cells occurs via mitotic division with differentiation into primary oocytes occurring as early as the 11th week of gestation. By the 14th week of gestation, a portion of these oocytes will have entered meiosis, and replication is arrested in the diplotene stage of prophase I. A single flattened layer of granulosa cells will eventually surround these oocytes giving rise to primordial follicles. By midgestation, primary follicles are discernable in the fetal ovary. Mitotic growth continues and the number of oocytes peaks at a total of 6–7 million by 16–20 weeks of gestation [51, 52]. Rapid atresia follows, with approximately 1–2 million oocytes remaining in the ovary at birth. Germ cells that fail to enter meiosis by this stage are among those that undergo cell death [53]. An example of this clinical scenario can be found in Turner syndrome (45,X), whereby accelerated loss of fetal oocytes due to failure to undergo meiosis frequently leads to the formation of streak gonads. Additionally, terminal deletions from Xp11 to Xp22.1 and X13 to Xq26 are associated with primary amenorrhea and premature ovarian failure [54, 55]. Postnatally, additional oocyte loss ensues, with 300,000–500,000 oocytes remaining at the beginning of puberty. Of the remaining oocytes, approximately 400–500 will ovulate during the reproductive years.

Transcription of proteins such as bone morphogenic protein-4 (BMP-4), steel factor (c-kit ligand), TIAR (an RNA recognition motif/ribonucleoprotein-type RNA-binding protein), and leukemia inhibitor factor (LIF) is required for successful proliferation and migration of germ cells [56, 57]. In addition, distribution of fibronectin appears to play a role in the migratory route [58]. Successful migration is critical for gonadal development, as germ cells that fail to migrate undergo apoptosis.

Ovarian Anatomy

The ovary lies in the peritoneum attached to the uterus through ovarian ligament. Grossly, the ovary consists of the outer cortex, medulla, and hilum. The cortex can be further divided into the overlying tunica albuginea and the inner cortex. Surrounded by stromal tissue, oocytes are located in the inner cortex. Innervation and blood flow to ovarian tissue occur through the hilum [59]. The suspensory ligament of the ovary, through which the vascular flow and innervation to the ovary occur, also serves to tether the ovary to the pelvic sidewall. The ovarian artery originates from the aorta and provides oxygenated blood flow to the organ. Venous blood return occurs by way of ovarian veins, with drainage directly to the inferior vena cava on the right and to the renal vein on the left. The autonomic nervous system provides ovarian innervation. Interestingly, alterations in ovarian autonomic tone may affect ovarian function by predisposing females to the formation of ovarian cysts (reduced tone) or a polycystic ovarian phenotype [60]. In culture, addition of sympathomimetics enhances theca-interstitial androgen production by 100–300% in response to hCG [61]. Animal studies suggest a role for vasoactive intestinal peptide from nerve fibers in granulosa cell development and follicular atresia [62–64].

Follicular Development and Atresia

The menstrual cycle has classically been described as consisting of a 28-day cycle characterized by an early follicular phase with multifollicular development, mid-follicular stage with selection of a dominant follicle, followed by ovulation before transition of the remnant follicle into a corpus luteum. Follicles not destined for dominance experience developmental arrest and atresia. Growth from the secondary follicle into preovulatory follicles occurs in approximately 85 days [65], with complete development from the primary to the preovulatory follicle requiring approximately 220 days [66].

Early Follicular Development

As previously described, follicular growth begins mid-gestation with formation of primary follicles and arrest of the oocyte in the diplotene stage of meiosis I. Follicular growth and development begins with a gonadotropin *independent* stage, as granulosa cells change from flattened to cuboidal shape, with a subsequent fivefold increase in proliferation [67]. These changes are followed shortly thereafter with an increase in oocyte diameter, and formation of the zona pellucida [65]. To differentiate it from *cyclic recruitment*, which occurs post-puberty through direct stimulation by FSH, this process is also called the *initial recruitment* [66].

Following transformation of granulosa cells from flattened to cuboidal shape, oocyte growth proceeds without resumption of meiosis. Theca interna formation occurs at the end of the primary follicle stage; apparent paracrine regulation occurs from the oocyte-derived growth differentiation factor-9 (GDF9) as, in its absence, the theca layer fails to develop [12, 68]. Other necessary paracrine regulators of both granulosa and oocyte growth include kit ligand (expressed in granulosa cells), BMP-15 (oocyte-derived), connexin 37 (found at oocyte-granulosa gap junctions), and cyclin D2 (expressed in granulosa cells) [66]. At this stage, FSH and activin appear to have little role in follicular progression as mouse models and case reports of novel human FSH receptor mutations demonstrate development through the secondary follicle stage [69, 70]. Nevertheless, preparation for future response to

FSH does occur as primordial and primary follicles respond to cAMP activation with increased expression of aromatase and FSH receptors [64].

Secondary Follicles

During the secondary follicle or preantral stage, granulosa cells continue to develop receptors for FSH, estradiol, and androgens [12, 66]. Progression to the antral stage is marked by cell proliferation and oocyte growth. Although alternate signaling pathways have been described, FSH induces aromatization in granulosa cells primarily through an adenylate cyclase-mediated mechanism. Elevated levels of estradiol, in turn, act to upregulate the FSH receptors, thereby increasing the sensitivity to FSH. FSH induces granulosa cell proliferation and communication by increasing the number of gap junctions. FSH also upregulates transcription of LH receptors in granulosa cells of the preovulatory follicle [59].

Theca cells arise from mesenchymal cells of the stroma and are primarily responsible for androgen synthesis in the ovary. Theca layer development continues to progress as secondary follicles develop. Interactions with granulosa cells occur through growth factors such as keratinocyte growth factor (KGF) and hepatocyte growth factor (HGF). Kit ligand produced by granulosa cells then stimulates further organization of the theca layer by way of a positive feedback loop [71].

Antral Follicle

Formation of the antral follicle requires an increase in transcellular permeability followed by a rapid influx of water mediated through channels formed by aquaporins [72]. Evidence also suggests a change in the collagen composition of the follicular extracellular matrix [73]. Within the antral cavity, granulosa cells surrounding the oocyte become a morphologically distinct layer of cumulus cells.

During the menstrual cycle, circulating FSH allows a cohort of antral follicles to escape apoptosis; however, through a mechanism not fully elucidated, a dominant follicle emerges early in the follicular phase; FSH receptor concentration, aromatase activity, and intrafollicular levels of estrogen all increase in the chosen follicle. Selection of a dominant follicle allows a progressive increase in the concentration of estrogen that results in estrogen negative feedback on gonadotropin release and atresia of the remainder of the previously responsive cohort. The subsequent decline in FSH results in decreased estrogen production, with a further decrease in responsiveness to gonadotropins by nondominant follicles that progressed into the preantral stage. In a natural cycle, this process may be detected as early as day 5 of the menstrual cycle [74].

The mid-cycle LH surge precedes ovulation and completion of meiosis I by approximately 24–36 h. Cumulus cell expansion occurs in response to increased synthesis of hyaluronic acid [59]. Mural granulosa cells express high levels of LH receptors; however few, if any, LH receptors proliferate in cumulus cells [75].

Instead, a complex signaling cascade of LH and epidermal growth factor-like growth factors such as amphiregulin, epiregulin, and betacellulin likely plays a role in cumulus cell differentiation [76]. Proteolytic enzymes, produced by granulosa and theca cells, are ultimately responsible for follicular rupture [59]. Prostaglandin synthesis is required for ovulation and appears to act through promotion of protease function [77].

Ovarian Physiology

Estrogen

Estradiol is the major form of circulating estrogen and is produced in its highest concentrations by the antral follicle during the follicular phase. Theca cell response to LH results in increased androgen production through transcription of P450scc, P450c17, and 3β-hydroxysteroid dehydrogenase. The classic two-cell model of steroid production describes the aromatization of androgens produced by theca cells and androgen diffusion into adjacent granulosa cells where FSH regulates aromatase synthesis of estradiol. Thus, the follicular phase of the menstrual cycle is marked by granulosa cell-mediated increased production of estradiol. Elevated estrogen levels act through negative feedback at the hypothalamic and pituitary level to inhibit pituitary release of FSH. As previously mentioned, increasing concentrations of estrogen also affect FSH isoform production, a physiological change with an unknown clinical relevance.

The majority of estradiol lies bound either to sex hormone binding hormone (SHBG; 69%) or albumin (30%); only approximately 1% circulates freely. Estrone, a weak estrogen, circulates more freely (8% bound to SHBG, 85% to albumin). Multiple factors affect SHBG levels, with subsequent changes to the amount of free estradiol to follow. These include body mass index, tobacco use, modulators of hepatic P450 enzymes, and diabetes.

Estrogen is primarily metabolized in the liver through the P450 cytochrome mechanism. The major metabolite progesterone imposes in urine is 3-methoxy-2-hydroxyestrone glucuronide; however, up to 20% may be excreted in the feces.

Progesterone

In addition to preparing the endometrium for implantation, luteal phase progesterone mediates negative feedback at the hypothalamic-pituitary level primarily by inhibiting GnRH neurons [78–80]. Progesterone also plays an obligate role in ovulation, with a small increase in synthesis noted in the periovulatory period [81]. Like estradiol, circulating free progesterone makes up a small percentage of the total concentration. Less than 2% of progesterone circulates as free hormone, with the remainder bound primarily to albumin (80%). Progesterone is principally metabolized in the liver by the 5α-reductase pathway, resulting in pregnanediol and pregnanetriol and conjugation with glucuronide. Pregnanediol glucuronide is excreted in the urine and can be used in research to assess ovulation.

Inhibin

Isolated in the 1980s, inhibin A and inhibin B are disulphide-linked dimers and members of the transforming growth factor-β family. Similar to other glycoproteins, they share a common α-subunit with one of two distinct β-subunits (β_A and β_B) [82, 83]. Inhibin is primarily secreted by granulosa cells; however, mRNA for both subunits has been identified in gonadotropes [84, 85]. Both inhibins affect gonadotropins almost exclusively through suppression of FSH secretion and augmentation of LH-stimulated androgen production [12].

Activin

Activin is a heterodimer composed of β-subunits of inhibin (β_{AB}, β_{AA}, β_{BB}). The β-subunits are relatively ubiquitous; however, the α-subunit is restricted to the pituitary, gonads, and adrenal glands. Activin is synthesized in granulosa cells and also appears to have an autocrine function in the pituitary through its effects on gonadotropin synthesis. It stimulates FSH secretion in cultured pituitary cells by upregulation of β-subunit mRNA levels and augments LH- and IGF-stimulated androgen production by theca cells [59, 86]. Activin is required for adequate pituitary response to GnRH.

Follistatin

Follistatin is a relatively ubiquitous protein that directly affects FSH by inhibition of its synthesis and GnRH responsiveness [87]. Follistatin is upregulated by activin and downregulated by inhibin [88]. FoxL2 (associated with the syndrome of blepherophimosis, ptosis, and epicanthus inversus as well as premature ovarian failure) has been implicated in the enhancement of follistatin gene transcription [89].

Summary

Female reproduction is a complex process that involves the integration of messages directly and indirectly received by the hypothalamus about the nutrient status, stress, and hormone exposure from external and internal environments. Information processed by GnRH neurons affects the pulse amplitude and frequency of gonadotropin release from the pituitary. This in turn affects gonadal steroidal production, and ovarian folliculogenesis and ovulation. The failure of any one organ in this triad results in disruption of female reproduction. The remaining chapters in this book will expound on factors that disrupt the function of the hypothalamic-pituitary-ovarian axis and give rise to reproductive dysfunction or amenorrhea.

References

1. Kandel E, Schwartz J, Jessel T (eds) (2000) Principles of neural science. McGraw-Hill, New York
2. Soussi-Yanicostas N, Faivre-Sarrailh C, Hardelin JP, Levilliers J, Rougon G, Petit C (1998) Anosmin-1 underlying the X chromosome-linked Kallmann syndrome is an adhesion molecule that can modulate neurite growth in a cell-type specific manner. J Cell Sci 111(pt 19): 2953–2965
3. Tsai PS, Moenter SM, Postigo HR, El Majdoubi M, Pak TR, Gill JC, Paruthiyil S, Werner S, Weiner RI (2005) Targeted expression of a dominant-negative fibroblast growth factor (FGF) receptor in gonadotropin-releasing hormone (GnRH) neurons reduces FGF responsiveness and the size of GnRH neuronal population. Mol Endocrinol 19:225–236
4. Clarke IJ (1993) Variable patterns of gonadotropin-releasing hormone secretion during the estrogen-induced luteinizing hormone surge in ovariectomized ewes. Endocrinology 133: 1624–1632
5. Skynner MJ, Sim JA, Herbison AE (1999) Detection of estrogen receptor alpha and beta messenger ribonucleic acids in adult gonadotropin-releasing hormone neurons. Endocrinology 140: 5195–5201
6. Ojeda SR, Ma YJ (1999) Glial-neuronal interactions in the neuroendocrine control of mammalian puberty: facilitatory effects of gonadal steroids. J Neurobiol 40:528–540
7. Morris BJ (1989) Neuronal localisation of neuropeptide Y gene expression in rat brain. J Comp Neurol 290:358–368
8. Coiro V, Chiodera P, Melani A, Manfredi G, Saccani Jotti G, Casti A (2006) Different plasma neuropeptide Y concentrations in women athletes with and without menstrual cyclicity. Fertil Steril 85:767–769
9. Haas DA, George SR (1989) Neuropeptide Y-induced effects on hypothalamic corticotropin-releasing factor content and release are dependent on noradrenergic/adrenergic neurotransmission. Brain Res 498:333–338
10. Hanson ES, Dallman MF (1995) Neuropeptide Y (NPY) may integrate responses of hypothalamic feeding systems and the hypothalamo-pituitary-adrenal axis. J Neuroendocrinol 7:273–279
11. Dhillon SS, Gingerich S, Belsham DD (2009) Neuropeptide Y induces gonadotropin-releasing hormone gene expression directly and through conditioned medium from mHypoE-38 NPY neurons. Regul Pept 156:96–103
12. Strauss JF, Barbieri RL (eds) (2004) Yen and Jaffe's reproductive endocrinology, 5th edn. Elsevier, Philadelphia, PA
13. Neal-Perry G, Lebesgue D, Lederman M, Shu J, Zeevalk GD, Etgen AM (2009) The excitatory peptide kisspeptin restores the luteinizing hormone surge and modulates amino acid neurotransmission in the medial preoptic area of middle-aged rats. Endocrinology 150:3699–3708
14. Kaiser UB, Kuohung W (2005) KiSS-1 and GPR54 as new players in gonadotropin regulation and puberty. Endocrine 26:277–284
15. Navarro VM, Castellano JM, Fernandez-Fernandez R, Tovar S, Roa J, Mayen A, Nogueiras R, Vazquez MJ, Barreiro ML, Magni P, Aguilar E, Dieguez C, Pinilla L, Tena-Sempere M (2005) Characterization of the potent luteinizing hormone-releasing activity of KiSS-1 peptide, the natural ligand of GPR54. Endocrinology 146:156–163
16. Dungan HM, Gottsch ML, Zeng H, Gragerov A, Bergmann JE, Vassilatis DK, Clifton DK, Steiner RA (2007) The role of kisspeptin-GPR54 signaling in the tonic regulation and surge release of gonadotropin-releasing hormone/luteinizing hormone. J Neurosci 27:12088–12095

17. Downs JL, Wise PM (2009) The role of the brain in female reproductive aging. Mol Cell Endocrinol 299:32–38
18. Jarry H, Leonhardt S, Schwarze T, Wuttke W (1995) Preoptic rather than mediobasal hypothalamic amino acid neurotransmitter release regulates GnRH secretion during the estrogen-induced LH surge in the ovariectomized rat. Neuroendocrinology 62:479–486
19. Jarry H, Leonhardt S, Wuttke W (1990) A norepinephrine-dependent mechanism in the preoptic/anterior hypothalamic area but not in the mediobasal hypothalamus is involved in the regulation of the gonadotropin-releasing hormone pulse generator in ovariectomized rats. Neuroendocrinology 51:337–344
20. Jennes L, Lin W, Lakhlani S (2002) Glutamatergic regulation of gonadotropin-releasing hormone neurons. Prog Brain Res 141:183–192
21. Neal-Perry GS, Zeevalk GD, Shu J, Etgen AM (2008) Restoration of the luteinizing hormone surge in middle-aged female rats by altering the balance of GABA and glutamate transmission in the medial preoptic area. Biol Reprod 79:878–888
22. Terasawa E, Luchansky LL, Kasuya E, Nyberg CL (1999) An increase in glutamate release follows a decrease in gamma aminobutyric acid and the pubertal increase in luteinizing hormone releasing hormone release in the female rhesus monkeys. J Neuroendocrinol 11:275–282
23. Mohankumar PS, Thyagarajan S, Quadri SK (1994) Correlations of catecholamine release in the medial preoptic area with proestrous surges of luteinizing hormone and prolactin: effects of aging. Endocrinology 135:119–126
24. Mohankumar PS, Thyagarajan S, Quadri SK (1995) Cyclic and age-related changes in norepinephrine concentrations in the medial preoptic area and arcuate nucleus. Brain Res Bull 38:561–564
25. Weiland NG, Wise PM (1986) Effects of age on beta 1- and beta 2-adrenergic receptors in the brain assessed by quantitative autoradiography. Brain Res 398:305–312
26. Wise PM (1982) Norepinephrine and dopamine activity in microdissected brain areas of the middle-aged and young rat on proestrus. Biol Reprod 27:562–574
27. Kelberman D, Dattani MT (2007) Hypothalamic and pituitary development: novel insights into the aetiology. Eur J Endocrinol 157(suppl 1):S3–S14
28. Kelberman D, Turton JP, Woods KS, Mehta A, Al-Khawari M, Greening J, Swift PG, Otonkoski T, Rhodes SJ, Dattani MT (2009) Molecular analysis of novel PROP1 mutations associated with combined pituitary hormone deficiency (CPHD). Clin Endocrinol (Oxf) 70:96–103
29. Gage PJ, Suh H, Camper SA (1999) Dosage requirement of Pitx2 for development of multiple organs. Development 126:4643–4651
30. Navratil AM, Knoll JG, Whitesell JD, Tobet SA, Clay CM (2007) Neuroendocrine plasticity in the anterior pituitary: gonadotropin-releasing hormone-mediated movement in vitro and in vivo. Endocrinology 148:1736–1744
31. Suganuma N, Furui K, Furuhashi M, Asada Y, Kikkawa F, Tomoda Y (1995) Screening of the mutations in luteinizing hormone beta-subunit in patients with menstrual disorders. Fertil Steril 63:989–995
32. Meduri G, Touraine P, Beau I, Lahuna O, Desroches A, Vacher-Lavenu MC, Kuttenn F, Misrahi M (2003) Delayed puberty and primary amenorrhea associated with a novel mutation of the human follicle-stimulating hormone receptor: clinical, histological, and molecular studies. J Clin Endocrinol Metab 88:3491–3498
33. Burger HG, Yamada Y, Bangah ML, McCloud PI, Warne GL (1991) Serum gonadotropin, sex steroid, and immunoreactive inhibin levels in the first two years of life. J Clin Endocrinol Metab 72:682–686
34. Greaves RF, Hunt RW, Chiriano AS, Zacharin MR (2008) Luteinizing hormone and follicle-stimulating hormone levels in extreme prematurity: development of reference intervals. Pediatrics 121:e574–e580
35. Winter JS, Faiman C (1972) Serum gonadotropin in concentrations in agonadal children and adults. J Clin Endocrinol Metab 35:561–564
36. Ulloa-Aguirre A, Espinoza R, Damian-Matsumura P, Chappel S (1988) Immunological and biological potencies of the different molecular species of gonadotrophins. Hum Reprod 3:491–501

37. Wide L, Eriksson K, Sluss PM, Hall JE (2009) Serum half-life of pituitary gonadotropins is decreased by sulfonation and increased by sialylation in women. J Clin Endocrinol Metab 94:958–964
38. Weiss J, Axelrod L, Whitcomb RW, Harris PE, Crowley WF, Jameson JL (1992) Hypogonadism caused by a single amino acid substitution in the beta subunit of luteinizing hormone. N Engl J Med 326:179–183
39. Abell AN, McCormick DJ, Segaloff DL (1998) Certain activating mutations within helix 6 of the human luteinizing hormone receptor may be explained by alterations that allow transmembrane regions to activate Gs. Mol Endocrinol 12:1857–1869
40. Beck-Peccoz P, Persani L, Romoli R, Asteria C, Borgato S (1998) Activating mutations of the gonadotrophin receptors. Arch Pediatr 5(suppl 4):380S–384S
41. Rajkhowa M, Talbot JA, Jones PW, Pettersson K, Haavisto AM, Huhtaniemi I, Clayton RN (1995) Prevalence of an immunological LH beta-subunit variant in a UK population of healthy women and women with polycystic ovary syndrome. Clin Endocrinol (Oxf) 43:297–303
42. Horseman ND, Zhao W, Montecino-Rodriguez E, Tanaka M, Nakashima K, Engle SJ, Smith F, Markoff E, Dorshkind K (1997) Defective mammopoiesis, but normal hematopoiesis, in mice with a targeted disruption of the prolactin gene. EMBO J 16:6926–6935
43. Ormandy CJ, Camus A, Barra J, Damotte D, Lucas B, Buteau H, Edery M, Brousse N, Babinet C, Binart N, Kelly PA (1997) Null mutation of the prolactin receptor gene produces multiple reproductive defects in the mouse. Genes Dev 11:167–178
44. Milenkovic L, D'Angelo G, Kelly PA, Weiner RI (1994) Inhibition of gonadotropin hormone-releasing hormone release by prolactin from GT1 neuronal cell lines through prolactin receptors. Proc Natl Acad Sci U S A 91:1244–1247
45. Sauder SE, Frager M, Case GD, Kelch RP, Marshall JC (1984) Abnormal patterns of pulsatile luteinizing hormone secretion in women with hyperprolactinemia and amenorrhea: responses to bromocriptine. J Clin Endocrinol Metab 59:941–948
46. Klibanski A, Beitins IZ, Merriam GR, McArthur JW, Zervas NT, Ridgway EC (1984) Gonadotropin and prolactin pulsations in hyperprolactinemic women before and during bromocriptine therapy. J Clin Endocrinol Metab 58:1141–1147
47. Sartorio A, Pizzocaro A, Liberati D, De Nicolao G, Veldhuis JD, Faglia G (2000) Abnormal LH pulsatility in women with hyperprolactinaemic amenorrhoea normalizes after bromocriptine treatment: deconvolution-based assessment. Clin Endocrinol (Oxf) 52:703–712
48. Cook CB, Nippoldt TB, Kletter GB, Kelch RP, Marshall JC (1991) Naloxone increases the frequency of pulsatile luteinizing hormone secretion in women with hyperprolactinemia. J Clin Endocrinol Metab 73:1099–1105
49. Matera C, Freda PU, Ferin M, Wardlaw SL (1995) Effect of chronic opioid antagonism on the hypothalamic-pituitary-ovarian axis in hyperprolactinemic women. J Clin Endocrinol Metab 80:540–545
50. Kuwana T, Fujimoto T (1983) Active locomotion of human primordial germ cells in vitro. Anat Rec 205:21–26
51. Baker TG (1963) A quantitative and cytological study of germ cells in human ovaries. Proc R Soc Lond B Biol Sci 158:417–433
52. Peters H (1976) Intrauterine gonadal development. Fertil Steril 27:493–500
53. Abir R, Orvieto R, Dicker D, Zukerman Z, Barnett M, Fisch B (2002) Preliminary studies on apoptosis in human fetal ovaries. Fertil Steril 78:259–264
54. Zinn AR, Ross JL (2001) Molecular analysis of genes on Xp controlling Turner syndrome and premature ovarian failure (POF). Semin Reprod Med 19:141–146
55. Zinn AR, Tonk VS, Chen Z, Flejter WL, Gardner HA, Guerra R, Kushner H, Schwartz S, Sybert VP, Van Dyke DL, Ross JL (1998) Evidence for a Turner syndrome locus or loci at Xp11.2-p22.1. Am J Hum Genet 63:1757–1766
56. Fujimoto T, Miyayama Y, Fuyuta M (1977) The origin, migration and fine morphology of human primordial germ cells. Anat Rec 188:315–330
57. Pereda J, Zorn T, Soto-Suazo M (2006) Migration of human and mouse primordial germ cells and colonization of the developing ovary: an ultrastructural and cytochemical study. Microsc Res Tech 69:386–395

58. Fujimoto T, Yoshinaga K, Kono I (1985) Distribution of fibronectin on the migratory pathway of primordial germ cells in mice. Anat Rec 211:271–278
59. Speroff L, Fritz M (eds) (2005) Clinical gynecologic endocrinology and infertility, 7th edn. Lippincott Williams & Wilkins, Philadelphia, PA
60. Greiner M, Paredes A, Rey-Ares V, Saller S, Mayerhofer A, Lara HE (2008) Catecholamine uptake, storage, and regulated release by ovarian granulosa cells. Endocrinology 149:4988–4996
61. Dyer CA, Erickson GF (1985) Norepinephrine amplifies human chorionic gonadotropin-stimulated androgen biosynthesis by ovarian theca-interstitial cells. Endocrinology 116:1645–1652
62. Ottesen B, Fahrenkrug J (1995) Vasoactive intestinal polypeptide and other preprovasoactive intestinal polypeptide-derived peptides in the female and male genital tract: localization, biosynthesis, and functional and clinical significance. Am J Obstet Gynecol 172:1615–1631
63. Flaws JA, DeSanti A, Tilly KI, Javid RO, Kugu K, Johnson AL, Hirshfield AN, Tilly JL (1995) Vasoactive intestinal peptide-mediated suppression of apoptosis in the ovary: potential mechanisms of action and evidence of a conserved antiatretogenic role through evolution. Endocrinology 136:4351–4359
64. Mayerhofer A, Dissen GA, Costa ME, Ojeda SR (1997) A role for neurotransmitters in early follicular development: induction of functional follicle-stimulating hormone receptors in newly formed follicles of the rat ovary. Endocrinology 138:3320–3329
65. Gougeon A (1986) Dynamics of follicular growth in the human: a model from preliminary results. Hum Reprod 1:81–87
66. McGee EA, Hsueh AJ (2000) Initial and cyclic recruitment of ovarian follicles. Endocr Rev 21:200–214
67. Da Silva-Buttkus P, Jayasooriya GS, Mora JM, Mobberley M, Ryder TA, Baithun M, Stark J, Franks S, Hardy K (2008) Effect of cell shape and packing density on granulosa cell proliferation and formation of multiple layers during early follicle development in the ovary. J Cell Sci 121:3890–3900
68. Dong J, Albertini DF, Nishimori K, Kumar TR, Lu N, Matzuk MM (1996) Growth differentiation factor-9 is required during early ovarian folliculogenesis. Nature 383:531–535
69. Fortune JE, Cushman RA, Wahl CM, Kito S (2000) The primordial to primary follicle transition. Mol Cell Endocrinol 163:53–60
70. Meduri G, Bachelot A, Cocca MP, Vasseur C, Rodien P, Kuttenn F, Touraine P, Misrahi M (2008) Molecular pathology of the FSH receptor: new insights into FSH physiology. Mol Cell Endocrinol 282:130–142
71. Parrott JA, Skinner MK (1998) Thecal cell-granulosa cell interactions involve a positive feedback loop among keratinocyte growth factor, hepatocyte growth factor, and Kit ligand during ovarian follicular development. Endocrinology 139:2240–2245
72. McConnell NA, Yunus RS, Gross SA, Bost KL, Clemens MG, Hughes FM Jr (2002) Water permeability of an ovarian antral follicle is predominantly transcellular and mediated by aquaporins. Endocrinology 143:2905–2912
73. Rodgers RJ, Irving-Rodgers HF, Russell DL (2003) Extracellular matrix of the developing ovarian follicle. Reproduction 126:415–424
74. Chikazawa K, Araki S, Tamada T (1986) Morphological and endocrinological studies on follicular development during the human menstrual cycle. J Clin Endocrinol Metab 62:305–313
75. Peng XR, Hsueh AJ, LaPolt PS, Bjersing L, Ny T (1991) Localization of luteinizing hormone receptor messenger ribonucleic acid expression in ovarian cell types during follicle development and ovulation. Endocrinology 129:3200–3207
76. Conti M, Hsieh M, Park JY, Su YQ (2006) Role of the epidermal growth factor network in ovarian follicles. Mol Endocrinol 20:715–723
77. Lim H, Paria BC, Das SK, Dinchuk JE, Langenbach R, Trzaskos JM, Dey SK (1997) Multiple female reproductive failures in cyclooxygenase 2-deficient mice. Cell 91:197–208
78. Araki S, Chikazawa K, Motoyama M, Ijima K, Abe N, Tamada T (1985) Reduction in pituitary desensitization and prolongation of gonadotropin release by estrogen during continuous administration of gonadotropin-releasing hormone in women: its antagonism by progesterone. J Clin Endocrinol Metab 60:590–598

79. Wildt L, Hutchison JS, Marshall G, Pohl CR, Knobil E (1981) On the site of action of progesterone in the blockade of the estradiol-induced gonadotropin discharge in the rhesus monkey. Endocrinology 109:1293–1294
80. McCartney CR, Gingrich MB, Hu Y, Evans WS, Marshall JC (2002) Hypothalamic regulation of cyclic ovulation: evidence that the increase in gonadotropin-releasing hormone pulse frequency during the follicular phase reflects the gradual loss of the restraining effects of progesterone. J Clin Endocrinol Metab 87:2194–2200
81. Chaffin CL, Stouffer RL (2002) Local role of progesterone in the ovary during the periovulatory interval. Rev Endocr Metab Disord 3:65–72
82. Demura R, Suzuki T, Tajima S, Mitsuhashi S, Odagiri E, Demura H, Ling N (1993) Human plasma free activin and inhibin levels during the menstrual cycle. J Clin Endocrinol Metab 76:1080–1082
83. Risbridger GP, Schmitt JF, Robertson DM (2001) Activins and inhibins in endocrine and other tumors. Endocr Rev 22:836–858
84. Roberts VJ, Peto CA, Vale W, Sawchenko PE (1992) Inhibin/activin subunits are costored with FSH and LH in secretory granules of the rat anterior pituitary gland. Neuroendocrinology 56:214–224
85. Roberts V, Meunier H, Vaughan J, Rivier J, Rivier C, Vale W, Sawchenko P (1989) Production and regulation of inhibin subunits in pituitary gonadotropes. Endocrinology 124:552–554
86. Blumenfeld Z (2001) Response of human fetal pituitary cells to activin, inhibin, hypophysiotropic and neuroregulatory factors in vitro. Early Pregnancy 5:41–42
87. Kogawa K, Ogawa K, Hayashi Y, Nakamura T, Titani K, Sugino H (1991) Immunohistochemical localization of follistatin in rat tissues. Endocrinol Jpn 38:383–391
88. Kogawa K, Nakamura T, Sugino K, Takio K, Titani K, Sugino H (1991) Activin-binding protein is present in pituitary. Endocrinology 128:1434–1440
89. Blount AL, Schmidt K, Justice NJ, Vale WW, Fischer WH, Bilezikjian LM (2009) FoxL2 and Smad3 coordinately regulate follistatin gene transcription. J Biol Chem 284:7631–7645

Chapter 2
The Mechanism of Menstruation

Anjana R. Nair and Hugh S. Taylor

Menstruation is a result of the profound tissue remodeling that occurs each month in reproductive-aged women. After withdrawal of steroid hormone support, the functionalis layer of the endometrium undergoes extensive changes, resulting in complete tissue breakdown. With each menstrual cycle, most of the endometrium is completely shed at menses and subsequently regenerated. Menstruation is seen in only a few animals that have hemochorial placentation. In hemochorial placentation, trophoblasts invade the maternal blood vessels and chorionic villi are in direct contact with maternal blood. Thus the invasive nature of hemochorial placenta requires a correspondingly defensive uterus. In pregnancy, under the influence of progesterone, the endometrial stroma undergoes extensive decidualization. Decidualization limits trophoblastic invasion; however, protection from invasive trophoblasts requires the development of a barrier, a process that results in terminal differentiation. This differentiated state is renewable only by regeneration from progenitor cells located in the basalis layer of the endometrium; a strategy that requires monthly bleeding events and introduces multiple potential opportunities for mechanistic failure and the emergence of abnormal uterine bleeding. An appreciation of normal endometrial physiology as it pertains to the regulation of menstruation is essential to understand disorders of menstruation.

The Endometrium During the Menstrual Cycle

The endometrium is composed of the basalis and functionalis layers. The basalis layer is deep and adjacent to the myometrium, while the functionalis layer comprises the superficial two-thirds of the endometrium. The functionalis is divided into stratum compactum and stratum spongiosum. The stratum compactum

H.S. Taylor (✉)
Division of Reproductive Endocrinology and Infertility, Department of Obstetrics and Gynecology Yale University School of Medicine, 333 Cedar Street, New Haven, CT 06510, USA
e-mail: hugh.taylor@yale.edu

N.F. Santoro and G. Neal-Perry (eds.), *Amenorrhea: A Case-Based, Clinical Guide*, Contemporary Endocrinology, DOI 10.1007/978-1-60327-864-5_2,

is a superficial thin layer with gland necks and dense stroma, while the stratum spongiosum is the deeper part of functionalis composed of glands and loosely arranged stroma. Only the functionalis layer of endometrium is shed with each cycle. The basalis layer contains the progenitor cells that regenerate the functionalis layer in each cycle. Endometrial tissue responds to sex steroid hormones produced in the follicular and luteal phases of the ovarian cycle. The menstrual cycle is divided into proliferative and secretory phases, and cytoarchitectural and molecular differences between the phases reflect endometrial responses to cyclic changes in ovarian hormone exposure.

Proliferative Phase

The functional layer (upper 2/3) of the endometrium is shed during each menstrual cycle. By the end of menstruation, the endometrial lining is about 2 mm thick and is composed of epithelial cells that arise from the glands in the basalis layer and migrate to the denuded surface of the endometrium. Of note, the thin epithelialized basalis layer seen in early menstrual cycle is similar to the endometrial cytoarchitecture observed in postmenopausal women and also in women with hypothalamic amenorrhea. The initial repair of the endometrial surface, an event critical for the regeneration, occurs before cessation of menses and prior to the rise in estradiol [1, 2]. A measurable increase in endometrial thickness does not commence until this process is complete.

Estradiol, produced by the ovaries on approximately day 4 or 5 (D4 or 5) of the cycle, induces growth and proliferation of the endometrium. The epithelial and stromal cells undergo mitoses and multiply, thus causing the glands to increase in length, while the stromal cells grow and expand the extracellular matrix [3]. Some of the surface epithelial cells commonly seen near the tubal ostia and endocervix become ciliated at this time.

Endometrial growth can be viewed using ultrasound, measuring the total width of the opposed endometrial epithelial surfaces (also known as the trilaminar endometrial stripe). There is rapid growth of the endometrium from cycle D4 or 5. Endometrial thickness begins from a nadir of approximately 4.5 mm on cycle D4 and increases linearly to a plateau of approximately 10 mm on cycle D9 or 10 [4]. The cessation of endometrial growth occurs before estradiol levels reach their peak and prior to the onset of secretory phase progesterone production, thereby indicating that nonsteroidal factors limit the growth of endometrium.

Amenorrhea in some women results from chronic anovulation, which can be associated with unopposed estrogen exposure and disordered endometrial growth. Although some anovulatory women may have thickened endometrium, they do not experience the continued rapid growth of endometrial tissue seen in the normal proliferative phase. The endometrium does not grow indefinitely and the average endometrial thickness is rarely greater than 11 mm [5]. Obviously, unopposed estrogen is not sufficient to produce continued endometrial growth, again suggesting the existence of factors that limit the extent of proliferation. The cellular mechanisms responsible for dysfunctional endometrial growth observed in anovulatory women are still poorly understood. Nonetheless, the observed pathophysiology of the endometrium in anovulatory women likely reflects dysregulation of modulators of endometrial repair and growth cessation which promotes long-term stabilization under anovulatory conditions or estrogen deficiency.

Secretory Phase

Secretion of progesterone after ovulation causes complete cessation of endometrial epithelial proliferation. Estrogen receptors expressed by the endometrial epithelial cells during the proliferative phase are downregulated by progesterone action, thus attenuating estrogen's proliferative effect. Progesterone exposure induces sub-nuclear glycogen-rich vacuoles to appear on approximately (D16) of the cycle and inhibits epithelial cell mitosis by D17. The vacuoles become supranuclear on D18 and secretions are found in the gland lumen by D19–20. Peak secretory activity is seen by D20–21 [6–10]. These changes are essential for conception and the generation of an endometrial surface receptive to blastocyst attachment.

Progesterone provokes profound stromal fibroblast changes characterized by cellular enlargement, as well as laminin and type 4 collagen accumulation [11, 12]. In the luteal phase, type 4 collagen and laminin are present in the extracellular space of the endometrial stroma and the basement membrane of glands and blood vessel walls. Even though Collagen types 1, 3, and 6, and laminin are present in the endometrium throughout the menstrual cycle, their ratios change with prolonged exposure to progesterone (i.e., type 3:1 decreases and type 5:1 increases) [13]. The endometrium also makes large quantities of prolactin and IGF-binding proteins (IGFBP-1). These changes in response to progesterone result in dramatic alterations in both the extracellular matrix and secretory products of the endometrium.

Stromal edema is apparent by D20–23 and in the few days immediately preceding menstruation, the stroma becomes infiltrated by natural killer cells, macrophages, and T cells. In contrast, continuous progesterone exposure results in endometrial atrophy and thinning, gland narrowing, and vasculature abnormalities characterized by the creation of sinusoids and hyperplasic endothelial cells. This endometrial histology characterizes women with amenorrhea due to chronic progestin exposure.

Endometrial Growth Regulation

Numerous growth factors as well as ovarian steroid hormones regulate the growth of the endometrium during the menstrual cycle.

Ovarian Steroids

The endometrium responds to the ovarian steroids estrogen and progesterone; these two hormones are the only extrinsic signals necessary to drive a normal uterine menstrual cycle and are in fact sufficient to do so. The proliferative phase of the cycle is mainly mediated by the effects of estrogens. Estrogen receptor alpha (ERα, also known as ESR1) and estrogen receptor beta (ERβ, also known as ESR2) are transcribed from different genes and have distinct expression patterns. ESR2 is expressed in the endometrium throughout the menstrual cycle [14]. ERS1 varies throughout the menstrual cycle and is expressed by both epithelial and stromal cells during the proliferative phase [14]. Estrogen receptors are largely lost in the epithelium after progesterone exposure. There is also evidence that estrogen signaling may be transmitted through non-classic estrogen receptors, including the membrane receptor G-coupled receptor 30 (GRP30); however, this remains controversial.

The effects of progesterone on the uterus are mediated through progesterone receptors A (PR-A), B (PR-B), and C (PR-C). Each is a homologous protein transcribed from different promoters of the same gene [15–17]. Epithelial and stromal cells express PR-A and PR-B in the proliferative phase. In the luteal phase, only the stromal cells express PR-A and PR-B (PR-A is predominant), while the expression of both the receptors are downregulated in the epithelial cells [18, 19]. PR expression in stromal cells is unaffected by chronic exposure to long-acting progestational agents [20].

Growth Factors

A large number of mitogenic growth factors are secreted by the endometrium, modulating sex steroid action on the endometrium. These peptide molecules can initiate the activation of a cascade of intracellular pathways by binding to their cognate membrane bound receptors (Fig. 2.1).

Epidermal growth factor (EGF) is expressed by the epithelial cells during the proliferative phase and by stromal cells during secretory phase of the cycle [21, 22]. The levels of EGF are stable throughout the menstrual cycle. EGF can either synergize with estradiol or act independently to stimulate epithelial cell growth. EGF stimulation indirectly leads to ERα activation and the expression of downstream targets of this receptor [23, 24]. EGF may mediate the proliferative effects on epithelial cells seen in the endometrium during the early follicular phase when estradiol levels are generally very low. Transforming growth factor alpha (TGFα), a member of the EGF family, binds the same receptor as EGF and achieves peak levels during the mid-cycle. TGFα is also thought to mediate the proliferative actions of estrogen on the endometrium.

Fibroblast growth factors (FGF) comprise a family of approximately nine members and of these, FGF-1, -2, -4, and -7 are expressed in human endometrium.

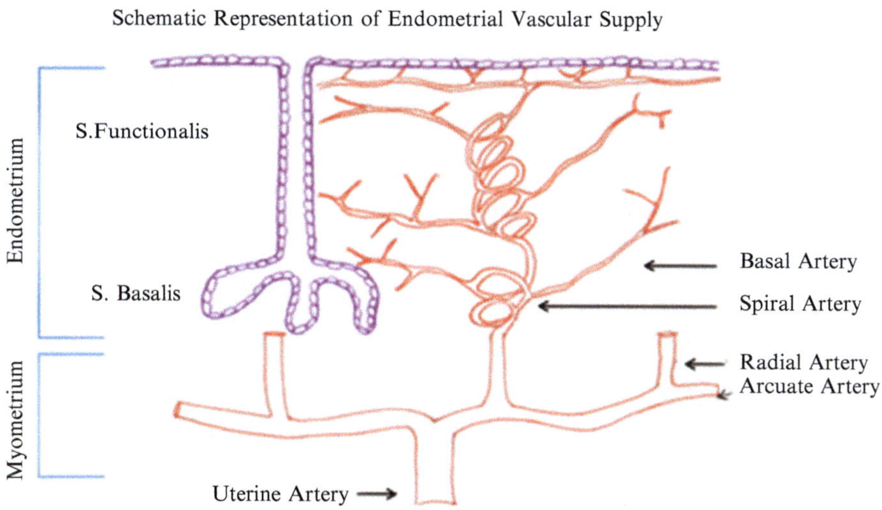

Fig. 2.1 Schematic presentation of the endometrial vascular system. The primate endometrium is comprised of the stratum basalis (s. basilis) and stratum functionalis (s. functionalis). Uterine arteries branch within the myometrium to yield the arcuate and radial arteries. The radial artery branches within the s. basilis to yield numerous straight and spiral arterioles in the lower third of the endometrium. Spiral arterioles provide the vascular blood supply to the s. functionalis through a vast network of fenestrated capillaries

Epithelial cells produce FGF-1 and -2 during the proliferative and secretory phases of the menstrual cycle. Stromal cells express FGF-2 in the proliferative phase, where it is proposed to induce mitosis and DNA synthesis [25–28].

Insulin-like growth factors (IGF)-1 and -2 are produced at high levels by epithelial and stromal cells throughout the menstrual cycle. Endometrial stromal fibroblast proliferation is induced by IGF-1 [29, 30]; however, both IGF-1 and -2 can also promote differentiation. IGF-1 production is upregulated by estradiol and it mediates estrogen's effect on endometrial growth. IGF-2 is involved in mediating differentiation of cells in response to progesterone effects. Their effects are mediated by binding to IGFBP-1. IGFBP-1 is one of six homologous proteins that specially modulate the mitogenic and metabolic effects of IGF-1 and -2. Both IGFBP-I protein and mRNA have been localized to the pre-decidual stromal cells in late secretory-phase endometrium and to decidual cells during pregnancy.

Multiple other relevant cytokines and growth factors have been described including keratinocyte growth factor (KGF), a member of the FGF family. KGF is expressed at higher levels in the stromal cells and during the secretory phase. It is proposed to mediate epithelial–stromal signaling [31]. Platelet-derived growth factor (PDGF) is secreted by stromal cells and platelets. It is localized to the stromal cells and stimulates stromal cell proliferation and angiogenesis. Tumor necrosis factor α (TNFα) activity in the endometrium is higher in the proliferative and mid-secretory phases. It has multiple influences on cell growth. TNFβ is mitogenic, angiogenic, immunomodulatory, and inflammatory in its actions.

While the list provided is far from complete, it serves to illustrate the complexity of cellular communication that is needed to maintain normal endometrial physiology. It makes sense that disequilibrium within this intricate network of cellular pathways could result in devastating consequences that affect menstrual cycles and implantation, and/or predispose some women to the development of neoplasia.

Endometrial Stem cells

In order for the epithelium and stroma to be completely renewed in each menstrual cycle, there must be a continuous pool of progenitor cells available to replenish and rebuild the endometrium. Hormonally, responsive stem cells residing in the basalis are hypothesized to be the source of progenitor cells that are committed to developing into specific types of differentiated cells, e.g., epithelial, stromal, and vascular. These resident stem cells are hypothesized to allow the rapid cyclic regeneration of the endometrium. However, there was no direct evidence to confirm this hypothesis until 2004. In that year, two reports from different laboratories provided evidence to support the hypothesis that local stem cells provided progenitor cells for cyclic endometrial renewal [32–34].

Human endometrium contains small populations of epithelial and stromal stem cells responsible for cyclic regeneration of endometrial glands and stroma. Notably, these cells exhibit clonogenicity. Consistent with this concept, small numbers of epithelial (0.22%) and stromal cells (1.25%) will initiate colonies and exhibit high proliferative potential in vitro. These cells comprise the local progenitor stem cells that are destined to give rise to most of the endometrium in each menstrual cycle.

Endometrial regeneration from multipotent stem cells derived from the bone marrow was recently demonstrated in bone marrow transplant recipients; donor-derived endometrial epithelial cells and stromal cells were detected in endometrial samples of bone marrow recipients. Histologically, these cells appeared to be endometrial epithelial and stromal cells and they also express appropriate markers of endometrial cell differentiation. These findings strongly suggest that bone marrow may also be an extrauterine source for endometrial stem cells [33, 35–37]. Moreover, these observations suggest that cyclic mobilization of bone marrow-derived stem cells may be a normal physiologic process. Interestingly, male donor-derived bone marrow transplant cells were found in the uterine endometrium of recipient female mice, and although rare, these cells differentiated into epithelial and stromal cells [38]. Endometrial stem cells are likely derived from a common stem cell found in both men and women. More recently, another group showed that bone marrow transplants-derived endothelial progenitors also contribute to the formation of new blood vessels in the endometrium [39].

The repopulation of endometrium with bone marrow-derived stem cells may be important to normal endometrial physiology and may also help to explain the cellular basis for the high rates of long-term failure following conservative alternatives to hysterectomy such as endometrial ablation or resection. Alternatively, endometrial regeneration may be incomplete in women with deficient stem cell reserves or defective recruitment of stem cells after injury, thereby increasing the risk for poor outcomes including Asherman's syndrome.

Endometrial Vessels

Since menstruation is a form of tissue remodeling where the lining of the uterine cavity is shed regularly, it is of utmost importance that the vasculature of the endometrium also be capable of regeneration. Nowhere outside the reproductive tract do vessels undergo this dramatic and regular regeneration. Angiogenesis and development of the microvasculature system within the endometrium may be the key event for normal endometrial cycling, as proliferation and subsequent maturation of the endometrium are dependent on delivery of local oxygen and nutrients to the tissue [40].

Endometrial Vascular Supply

Arcuate arteries arise from the uterine arteries in the myometrium. The arcuate arteries divide just inside the border of the endometrium and give rise to numerous straight arterioles that supply the lower third of the endometrium. These vessels continue as the spiral arteriole and supply the functional two-thirds of the endometrium. Endometrial blood vessels have abundant smooth muscle cells and just beneath the surface of the endometrium, the capillaries are fenestrated. The venules from the area drain into the uterine vein [41–44]. A sketch of the endometrial vascular system can be found in Fig. 2.1.

Regulation of Endometrial Vessel Growth

Menstruation results in open vessels that need to be repaired in order to control bleeding. The blood vessels begin to regenerate at the end of menstruation and continue into the proliferative phase of the menstrual cycle. Balances between factors that stimulate and inhibit angiogenesis regulate endometrial shedding and regeneration. Numerous angiogenic factors have been described by several investigators and include EGF [23], TGFα, TGFβ, TNFα, FGF-1, FGF-2, PDGF, and vascular endothelial growth factor (VEGF) [45, 46] Fig. 2.2. Appropriate angiogenesis is required for cessation and regulation of menstrual flow . Disorders of blood vessel function and repair may contribute to abnormal uterine bleeding.

Several specific factors involved in endometrial endothelial regeneration are well studied. VEGFs are heparin-binding 30–45 kDa molecules that are potent

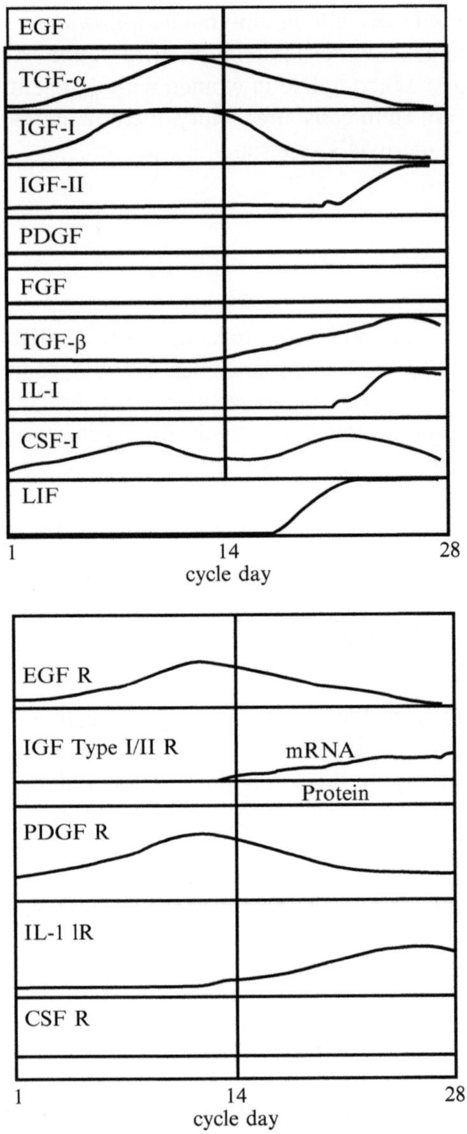

Fig. 2.2 Endometrial growth factors. Relative amounts of growth factor (*top*) and growth factors receptor (*bottom*) mRNA and protein levels in the human endometrium during the menstrual cycle. Levels illustrated are relative to levels during the early proliferative phase. *CSF-1* colony-stimulating factor-1; *EGF* epidermal growth factor; *FGF* fibroblast growth factor; *IGF-1* insulin-like growth factor-1; *IL-1* interleukin-1; *LIF* leukemia-inhibiting factor; *PDGF* platelet-derived growth factor; *TGF* transforming growth factor. From Guidice L, Saleh W (Trends Endocrinol Metab 1995;6:60–69) with permission

mitogens. VEGFs are proposed to have a crucial role in the development of vascular endothelium and thus formation of new blood vessels [47, 48]. Of the five different variants of VEGF, VEGF 121 and 165 isoforms are the predominant forms that regulate endometrial angiogenesis.

VEGF-A is produced in the glandular and luminal epithelium as well as in the stroma in the proliferative phase of the cycle. In the secretory phase of the menstrual cycle, only the epithelial cells continue to express VEGF-A [49, 50]. Several studies suggest that VEGF is hormonally regulated. Estradiol is thought to increase VEGF release; however, the exact role of ovarian hormones in the regulation of VEGF expression and function is not clear. [51]

Menstruation

Menstruation is the occurrence of bleeding when progesterone is withdrawn from an estrogen- and progestin-primed uterus. While progesterone withdrawal occurs in all species with an estrus cycle, only a very few menstruate, suggesting the existence of unique regulatory mechanisms in the endometrium of these species. The cellular events that follow withdrawal of steroid support can be divided into four types and are described below.

Loss of Vascular Integrity

Spiral arterioles are unique to menstruating species. The classic studies conducted more than 50 years ago by Markee demonstrated that steroid (estrogen/progesterone) withdrawal produced severe vasoconstriction of the endometrial spiral arterioles lasting 4–24 h [52]. The vasoconstriction is followed by vasodilatation in these vessels, causing increased blood flow. Ischemic damage induced by the vasoconstriction causes blood to flow out of the vessels to the epithelial surface. The interruption of blood supply and the acute tissue hemorrhage culminate in shedding of the superficial functional layer of the endometrium.

Several vasoactive agents likely mediate the response to steroid withdrawal. Local prostaglandin (PG) production is proposed to affect endometrial vasoregulation by increasing the ratio of the vasodilatory PGE2 relative to the vasoconstrictor PGF2α at menstruation [53]. Nitric oxide (NO), a vasodilator, is also locally synthesized in the endometrium and may have a role in regulating vascular tone [54]. VEGF may affect the induction of NO synthesis. Molecular studies of endometrial NOS expression, as well as animal experiments with NOS inhibitors, indicate that NO plays an important role in endometrial functions such as endometrial receptivity, implantation, and menstruation. Endothelins are also potent vasoconstrictors. Cameron et al. have shown that endometrium is rich in these molecules as well as their cognate receptors, thereby regulating bleeding during menstruation [55]. Many of these agents have yet to be explored in the treatment of abnormal uterine bleeding.

It is important to appreciate that prior to overt vascular breakdown and menstruation, an inflammatory process ensues and vasospasm prompts tissue degeneration. Leukocytes are recruited to the endometrium, where they make up nearly 50% of the tissue just prior to menstruation. Chemokines involved in endometrial tissue breakdown include molecules such as IL-8, which are produced by the endometrium after progesterone withdrawal. These molecules in turn attract various leukocytes to the uterus. Myeloid cells are particularly abundant and release pro-inflammatory cytokines at this time, as well as multiple other molecules involved in tissue degradation.

Matrix Metalloproteins (MMPs) and Tissue Breakdown

The endometrial matrix consists of the collagen, laminin, gelatin, fibronectin, proteoglycans, and hyaluronic acid. In addition to spiral arteriolar vasoconstriction, enhanced matrix degradation is a key mechanism that contributes to the onset of menstruation. MMPs regulate the degradation of all of the components of the extracellular matrix. Endometrial stroma expresses MMP 1, 2, 3, and 10, while epithelium expresses MMP 7. A plethora of MMPs are produced by leukocytes as well. MMPs are generally secreted in an inactive form. Pro-MMPs are made in increasing numbers prior to menstruation in response to local signals as well as progesterone withdrawal. A tightly regulated balance among MMP production, activation, and inhibition controls the activity of MMPs and hence tissue integrity. MMPs are also regulated by tissue inhibitors of MMPs (TIMPs). Withdrawal of progesterone at menstruation leads to increased MMP production and activation as well as release of TIMPs, thus causing matrix degradation. The degradation of tissue matrix results in massive tissue destruction, loss of structural integrity, and vascular disruption. These events have an even more profound effect than the vascular events previously described. The endometrium is sloughed along with blood coming from the destroyed endometrial vasculature [56].

Mechanisms have evolved to prevent premature clotting during the initial phase of endometrial shedding [57]. Hemostasis is achieved after menstruation by coagulation in the basal endometrium. Tissue breakdown induced by MMPs activates endometrial platelets and results in coagulation of blood. Coagulation abnormalities in various disease states will lead to an increase in menstrual blood loss.

Endometrial Re-epithelialization

Endometrial epithelial cells from the basal glands cover the denuded surface of the endometrium on D2 of the cycle. The epithelial cells migrate and spread to cover the endometrial surface. Of note, re-epithelialization at this time does not reflect mechanisms that involve clonal expansion or a significant effect of estrogen. It is unclear if migrating cells are epithelial stem cells and whether loss of cell–cell contact stimulates this migration.

Vascular Repair

Repair of the endometrial vessels is a crucial event in cyclic shedding of the uterine lining. Endothelial cells sprout from the ruptured arterioles and venules in the basal layer of endometrium and recruit pericytes and smooth muscle cells [58, 59]. VEGF plays an important initial role, inducing recruitment and proliferation of endothelial cells, and forming tubules and tight junctions between cells [60, 61]. Intense vasoconstriction of spiral arterioles prior to onset of bleeding induces local tissue ischemia in the endometrium. This hypoxia induces VEGF expression via hypoxia-inducible factor α [62]. Recruitment of pericytes and smooth muscle cells for maturation of the vessels follows endothelial cell recruitment.

Summary

An endometrium, receptive to embryo implantation, is prepared and shed each month during the menstrual cycle. A woman typically will have about 500 menstrual cycles in her lifetime. Disorders of the menstruation are a common problem and one of the most frequent indications for medical care in a reproductive-aged woman. Precisely regulated tissue degradation, controlled hemorrhage, and rapid hemostasis and repair are required for normal menstruation. A thorough understanding of the mechanisms that underlie this process is important to understand the basis and treatment of disorders in this complex physiologic process.

References

1. Ferenczy A (1979) Diagnostic electron microscopy in gynecologic pathology. Pathol Annu 14(1):353–381
2. Ferenczy A (1979) Regeneration of the human endometrium. In: Fenoglio CM, Wolff M (eds) Progress in surgical pathology. Mason, New York, pp 157–172
3. Casanas-Roux F, Nisolle M, Marbaix E et al (1996) Morphometric, immunohistological and three-dimensional evaluation of the endometrium of menopausal women treated by oestrogen and crinone, a new slow release vaginal progesterone. Hum Reprod 11:357–363
4. Bromer JG, Aldad TS, Taylor HS (2009) Defining the proliferative phase endometrial defect. Fertil Steril 91(3):698–704
5. Balen AH, Conway GS, Kaltsas G et al (1995) Polycystic ovary syndrome: the spectrum of the disorder in 1741 patients. Hum Reprod 10:2107–2111

6. Cornillie FJ, Lauweryns JM, Brosens IA (1985) Normal human endometrium: an ultra structural survey. Gynecol Obstet Invest 20:113–129
7. Dockery P, Li TC, Rogers AW et al (1988) The ultrastructure of the glandular epithelium in the timed endometrial biopsy. Hum Reprod 3:826–834
8. Wilkinson N, Buckley CH, Chawner L et al (1990) Nucleolar organizer regions in normal, hyperplastic and neoplastic endometria. Int J Gynecol Pathol 9:55–59
9. Li TC, Rogers AW, Dockery P et al (1988) A new method of histologic dating of human endometrium in the luteal phase. Fertil Steril 50:52–60
10. Hey NA, Li TC, Devine PL et al (1995) MUC1 in secretory phase endometrium: expression in precisely dated biopsies and flushings from normal and recurrent miscarriage patients. Hum Reprod 10:2655–2662
11. Church HJ, Vicovac LM, Williams JDL et al (1996) Laminins 2 and 4 are expressed by human decidual cells. Lab Invest 74:21–32
12. Aplin JD, Charlton AK, Ayad S (1988) An immunohistochemical study of human endometrial extracellular matrix during the menstrual cycle and first trimester of pregnancy. Cell Tissue Res 253:231–240
13. Iwahashi M, Muragaki Y, Ooshima A et al (1996) Alterations in distribution and composition of the extracellular matrix during decidualization of the human endometrium. J Reprod Fertil 108:147–155
14. Rey JM, Pujol P, Dechaud H et al (1998) Expression of oestrogen receptor-alpha splicing variants and oestrogen receptor beta in endometrium of infertile patients. Mol Hum Reprod 4:641–647
15. Wei LL, Krett NL, Francis MD et al (1988) Multiple human progesterone receptor messenger ribonucleic acids and their auto regulation by progestin agonists and antagonists in breast cancer cells. Mol Endocrinol 2:62–72
16. Wen DX, YF XU, Mais DE et al (1994) The A and B isoforms of the human progesterone receptor operate through distinct signaling pathways within target cells. Mol Cell Biol 14:8356–8364
17. Ogle TF, Dai D, George P et al (1998) Regulation of the progesterone receptor and estrogen receptor in decidua basalis by progesterone and estradiol during pregnancy. Biol Reprod 58:1188–1198
18. Critchley HOD, Abberton KM, Taylor NH et al (1994) Endometrial sex steroid receptor expression in women with menorrhagia. Br J Obstet Gynecol 101:428–434
19. Wang H, Critchley HOD, Kelly RW et al (1998) Progesterone receptor subtype B is differentially regulated in human endometrial stroma. Mol Hum Reprod 4:407–412
20. Goodger AM, Rogers PAW (1994) Endometrial endothelial cell proliferation during the menstrual cycle. Hum Reprod 9:399–405
21. Haining REB, Cameron IT, Van Papendorp C et al (1991) Epidermal growth factor in human endometrium: proliferative effects in culture and immunocytochemical localization in normal and endometriotic tissues. Hum Reprod 6:1200–1205
22. Haining REB, Schofield JP, Jones DSC et al (1991) Identification of mRNA for epidermal growth factor and transforming growth factor α present in low copy number in human endometrium and decidua using reverse transcriptase polymerase chain reaction. J Mol Endocrinol 6:207–214
23. Nelson KG, Takahashi T, Bossert NL et al (1991) Epidermal growth factor replaces estrogen in the stimulation of female genital-tract growth and differentiation. Proc Natl Acad Sci U S A 88:21–25
24. Ignar-Trowbridge DM, Teng CT, Ross KA et al (1993) Peptide growth factors elicit estrogen receptor-dependent transcriptional activation of an estrogen-responsive element. Mol Endocrinol 7:992–998
25. Presta M (1988) Sex hormones modulate the synthesis of basic fibroblast growth factor in human endometrial adenocarcinoma cells: implications for the neovascularization of normal and neoplastic endometrium. J Cell Physiol 137:593–597
26. Ferriani RA, Charnock-Jones DS, Prentice A et al (1993) Immunohistochemical localization of acidic and basic fibroblast growth factors in normal human endometrium and endometriosis and the detection of their mRNA by polymerase chain reaction. Hum Reprod 8:11–16

27. Sangha RK, Xiao Feng L, Shams M et al (1997) Fibroblast growth factor receptor 1 is a critical component for endometrial remodeling: localization and expression of basic fibroblast growth factor and FGF R1 in human endometrium during the menstrual cycle and decreased FGF R1 expression in menorrhagia. Lab Invest 77:389–402
28. Siegfried S, Pekonen F, Nyman T et al (1997) Distinct patterns of expression of keratinocyte growth factor and its receptor in endometrial carcinoma. Cancer 79:1166–1171
29. Roy RN, Cecutti A, Gerulath AH et al (1997) Endometrial transcripts of human insulin-like growth factors arise by differential promoter usage. Mol Cell Endocrinol 135:11–19
30. Irwin JC, De Las Fuentes L, Dsupin BA et al (1993) Insulin-like growth factor regulation of human endometrial stromal cell function: coordinate effects of insulin-like growth factor binding protein-1, cell proliferation and prolactin secretion. Regul Pept 48:165–177
31. Matsui H, Taga M, Kurogi K et al (1997) Gene expression of keratinocyte growth factor and its receptor in the human endometrium/decidua and chorionic villi. Endocr J 44:867–871
32. Chan RW, Schwab KE, Gargett CE (2004) Clonogenicity of human endometrial epithelial and stromal cells. Biol Reprod 70:1738–1750
33. Cervelló I, Simón C (2009) Somatic stem cells in the endometrium. Reprod Sci 16(2):200–205
34. Chan RW, Gargett CE (2006) Identification of label-retaining cells in mouse endometrium. Stem Cells 24:1529–1538
35. Taylor HS (2004) Endometrial cells derived from donor stem cells in bone marrow transplant recipients. JAMA 292:81–85
36. Du H, Taylor HS (2009) Stem cells and female reproduction. Reprod Sci 16(2):126–139
37. Dimitrov R, Timeva T, Kyurkchiev D et al (2008) Characterization of clonogenic stromal cells isolated from human endometrium. Reproduction 135:551–558
38. Du H, Taylor HS (2007) Contribution of bone marrow-derived stem cells to endometrium and endometriosis. Stem Cells 25:2082–2086
39. Mints M, Jansson M, Sadeghi B et al (2008) Endometrial endothelial cells are derived from donor stem cells in a bone marrow transplant recipient. Hum Reprod 23:139–143
40. Klauber N, Rohan RM, Flynn E et al (1997) Critical components of the female reproductive pathway are suppressed by the angiogenesis inhibitor AGM-1470. Nat Med 3:443–446
41. Markee JE (1940) Menstruation in intraocular endometrial transplants in the rhesus monkey. Contrib Embryol Carnegie Inst 28:219–308
42. Ramsey EM (1982) In: Biology of the uterus. Plenum Press, New York, pp 59–76
43. Ferenczy A (1987) In: Blaustein's pathology of the genital tract. Springer, New York, pp 257–291
44. Abberton KM, Taylor NH, Healy DL (1996) Vascular smooth muscle α-actin distribution around endometrial arterioles during the menstrual cycle: increased expression during the perimenopause and lack of correlation with menorrhagia. Hum Reprod 11:204–211
45. Ferrara N, Henzel WJ (1989) Pituitary follicular cells secrete a novel heparin-binding growth factor specific for vascular endothelial cells. Biochem Biophys Res Commun 161:851–858
46. Esch F, Ueno N, Baird A (1985) Primary structure of bovine brain acidic fibroblast growth factor (FGF). Biochem Biophys Res Commun 133:554–562
47. Kech PJ, Hauser SD, Krivi G et al (1989) Vascular permeability factor, an endothelial cell mitogen related to platelet-derived growth factor. Science 246:1309–1312
48. Leung DW, Cachianes G, Kuang WJ et al (1989) Vascular endothelial growth factor is a secreted angiogenic mitogens. Science 246:1306–1309
49. Charnock-Jones DS, Sharkey AM, Rajput-Williams J et al (1993) Identification and localization of alternately spliced mRNAs for vascular endothelial growth factor in human uterus and estrogen regulation in endometrial carcinoma cell lines. Biol Reprod 48:1120–1128
50. Li XF, Gregory J, Ahmed A (1994) Immunolocalisation of vascular endothelial growth factor in human endometrium. Growth Factors 11:277–282
51. Krikun G, Schatz F, Lockwood CJ (2004) Endometrial angiogenesis: from physiology to pathology. Ann N Y Acad Sci 1034:27–35
52. Lockwood CJ, Krikun G, Hausknecht V, Wang EY, Schatz F (1997) Decidual cell regulation of hemostasis during implantation and menstruation. Ann N Y Acad Sci 828:188–193
53. Smith SK (1989) Prostaglandins and growth factors in the endometrium. Baillieres Clin Obstet Gynaecol 3:249–270

54. Chwalisz K, Garfield RE (2000) Role of nitric oxide in implantation and menstruation. Hum Reprod 15:96–111
55. Collett GP, Kohnen G, Campbell S, Davenport AP, Jeffers MD, Cameron IT (1996) Localization of endothelin receptors in human uterus throughout the menstrual cycle. Mol Hum Reprod 2:439–444
56. Rogers PA, Abberton KM (2003) Endometrial arteriogenesis: vascular smooth muscle cell proliferation and differentiation during the menstrual cycle and changes associated with endometrial bleeding disorders. Microsc Res Tech 60:412–419
57. Lockwood CJ, Schatz F (1996) A biological model for the regulation of peri-implantational hemostasis and menstruation. J Soc Gynecol Investig 3(4):159–165
58. Folkman J, D'Amore PA (1996) Blood vessel formation: what is its molecular basis? Cell 87:1153–1155
59. Hanahan D (1997) Signaling vascular morphogenesis and maintenance. Science 277:48–50
60. Shalaby F, Rossant J, Yamaguchi TP et al (1995) Failure of blood island formation and vasculogenesis in Flk 1 deficient mice. Nature 376:62–66
61. Fong GH, Rossant J, Gertsenstein M et al (1995) Role of the Flt-1 receptor tyrosine kinase in regulating the assembly of vascular endothelium. Nature 376:66–70
62. Wang GL, Semenza GL (1993) Characterization of hypoxia-inducible factor 1 and regulation of DNA binding activity by hypoxia. J Biol Chem 268:21513–21518

Chapter 3
Amenorrhea Due to Idiopathic Hypogonadotropic Hypogonadism and Kallmann Syndrome

Lawrence C. Layman

Case Study

The patient is a 17-year-old white female who was seen for primary amenorrhea. Her mother states that she was healthy during her childhood years other than having several surgeries for repair of cleft lip and palate. Upon further questioning, she is not able to smell foods or other common smells. Her mother had normal puberty but she also has diminished sense of smell. Her mother's brother reportedly had delayed puberty, cleft palate, and subsequent infertility.

On physical exam, she is 5′1″ tall with Tanner 1 breasts and Tanner 3 pubic hair. By bimanual exam, the physician is able to place a finger into the vagina and palpate a cervix. Laboratory studies include a prolactin = 10ng/ml (3–20), TSH = 1.7 μU/ml (0.4–4), total T4 = 8.1 μg/dl (4.5–12.5), LH = 1 mIU/ml (1–11), and FSH = 1.5 mIU/ml (1–11). An MRI reveals no tumor in the brain, but the olfactory bulbs are not seen. Following these studies, additional laboratory studies are obtained: an 8:00 a.m. cortisol is 17ug/dl (8–20) and a growth hormone level rises from 1 to 8 ng/ml after 30 min of exercise.

Development of the Hypothalamic-Pituitary-Gonadal Axis

During embryological development, gonadotropin releasing hormone (GnRH) and olfactory neurons migrate from the olfactory placode region into the brain [1]. Once the olfactory neurons cross the cribriform plate into the brain, a dorsal branch migrates dorsally to reach the olfactory bulbs while a ventral branch migrates to the hypothalamus along with GnRH neurons. GnRH is secreted in a pulsatile fashion

L.C. Layman (✉)
Section of Reproductive Endocrinology, Infertility, and Genetics, Department of Obstetrics and Gynecology, Developmental Neurobiology Program, Institute of Molecular Medicine and Genetics, Medical College of Georgia, Augusta, GA 30912-3360, USA
e-mail: llayman@mcg.edu

N.F. Santoro and G. Neal-Perry (eds.), *Amenorrhea: A Case-Based, Clinical Guide*, Contemporary Endocrinology, DOI 10.1007/978-1-60327-864-5_3,

from the arcuate nucleus of the hypothalamus, where it is released into the hypophyseal-portal system to affect pituitary synthesis and secretion of gonadotropins luteinizing hormone (LH) and follicle stimulating hormone (FSH). Pituitary gonadotropins then stimulate the ovary to produce sex steroids and oocytes.

Without the use of green fluorescence protein labeling, it is very difficult to study the neurophysiology of individual GnRH neurons in the laboratory. The main reason that it is so difficult to study individual GnRH neurons is because they are widely dispersed throughout the hypothalamus and they are few in number – mice have only 800–1,000 and primates have only 1,000–2,000 [1]. Fortunately, there are two types of immortalized GnRH neurons commonly studied in the literature that are easily manipulated experimentally and maintain important characteristics of GnRH neurons (express GnRH mRNA and release peptide in a pulsatile pattern). GT1–7 cells represent one such group of immortalized GnRH neurons. These immortalized GnRH neurons were generated by cloning the rat GnRH promoter upstream to the T-antigen, which was then injected into single cell embryos [2]. This technique resulted in hypothalamic tumors which were harvested, cultured, and subsequently named GT1–7 cells. These cells are of neuronal origin (but not glia) and are postmigratory.

When the human GnRH promoter was cloned upstream to the T-antigen and injected into single cell embryos to create transgenic mice, tumors were observed along the migratory pathway. These GN11 and NLT cells not only express GnRH, albeit, at lower levels than GT1–7 cells, but they also display migratory properties in vitro [3].

The Diagnosis of Delayed Puberty

Following the childhood period and for reasons not completely understood, central inhibition of GnRH pulses is reduced, and GnRH pulses stimulate first nocturnal LH pulses, which then later occur throughout the 24-h period. These LH pulses stimulate ovarian estrogen production and initiate the onset of the pubertal transition. Normal puberty is usually a progression of events. Once the pubertal process is initiated, it is generally completed within 3–4 years. Thelarche is typically the first sign of estrogen production, and occurs at about age 10.5 years, while pubarche (pubic hair growth) generally occurs about 6 months later. In 10–20% of girls, pubarche precedes thelarche. The peak height velocity occurs at about age 12, and on the descending arm of the growth spurt, menarche occurs at age 12–13 [4].

In girls, delayed puberty is defined as either the absence of thelarche by age 13 or menarche by age 15, which represents 2.5 standard deviations above the mean for North American children. The differential diagnosis is complex and may include hypogonadism, anatomic abnormalities, such as the absence or obstruction of the outflow tract, and certain disorders with ongoing estrogen production – most commonly polycystic ovary syndrome (PCOS). An overview is shown in Fig. 3.1. Although not discussed here, the evaluation and diagnostic categories are similar for males.

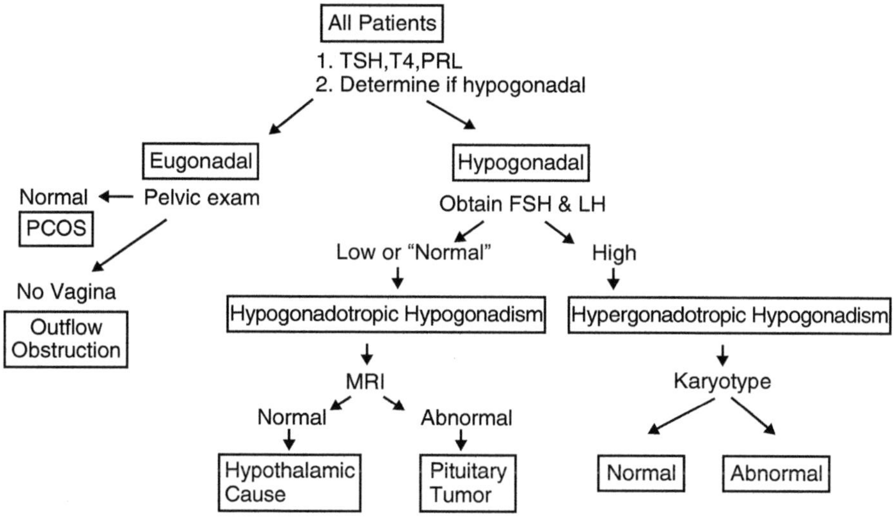

Fig. 3.1 An overview of the diagnostic steps in girls with delayed puberty. The two most common causes of outflow obstruction causing primary amenorrhea are complete androgen insensitivity syndrome and mullerian aplasia (Mayer–Rokitansky–Kuster–Hauser syndrome). *PCOS* polycystic ovary syndrome; *T4* thyroxin; *TSH* thyroid stimulating hormone; *PRL* prolactin

All patients who present with delayed puberty should have a TSH, total T4 (more robust assay than the problematic free T4 – unless it is done by dialysis and subsequent immunoassay), serum prolactin, and detailed psychosocial history. Hypothyroidism (central, rather than primary), hyperprolactinemia, and hypothalamic disorders (eating disorders/stress/exercise) may occur in patients who are eugonadal or hypogonadal depending upon how long the process has been ongoing.

A careful history and physical exam of the female with delayed puberty are extremely important. It is necessary to ascertain any initial signs of puberty and estrogen production. If there are no signs of breast development, the patient clearly has hypogonadism. If she has breast development, she has evidence of having estrogen exposure at some time in her life, but her estrogen status must be determined at the time of presentation (as she could be now hypogonadal).

Several different methods could be considered to determine estradiol exposure, but it should be remembered that estradiol levels are usually not very helpful because discrimination between low and low-normal levels is not easy. A vaginal maturation index can be determined with a vaginal smear performed at the first visit by inserting a Q-tip and rolling it in the fornices of the vagina. Collected cells are then gently rolled on to a slide and set with urine Sedi-Stain or another quick prep stain (liquid prep pap smear fixative may also be used) and the ratio of parabasal, intermediate, and superficial (P/I/S) cells counted in ~100 cells. A predominance of parabasal cells (such as 80:20:0 ratio) indicates that the patient is hypoestrogenic, and therefore, hypogonadal. It is important to remember that this does not tell anything about the etiology of the hypogonadism – just that hypogonadism is present.

If superficial cells are present (as in 0:20:80), the patient is probably making estrogen and is probably eugonadal.

Another method used to assess gonadal status is the progestin challenge test. It is usually performed by administering medroxyprogesterone acetate 10 mg for 5–10 days (after a negative pregnancy test if the patient has normal breast development). Progesterone could also be used, but norethindrone should probably not be used since it may be contaminated with and/or converted to estrogen (which could cause the hypogonadal patient to bleed) [5]. If the patient is hypogonadal, she may not bleed at all or have only minimal spotting. A normal menstrual bleed after the medication is completed indicates that sufficient endogenous estrogen is being produced to prime the endometrium. This test does not need to be performed in patients with no breast development, or who have a vaginal smear inconsistent with estrogen exposure (predominant parabasal cells).

Hypogonadism

If hypogonadism is suspected on the basis of physical exam (Tanner 1 breasts), vaginal maturation index, or negative progestin withdrawal, then serum gonadotropins should be obtained. If elevated, they should be repeated in several weeks for confirmation because of the pulsatile secretion of gonadotropins. If gonadotropins are elevated on several occasions, gonadal failure, also known as *hypergonadotropic hypogonadism*, is present. A karyotype should be performed in patients (boys and girls) with elevated gonadotropins to rule out a chromosomal abnormality (most commonly a 45,X with or without mosaicism or a pure 46,XY cell line in a girl; or a 47,XXY or 46,XX in a male) [6, 7]. If gonadotropins are low or normal in the face of hypogonadism, then the patient has *hypogonadotropic hypogonadism* (HH) due to hypothalamic or pituitary dysfunction or disease. It is usually taught that chromosome abnormalities are uncommon and hence unnecessary to evaluate in patients with HH. However, this presumption may be challenged by studies from our lab which found that as many as 2–3% of patients with HH have chromosomal rearrangements [8].

Sex steroids are necessary for growth therefore performing a bone age should be considered in hypogonadal patients. These patients can have delayed bone age compared to chronological age. They do not usually have a bone age beyond 11–12 years; however, if bone age is markedly delayed, growth hormone deficiency and/or hypothyroidism should strongly be considered.

Idiopathic Hypogonadotropic Hypogonadism

When the patient is hypogonadal with low serum gonadotropins (or "normal," an inappropriate finding on a background of hypogonadism), the diagnosis is HH. An MRI with and without gadolinium of the brain is necessary to exclude a CNS tumor, most commonly a prolactinoma or craniopharygioma. It is also reasonable to visualize the olfactory tracts and bulb – if they are absent or hypoplastic, this suggests Kallmann syndrome (KS). If a tumor is not present, the cause is usually considered to be hypothalamic by exclusion. Although it is possible to perform a triple test (insulin induced hypoglycemia, GnRH, and TRH stimulation and check baseline and hormone levels every 15 min for 1–2 h – TSH, prolactin, cortisol, LH, FSH, and GH), the cost is great and the yield is very low except in patients who have extreme short stature, which could suggest pituitary failure. However, cryptic adrenal failure is very serious and could indicate pituitary insufficiency with reduced ACTH, therefore, it is reasonable to obtain an 8:00 AM cortisol. If the patient has a height below the 5th percentile, particularly with a family history of pituitary failure, then combined pituitary hormone deficiency (CPHD) should be considered. Genetic counseling and testing for mutations in genes such as *PROP1*, *HESX1*, *SOX2*, *SOX3*, *LHX3*, or *LHX4* could be considered in these patients (Fig. 3.1) [9]. In the absence of a tumor, strong consideration must be given to the history and physical exam with particular attention to body mass index, eating and exercise patterns, and stress.

For patients with HH who have no pituitary tumor and are of normal weight, two diagnoses must be entertained. The first is constitutional delay of puberty (CDP), which really can only be documented in retrospect if girls subsequently initiate spontaneous puberty before age 17 (CDP is more common in boys). If girls remain hypogonadal by age 17, then the diagnosis is idiopathic or isolated hypogonadotropic hypogonadism (IHH). A history should be sought for anosmia/hyposmia, midline facial defects, associated neurologic deficits such as synkinesia (on exam she raises both arms when she is asked to raise one), hearing loss, or visual abnormalities. When IHH is combined with anosmia/hyposmia, she has KS. Certainly, a history for eating disorders (anorexia or bulimia), extreme stress, or strenuous exercise must be excluded (discussed in Chap. 8).

The Genetic Basis of IHH/KS

Chromosome Analysis

Although they do not occur as commonly as in women with hypergonadotropic hypogonadism, karyotype abnormalities may occur in several percent of IHH/KS patients [8]. Although their immediate significance is less obvious than a 45,X cell line in a patient with gonadal dysgenesis, a balanced chromosomal translocation could provide an indication of a new IHH/KS gene. These types of studies are being actively pursued in our molecular reproductive endocrinology laboratory. For example, it is possible that a chromosomal translocation could disrupt a gene at the breakpoint, which could cause IHH/KS in that patient. Then, this gene becomes a candidate gene to test in other patients with IHH/KS who do not have chromosome abnormalities. It is also very reasonable to karyotype patients with multiple anomalies and IHH/KS, as this could indicate an unbalanced chromosomal rearrangement with the loss of multiple genes. Prader-Willi syndrome, due to a 15q deletion by FISH, should be considered if associated anomalies are present.

Comparative genomic hybridization (CGH) could also be very helpful in ascertaining if deletions or duplications occur.

Molecular Analysis

Mutations have been identified in approximately 30% of IHH/KS families, including *KAL1, GNRHR, NR0B1, FGFR1, KISS1R, PROK2, PROKR2, CHD7, FGF8, TAC3, TAC3R, NELF*, and *GNRH1* (reviewed in Kim et al. [9] and summarized in Table 3.1). In this section, the more common genes, particularly those that have consequences for genetic counseling will be briefly reviewed. Mutations in the first identified gene – *KAL1* [10, 11] – on the X chromosome account for about 5–10% of the causes of KS in males (not females since it is X-linked recessive) [12]. If a clear X-linked recessive family history is present, 30–60% of these patients will have *KAL1* mutations [12]. Males with mutations in the *KAL1* gene may also have unilateral renal agenesis (50% in one series), which should be tested. To date *KAL1* mutations have only been reported in males with either anosmia or hyposmia – not normosmia. Mutations in the *FGFR1* (*KAL2*) gene occur in about 10% of patients with either KS or normosmic IHH [13, 14]. This autosomal dominant disorder can lead to individuals with mutations who are not affected (reduced penetrance) or to patients with a mild phenotype, such as anosmia only (variable expressivity), which can complicate the diagnosis. Midline facial defects and dental agenesis may occur in patients with *FGFR1* mutations.

Mutations in the *CHD7* gene cause CHARGE syndrome (*C*oloboma of the eye, *H*eart defects, choanal *A*tresia, *R*etardation in growth and development, *G*enito-urinary anomalies, and *E*ar – both vestibular and auditory) [15]. This disorder can be autosomal dominant or sporadic. Recently, *CHD7* mutations were found to be present in 6% of KS patients and 6% of those with normosmic IHH [16]. Mutations in *CHD7* and *FGFR1* are particularly important because they cause autosomal dominant disease with an attendant 50% risk to each pregnancy, indicating that the patient should be properly counseled prior to pregnancy.

For patients with normosmia, *FGFR1* and *CHD7* are the most common. *GNRHR* mutations [17, 18] comprise approximately 3–5% of the cases and are inherited in an autosomal recessive fashion [19]. They have only been reported in normosmic IHH – not KS. Although mutations in other genes have been reported, they are currently thought to be rare or the role of genetic counseling is marginally understood. There have also been some cases in which mutations in two different genes – digenic inheritance – has been reported [20, 21].

Currently, the molecular basis of IHH/KS usually relies upon research labs, including our own. Blood from the affected patient, parents, and siblings (both affected and unaffected) are obtained so that segregation studies can be performed. In this way, if a mutation is identified, other family members can be tested to see if the putative mutation is found in those affected and absent in those who are unaffected. Molecular analysis should be offered to any patient who desires to understand more about her disease, as well as for the risk of recurrence to her child if she elects to attempt conception.

Table 3.1 IHH/KS genes. The gene symbol and its chromosomal location are shown in addition to the phenotype, inheritance pattern, and frequency

Gene	Localization	Phenotype	Inheritance	Frequency
GnRH and olfactory neuron migration				
KAL1	Xp22.3	KS	XLR	5–10%; 30–70% familial
FGFR1	8p12	KS, IHH	AD	–10%
CHD7	8q12.2	KS, IHH, CHARGE syndrome	AD, sporadic	6%
FGF8	10q24	KS, IHH	AD	1.3%
NELF	9q34.3	IHH/KS	Digenic and monogenic	1–2%
PROK2	3p21.1	KS	Unknown	1–2%
PROKR2	20p13	KS	Unknown	5%
Hypothalamus				
KISS1R	19p13.3	IHH	AR	Low
LEP	7q31.3	Obesity, IHH	AR	Low
LEPR	1p31	Obesity, IHH	AR	Low
NROB1[a]	Xp21	Adrenal hypoplasia congenita and IHH	XLR	Low
PCSK1	5q15-q23	Obesity, IHH	AR	Rare
TAC3	12q13-q21	IHH	AR	Unknown
TACR3	4q25	IHH	AR	Unknown
GNRH1	8p21-p11.2	IHH	AR	0.3–0.8%
Pituitary				
GNRHR	4q21.2	IHH	AR	3–5%
FSHB	11p13	Isolated FSH deficiency	AR	Rare
LHB	19q13.3	Isolated LH deficiency	AR	Rare
HESX1	3p21.1–21.2	Septo-optic dysplasia, CPHD	AR, AD	Low
PROP1	5q	Short stature, hypothyroid, CPHD	AR	Low
LHX3	9q34.3	CPHD	AR	Low
LHX4	1q25	CPHD	AD	Low
SOX2	3q26.3-q27	Microphthalmia/ midline CNS defects, CPHD	AD, sporadic	2–3%
SOX3	Xq26.3	Midline CNS anomalies, CPHD	XLR	Low

FGFR1, CHD7, FGF8, PROKR2, and PROK2 mutations cause both normosmic IHH and KS. *XLR* X-linked recessive; *AD* autosomal dominant; *AR* autosomal recessive; *CPHD* combined pituitary hormone deficiency

[a]NROB1 has hypothalamic and pituitary effects

Treatment

Treatment for patients with IHH involves administration of estrogen for girls [22]. Usually, estrogen-only preparations are started at a low dose and increased gradually until normal breast development is reached (or she begins bleeding). This could be 0.3 mg of conjugated equine estrogens that are increased every 3–6 months to 1.25 mg/day. Alternatively, 0.5 mg of estradiol could be given and increased by 0.5 mg increments until the desired result is observed. This could take a year or longer. Then, a progestin is added, or for ease of administration, a combined estrogen–progestogen preparation could then be prescribed.

When pregnancy is desired the estrogen–progestogen is discontinued. Since clomiphene acts principally in the hypothalamus, and these patients have hypothalamic dysfunction, it usually will not work. In contrast to patients with gonadal failure, patients with IHH or KS can be treated with subcutaneous FSH and LH (usually 150 IU/day with monitoring of ovarian follicular development) for ovulation induction in females. These patients are at high risk for ovarian hyperstimulation syndrome and high-order multiple pregnancies. Therefore, it is prudent to be cautious and not aggressive with exogenous stimulation of the ovaries. Previously, this risk was circumvented with the use of a GnRH pump which supported monofollicular ovarian development. Unfortunately, this method of ovulation induction is not available at this time in the United States. Nonetheless, if tubal patency and normal semen parameters exist, ovulation induction as a therapeutic approach yields cycle fecundity that is similar with age-matched fertile women [22].

Case Discussion

This patient has no evidence of puberty – she has Tanner 1 breasts and primary amenorrhea. The fact that she does not demonstrate any stigmata of puberty and there is an absence of breast development strongly indicates hypoestrogenism. There is no reason to obtain a serum estradiol level in this case. In fact, most estradiol assays are not designed to distinguish between low (<30 pg/ml) and early follicular phase levels (30–60 pg/ml). Low or normal serum levels of gonadotropins in the presence of clinical evidence consistent with hypoestrogenism indicate that the patient has HH. An MRI excludes the presence of a tumor, which could be either a prolactinoma or a craniopharygioma. In this patient, as in many others, the cause is usually unknown; and it is often termed idiopathic hypogonadotropic hypogonadism (IHH). She has anosmia with absent olfactory bulbs, findings that strongly suggest that she has KS. If she were tested with a smell identification test, it is likely she would be anosmic or hyposmic. Midline facial defects may also be present in patients with IHH.

The findings of: (1) KS in the patient, (2) her mother who has anosmia only, and (3) an uncle who had delayed puberty and infertility suggest autosomal dominant inheritance. Mutations in either *FGFR1* or *CHD7* genes cause autosomal dominant KS and could be present in this family. DNA sequencing of first the *FGFR1* gene, which is more common (10%), and if negative, the *CHD7* gene (6%) could be considered in this patient. Autosomal dominant diseases may manifest either reduced penetrance (meaning that not all patients with a mutation manifest the disease), or as in this family, variable expressivity (indicating variable severity). The patient has KS; the mother has only anosmia; and an uncle probably has IHH without anosmia, but who had a more serious defect – cleft palate.

This patient can be treated with estrogen to induce breast development. Once breast development is adequate or she has menses, then adding a progestin or switching to a combined estrogen–progesterone combination preparation can be done. When she considers pregnancy, treatment with gonadotropins (both FSH and LH will be necessary) can be used for ovulation induction. It must be remembered that she should be counseled that there could be up to a 50% chance of having an affected child with the same disorder.

References

1. Wierman ME, Pawlowski JE, Allen MP, Xu M, Linseman DA, Nielsen-Preiss S (2004) Molecular mechanisms of gonadotropin-releasing hormone neuronal migration. Trends Endocrinol Metab 15:96–102
2. Mellon PL, Windle JJ, Goldsmith PC, Padula CA, Roberts JL, Weiner RI (1990) Immortalization of hypothalamic GnRH neurons by genetically targeted tumorigenesis. Neuron 5:1–10
3. Radovick S, Wray S, Lee E et al (1991) Migratory arrest of gonadotropin-releasing hormone neurons in transgenic mice. Proc Natl Acad Sci USA 88:3402–3406
4. Layman LC, Reindollar RH (1994) The diagnosis and treatment of pubertal disorders. Adolesc Med State Art Rev 5:37–55
5. Chu MC, Zhang X, Gentzschein E, Stanczyk FZ, Lobo RA (2007) Formation of ethinyl estradiol in women during treatment with norethindrone acetate. J Clin Endocrinol Metab 92:2205–2207
6. Layman LC (2002) Human gene mutations causing infertility. J Med Genet 39:153–161
7. Layman LC (2003) Genetic causes of human infertility. Endocrinol Metab Clin North Am 32:549–572
8. Bhagavath B, Podolsky RH, Ozata M et al (2006) Clinical and molecular characterization of a large sample of patients with hypogonadotropic hypogonadism. Fertil Steril 85:706–713
9. Kim HG, Bhagavath B, Layman LC (2008) Clinical manifestations of impaired GnRH neuron development and function. Neurosignals 16:165–182
10. Franco B, Guioli S, Pragliola A et al (1991) A gene deleted in Kallmann's syndrome shares homology with neural cell adhesion and axonal path-finding molecules. Nature 353:529–536
11. Legouis R, Hardelin JP, Levilliers J et al (1991) The candidate gene for the X-linked Kallmann syndrome encodes a protein related to adhesion molecules. Cell 67:423–435
12. Bhagavath B, Xu N, Ozata M et al (2007) KAL1 mutations are not a common cause of idiopathic hypogonadotrophic hypogonadism in humans. Mol Hum Reprod 13:25–30
13. Dode C, Levilliers J, Dupont JM et al (2003) Loss-of-function mutations in FGFR1 cause autosomal dominant Kallmann syndrome. Nat Genet 33:463–465
14. Pitteloud N, Acierno JS Jr, Meysing A et al (2006) Mutations in fibroblast growth factor receptor 1 cause both Kallmann syndrome and normosmic idiopathic hypogonadotropic hypogonadism. Proc Natl Acad Sci U S A 103:6281–6286
15. Vissers LE, van Ravenswaaij CM, Admiraal R et al (2004) Mutations in a new member of the chromodomain gene family cause CHARGE syndrome. Nat Genet 36:955–957

16. Kim HG, Kurth I, Lan F et al (2008) Mutations in CHD7, encoding a chromatin-remodeling protein, cause idiopathic hypogonadotropic hypogonadism and Kallmann syndrome. Am J Hum Genet 83:511–519
17. de Roux N, Young J, Misrahi M et al (1997) A family with hypogonadotropic hypogonadism and mutations in the gonadotropin-releasing hormone receptor. N Engl J Med 337:1597–1602
18. Layman LC, Cohen DP, Jin M et al (1998) Mutations in the gonadotropin-releasing hormone receptor gene cause hypogonadotropic hypogonadism. Nat Genet 18:14–15
19. Bhagavath B, Ozata M, Ozdemir IC et al (2005) The prevalence of gonadotropin-releasing hormone receptor mutations in a large cohort of patients with hypogonadotropic hypogonadism. Fertil Steril 84:951–957
20. Dode C, Teixeira L, Levilliers J et al (2006) Kallmann syndrome: mutations in the genes encoding prokineticin-2 and prokineticin receptor-2. PLoS Genet 2:e175
21. Pitteloud N, Quinton R, Pearce S et al (2007) Digenic mutations account for variable phenotypes in idiopathic hypogonadotropic hypogonadism. J Clin Invest 117:457–463
22. Layman LC (2007) Hypogonadotropic hypogonadism. Endocrinol Metab Clin North Am 36:283–296

Chapter 4
Polycystic Ovary Syndrome

Enrico Carmina

Introduction

Polycystic ovary syndrome (PCOS) is a heterogeneous disorder characterized by the pathogenetic importance of ovarian hyperandrogenism and insulin resistance and by the variable presence of four key features: (1) chronic anovulation; (2) hyperandrogenism; (3) abdominal obesity; and (4) polycystic ovaries [1].

These features were already described by Stein and Leventhal in 1935 [2] and, with the notable exception of the abdominal obesity, are the components of the newer diagnostic criteria of Rotterdam and of Androgen Excess and PCOS Society [3, 4]. The main difference between these two diagnostic approaches is that the first includes in the syndrome also patients with no clinical or biochemical hyperandrogenism while AEPCOS criteria consider essential the presence of hyperandrogenism.

Because it is sufficient that two of the key features are present to make the diagnosis; four different phenotypes may be found with Rotterdam criteria while with AEPCOS criteria three different phenotypes are observed [5]. In Table 4.1, the four main phenotypes according to Rotterdam criteria are reported.

Independently on diagnostic criteria, PCOS is a very common disorder. Studies on the prevalence of the classic form (chronic anovulation and hyperandrogenism) have shown that in most ethnic groups about 6% of adult women are affected by the disorder [6]. Including the milder or contested phenotypes, the prevalence of PCOS is probably around 10% of all adult women [7].

E. Carmina (✉)
Department of Medical and Biological Sciences, University of Palermo, Via delle Croci 47, 90139 Palermo, Italy
e-mail: enricocarmina@libero.it

N.F. Santoro and G. Neal-Perry (eds.), *Amenorrhea: A Case-Based, Clinical Guide*, Contemporary Endocrinology, DOI 10.1007/978-1-60327-864-5_4,

Table 4.1 Phenotypes of PCOS according to Rotterdam meeting

1. Classic PCOS
(a) With polycystic ovaries
(b) With normal ovaries
2. Ovulatory PCOS
3. Normoandrogenic PCOS

Clinical and Endocrine Characteristics of Main PCOS Phenotypes

Although only few studies have evaluated the clinical and endocrine characteristics of the four main Rotterdam phenotypes [8–12], the available data may be so summarized (Table 4.2):

1. Type I classic PCOS represents the most common and severe form of PCOS. These patients present as group an abdominal obesity, chronic anovulation with oligomenorrhea or amenorrhea, increased levels of LH and LH/FSH ratio, increased androgens, elevated insulin, insulin resistance, and polycystic ovaries. They represent almost 60% of all PCOS patients but in some settings may represent 80–90% of all PCOS patients.
2. Type II classic PCOS are very similar to other classic PCOS patients but are less common (only 5–10% of the total number of PCOS patients). These patients present normal ovaries and the main endocrine difference between type I and type II classic PCOS is related to LH levels and LH/FSH ratio. Although all patients with classic PCOS have increased LH and LH/FSH ratios when compared to controls, those patients with polycystic ovaries have significantly higher LH levels (and LH/FSH ratios) than patients with normal ovaries. It suggests that LH is important or in some way related to the morphologic appearance of the ovaries.
3. Ovulatory PCOS seems to be the mild form of classic PCOS. In fact, these patients present most endocrine characteristics of PCOS but in a milder form. In fact, patients with ovulatory PCOS have intermediate values (between classic PCOS and controls) of BMI, waist circumference, testosterone, insulin, and QUICKI. Only LH is generally normal, and it represents the main endocrine difference with the other phenotypes of PCOS. On the other hand, it is well known that in many patients with classic PCOS, it is possible to get ovulation by reducing body weight [13]. Passage from classic to ovulatory PCOS and vice versa may be possible and related to sociocultural and environmental influences [14, 15].
4. Patients with normoandrogenic PCOS represent a unique group. However, also these patients have a mild testosterone excess in spite of having androgen levels in the normal range [11]. This group of subjects is mostly characterized by increased LH and LH/FSH ratio but normal body weight, waist circumference, insulin, and insulin sensitivity. Probably, they are part of PCOS spectrum but may have different pathogenetic components. In fact, hyperandrogenism is very mild and insulin resistance is generally absent. Because of it, it may be correct to keep these patients separated from other PCOS patients as previously suggested by AEPCOS Committee [4].

Table 4.2 Main characteristics of PCOS phenotypes

	Androgen levels	LH/FSH	Insulin resistance	CV risk
Type I classic PCOS	Increased	Increased	Increased	Increased
Type II classic PCOS	Increased	Mild increase	Increased	Increased
Ovulatory PCOS	Increased	Normal	Mild increase	Mild increase
Normoandrogenic PCOS	Normal	Increased	Normal	Normal?

In conclusion, the different phenotypes of PCOS not only present similarities, but also important differences in their clinical and endocrine pattern.

Amenorrhea and PCOS: Prevalence and Clinical Significance

In the original paper of Stein and Leventhal [2], the patients presented with amenorrhea, and for many years amenorrhea has been considered prevalent in women with PCOS. In 1963, Goldzieher and Axelrod reviewing the clinical data of 1,079 patients, tabulated from 187 references, reported that amenorrhea was present in the majority (51%) of the patients with PCOS [16]. More recent studies have indicated that amenorrhea, while relatively common, is present in a minority of PCOS women, with a prevalence ranging between 10 and 20% of the patients [17, 18]. Probably, differences in diagnostic criteria have determined such differences in prevalence.

It is unclear that the motive of the occurrence of amenorrhea in PCOS patients. Probably, differences in estrogen production may explain these differences, but it is the opinion of the author that in some PCOS patients, amenorrhea may be linked also to psychological stress. In our experience, amenorrhea is present in 12% of classic PCOS and in 15% of patients with normoandrogenic PCOS.

Abdominal Obesity as the Main Determinant of the Severity of PCOS Phenotype

Abdominal obesity is probably the most important factor that may modify the PCOS phenotype [12, 19, 20]. In fact, the main difference between the different PCOS phenotypes is related to body weight and mostly to variations in abdominal adipose tissue. While some patients with mild PCOS phenotypes are obese, and at the contrary some patients with classic PCOS have normal body weight and no increased abdominal adipose tissue, only patients with classic PCOS have a significant increase of prevalence of obesity when compared to normal population [19]. In addition, changes in body weight may modify the phenotype of PCOS moving the patient from a severe to a mild phenotype and vice versa [12, 13]. Above all, it suggests that obesity may modify the androgenic phenotype and transform a mild androgenic phenotype (ovulatory or maybe normoandrogenic PCOS) in classic PCOS [12].

Of course, obesity is not the only one factor able to influence the PCOS phenotype. Many patients with classic PCOS have a normal body weight [14]. Although a proportion of normal weight patients with classic PCOS have increased abdominal fat quantity, in the majority of these patients abdominal fat quantity is normal [19, 20]. Other factors, maybe also genetic components influencing insulin resistance and/or ovarian androgen secretion may be important. However, it is probable that the phenotypic differences in PCOS are mostly related to environmental differences. The consequence is very important. Most women with classic PCOS may reverse to a mild PCOS phenotype by changing their lifestyle. It is a message that the doctor should always give to his patients.

Adolescent PCOS: Specific Problems and Diagnosis

In adolescent girls, the diagnosis of PCOS may be particularly difficult. In fact, all main diagnostic criteria that are used in adult women may be transitory or not well defined in adolescent girls. In particular, both menstrual irregularities and altered ovarian morphology may spontaneously reverse to normal pattern in few years.

In fact, several studies have shown that 40–50% of adolescent women with oligomenorrhea, or amenorrhea will have normal ovulatory menses during their adult life. Van Hoof et al. followed a cohort of 766 girls and observed that only 51% of the 67 subjects, who presented oligomenorrhea at the age of 15, had menstrual disorders at the age of 18 [21]. Similarly, in a Swedish study, 40% of 87 adolescent girls with menstrual irregularities followed for 6 years spontaneously normalized their menstrual cycles [22]. Normalization of menstrual cycles may depend on the changes in food assumption or on the maturation of ovulatory process, but it is a common phenomenon, and we should be careful in evaluating the results of treatments in adolescent girls.

In adolescent girls, also morphologic appearance of ovaries may not be definitive. On the contrary, it has been reported that multifollicular ovary is quite common during adolescence but generally reverses to normal after some years [23]. It has to be remembered that multifollicular ovary may not be easily differentiated by the polycystic ovary, in particular when, as stated in Rotterdam guidelines, hyperplasia of the stroma is not assessed. In fact, the simple count of follicular cysts does not permit to distinguish between multifollicular and polycystic ovaries. Probably, the assessment of ovarian volume or of theca hyperplasia is needed in adolescent girls [24].

Also hyperandrogenism may be transitory [23]. However, it has been reported that hyperandrogenism is relatively constant and may represent the most important symptom of PCOS during adolescence [25]. In addition, it has been suggested that progressive hirsutism may represent an important sign of PCOS [25].

Because of it, it has been suggested to delay the diagnosis of PCOS until the end of the adolescence. Others have suggested making the diagnosis on the presence of at least four out the following five criteria: clinical hyperandrogenism, biological hyperandrogenism, hyperinsulinism, oligo/amenorrhea, and polycystic ovaries [23].

However, these criteria look too much restrictive. It is probably better to diagnose PCOS in adolescence only in patients with the most severe phenotype (Type 1 classic PCOS). Also in patients with the severe phenotype, increased ovarian size and/or theca hyperplasia is probably needed to make the diagnosis. The other PCOS phenotypes cannot be diagnosed during adolescence, and girls who present incomplete symptoms should be included in a strict follow up and the final diagnosis should be determined only after 18.

Treatment of PCOS

There is not a specific treatment of PCOS, but lifestyle changes are the only form of management that may give prolonged results on all characteristics of the syndrome [13].

The other treatments depend on the main symptom or on specific requests of the patients. When fertility is the main concern, clomiphene should be preferred as the first-line therapy [26]. While some authors [27] claim the metformin is as effective as clomiphene, there is a large consensus that clomiphene is more effective for ovulation induction [26]. Probably, for ovulation induction, the better alternative to clomiphene is the use of aromatase inhibitors that shows a good safety profile and efficacy at least similar to clomiphene [28].

When hirsutism is the main concern estro-progestins (E-P) or spironolactone is the choice therapy [29, 30]. When using E-P, the progestin component is particularly important and products having antiandrogen activity such as cyproterone acetate (where available) or drospirenone should be preferred. In selected patients, with no or insufficient response to E-P, pure antiandrogens as flutamide may be used [29, 30]. Because of its potential hepatotoxicity, very low doses (125–250 mg/day) of flutamide have to be utilized and liver enzymes should be carefully monitored. In fact, the elevation of liver enzymes may be found with doses of flutamide as low as 250 mg/day.

When menstrual disorders, but no fertility, are the main concern, E-P or metformin may be used.

Finally, long-term treatment of PCOS women requires an individualization of the therapy. It is essential to know the possible risk factors and complications of the single patient, and treatments should be chosen according to it.

Clinical Case No. 1

History. A 16-year-old girl who from menarche complains of increased facial and body hair and menstrual disorders. Her menses are characterized by oligomenorrhea with phases of amenorrhea (of 4–6 months). Her past medical history and family history are unremarkable.

Examination. She is a girl with a mild diffuse hirsutism (Ferriman–Gallwey–Lorenzo scores 9) but no other physical abnormalities. She has a normal body weight (BMI 22) and waist circumference (82 cm). She has no increased skin pigmentation or striae. The blood pressure is 110/70 mm Hg and the pulse 90 per minute.

Laboratory data. In day 5 of the cycle, the following blood hormone levels are obtained.

LH 15 mUI/ml, FSH 8 mUI/ml, LH:FSH ratio 1.9
Testosterone 48 ng/dl, SHBG 46 nmol/ml, FAI 3.6, DHEAS 1 μg/ml, 17OHP 0.9 ng/ml
Insulin: 11.3 μU/ml, glucose: 74 mg/dl
Cholesterol 197 mg/dl, HDL-cholesterol 63 mg/dl, LDL-cholesterol 104 mg/dl, triglycerides 82 mg/dl

Ovarian sonography shows polycystic ovaries (15 microcysts with a diameter between 5 and 8 mm in each ovary) that present a normal size (mean ovarian size 6.8 cm^3) and no stromal hyperplasia.

Questions

1. The most likely diagnosis in this girl is:
   - PCOS?
   - HAIR-AN syndrome?
   - Androgen secreting tumor?
   - Idiopathic hirsutism?
   - Cushing syndrome?
2. What is the most appropriate treatment?
   (a) Estro-progestins
   (b) Metformin
   (c) Antiandrogens
   (d) Only esthetic measures and follow-up

Answer and Comment

1. The available data do not permit a sure diagnosis. PCOS or idiopathic hirsutism are both possible diagnoses. While HAIR-AN syndrome, androgen secreting tumor, and Cushing's syndrome may be ruled out because of the clinical history, the physical examination, and the values of androgens, it is impossible at the moment to make a diagnosis of PCOS or of another mild androgen excess disorder. In fact, while this adolescent patient presents all diagnostic criteria according to Rotterdam or AEPCOS guidelines, androgen levels and ovarian size are normal.

Because menstrual disorders and polycystic ovaries may reverse to normal in few years, only hirsutism should be considered a probably permanent symptom.

2. The correct answer is d: only esthetic measures and follow up. In fact, in the absence of a diagnosis, no specific therapy should be suggested. In addition, hirsutism is mild and circulating androgens are normal. Esthetic measures should be suggested to reduce the hirsutism until the diagnosis becomes clear.

Follow-Up

In another hospital, the diagnosis of PCOS was made and treatment with E-P containing cyproterone acetate was suggested. After 6 months of treatment, the following hormone and metabolic values were obtained:

- Fasting insulin 21 μU/ml, blood glucose 71 mg/dl
- Cholesterol 232 mg/dl, HDL-cholesterol 53 mg/dl, LDL-cholesterol 145 mg/dl, Triglycerides 145 mg/dl

Treatment with E-P was stopped

After 4 years (at age 20), the patient was reevaluated in our department. At the moment of the study, she referred normal menses and mild hirsutism (FGL scores: 9)

The following hormone and metabolic values were obtained:

- Serum P: 8.6 ng/ml, testosterone 42 ng/dl, SHBG 45 nmol/L, FAI 3
- Fasting insulin 10 μU/ml, blood glucose 86 mg/dl
- Cholesterol 197 mg/dl, HDL-cholesterol 69 mg/dl, LDL-cholesterol 123 mg/dl, Triglycerides 74 mg/dl
- Ovarian sonography showed a few microcysts but no polycystic ovaries. Ovarian size was normal and no theca hyperplasia was observed.

Conclusions

The patient presents with hirsutism and only esthetic measures (including laser therapy) were suggested.

The clinical history indicates the difficulties in making a correct diagnosis of PCOS in adolescent girls. If a diagnosis of PCOS were made, and the patient treated with a more aggressive agent (such as metformin), then the spontaneous improvement in menses and ovarian morphology would have been attributed to that therapy. In adolescence, only patients presenting with severe symptoms (hyperandrogenism, polycystic ovaries with increased ovarian size or theca hyperplasia and irregular menses) should have a diagnosis of PCOS and a specific treatment. In all other young girls, the diagnosis should be postponed until adulthood.

It is interesting to observe that this patient developed an altered lipid pattern when treated by an estroprogestin containing cyproterone acetate. Dyslipidemia is uncommon in women taking oral contraceptives (also containing cyproterone acetate) but may develop in patients presenting some hidden metabolic alterations. It indicates another interesting question. Does this patient also have subclinical insulin resistance? Will she develop a PCOS if the body weight increases? It is difficult to answer to these questions, but maintenance of normal body weight should be a primary objective in adolescents (and adult women) presenting with hirsutism or menstrual disorders.

References

1. Carmina E, Lobo RA (1999) Polycystic ovary syndrome (PCOS): arguably the most common endocrinopathy is associated with significant morbidity in women. J Clin Endocrinol Metab 84:1897–1899
2. Stein IF, Leventhal ML (1935) Amenorrhea associated with bilateral polycystic ovaries. Am J Obstet Gynecol 29:181–191
3. Rotterdam ESHRE/ASRM sponsored PCOS Consensus Workshop Group (2004) Revised 2003 consensus on diagnostic criteria and long-term health risks related to polycystic ovary syndrome. Fertil Steril 81:19–25
4. Azziz R, Carmina E, Dewailly D, Diamanti-Kandarakis E, Escobar-Morreale HF, Futterweit W, Janssen OE, Legro RS, Norman RJ, Taylor AE, Witchel SF (2006) Position statement: criteria for defining Polycystic Ovary Syndrome as a predominantly hyperandrogenic syndrome: an androgen excess society guideline. J Clin Endocrinol Metab 91:4237–4245
5. Carmina E, Azziz R (2006) Diagnosis, phenotype and prevalence of polycystic ovary syndrome. Fertil Steril 86(suppl 1):87–89
6. Azziz R, Woods KS, Reyna R et al (2004) The prevalence and features of the polycystic ovary syndrome in an unselected population. J Clin Endocrinol Metab 89:2745–2749
7. Carmina E, Rosato F, Jannì A, Rizzo M, Longo RA (2006) Relative prevalence of different androgen excess disorders in 950 women referred because of clinical hyperandrogenism. J Clin Endocrinol Metab 91:2–6
8. Chang WY, Knochenhauer ES, Bartolucci AA, Azziz R (2005) Phenotypic spectrum of polycystic ovary syndrome: clinical and biochemical characterization of the three major clinical subgroups. Fertil Steril 83:1717–1723
9. Carmina E, Longo RA, Rini GB, Lobo RA (2005) Phenotypic variation in hyperandrogenic women influences the finding of abnormal metabolic and cardiovascular risk parameters. J Clin Endocrinol Metab 90:2545–2549
10. Welt CK, Gudmundsson JA, Arsson G, Adams J, Palsdottir H, Gudlaugsdottir G, Ingadottir G, Crowley WF (2006) Characterizing discrete subsets of Polycystic Ovary Syndrome as defined by the Rotterdam criteria: the impact of weight on phenotype and metabolic features. J Clin Endocrinol Metab 91:4842–4848
11. Dewailly D, Catteau-Jonard S, Reyss AC, Leroy M, Pigny P (2006) Oligoanovulation with polycystic ovaries but not overt hyperandrogenism. J Clin Endocrinol Metab 91:3922–3927
12. Guastella E, Longo RA, Carmina E (2010) Clinical and endocrine characteristics of main PCOS phenotypes. Fertil Steril Epub March 10
13. Huber-Buckholz MM, Carey DG, Norman RJ (1999) Restoration of reproductive potential by lifestyle modification in obese polycystic ovary syndrome: role of insulin sensitivity and luteinizing hormone. J Clin Endocrinol Metab 84:1470–1474
14. Carmina E, Legro R, Stamets K, Lowell J, Lobo RA (2003) Differences in body weight between American and Italian women with the polycystic ovary syndrome: influence of the diet. Hum Reprod 11:2289–2293

15. Di Fede G, Mansueto P, Longo RA, Rini G, Carmina E (2009) Influence of sociocultural factors on the ovulatory status of polycystic ovary syndrome. Fertil Steril 91:1853–1856
16. Goldzieher JW, Axelrod LR (1963) Clinical and biochemical features of polycystic ovary disease. Fertil Steril 14:631–653
17. Balen A, Conway GS, Kaltsas G et al (1995) Polycystic ovary syndrome: the spectrum of the disorder in 1741 patients. Hum Reprod 10:2107–2111
18. Lobo RA, Carmina E (1997) Polycystic ovary syndrome. In: Lobo RA, Mishell DR Jr, Paulson RJ, Shoupe D (eds) Infertility, contraception and reproductive endocrinology. Blackwell, Malden, pp 362–383
19. Carmina E, Bucchieri S, Esposito A, Del Puente A, Mansueto P, Di Fede G, Rini GB (2007) Abdominal fat quantity and distribution in women with polycystic ovary syndrome and extent of its relation to insulin resistance. J Clin Endocrinol Metab 92:2500–2505
20. Carmina E, Bucchieri S, Mansueto P, Rini G, Ferin M, Lobo RA (2009) Circulating levels of adipose products and differences in fat distribution in the ovulatory and anovulatory phenotypes of polycystic ovary syndrome. Fertil Steril 91:1332–1335
21. Van Hoof MH, Voorhorst FJ, Kaptein MB, Hirasing RA, Koppenaal C, Schoemaker J (2004) Predictive value of menstrual cycle patter, body mass index, hormone levels and polycystic ovaries for oligo-amenorrhea at age 18 years. Hum Reprod 19:383–392
22. Wiksten-Almstromer M, Hirschberg AL, Hagenfeldt K (2007) Prospective follow-up of menstrual disorders in adolescence and prognostic features. Acta Obstet Gynecol Scand 87:1162–1168
23. Sultan C, Paris F (2006) Clinical expression of polycystic ovary syndrome in adolescent girls. Fertil Steril 86(Suppl 1):S6
24. Chen J, Yang D, Li L, Chen X (2008) The role of ovarian volume as a diagnostic criterion for Chinese adolescents with polycystic ovary syndrome. J Pediatr Adolesc Gynecol 21:347–350
25. Chang JR, Coffler MS (2007) Polycystic ovary syndrome: early detection in the adolescent. Clin Obstet Gynecol 50:178–187
26. Thessaloniki ESHRE/ASRM Sponsored PCOS Consensus Workshop Group (2008) Consensus on infertility treatment related to polycystic ovary syndrome. Hum Reprod 23:462–477
27. Palomba S, Pasquali R, Orio F Jr, Nestler JE (2009) Clomiphene citrate, metformin or both as first step approach in treating anovulatory infertility in patients with polycystic ovary syndrome (PCOS): a systematic review of head-to-head randomized controlled studies and meta-analysis. Clin Endocrinol (Oxf) 70:311–321
28. Begum MR, Ferdous J, Begum A, Qadir E (2009) Comparison of the efficacy of aromatase inhibitor and clomiphene citrate in induction of ovulation in polycystic ovarian syndrome. Fertil Steril 92:853–857
29. Martyn KA, Chang RJ, Ehrmann DA, Ibanez L, Lobo RA, Rosenfield RL, Shapiro J, Montori V, Swiglo BA (2008) Evaluation and treatment of hirsutism in premenopausal women: an endocrine society clinical practice guideline. J Clin Endocrinol Metab 93:1105–1120
30. Carmina E (2001) A risk-benefit assessment of pharmacological therapies for hirsutism. Drug Saf 24:267–276

Chapter 5
Primary Ovarian Insufficiency

Amber R. Cooper, Sharon N. Covington, and Lawrence M. Nelson

A Clinical Vignette

A 29-year-old G0 woman presented to her gynecologist with the complaints of an inability to get pregnant and abnormal menses. She married 1 year ago and immediately stopped her oral contraceptives with hopes to conceive. She had irregular light cycles the first 3–4 months off of OCPs, 1 menses 3 months later, and none since that time (about 4–5 months). Her past medical history was unremarkable and her review of systems was noncontributory except for a 10 lb weight loss in the last 6 months, which she attributes to stress from an inability to conceive and vaginal dryness. She is on no other medications but does smoke 5–10 cigarettes/day, although is trying to quit. She had normal puberty and menarche at age 13 years. Her cycles had previously been regular and she had been on oral contraceptives for 8 years. Her family history was remarkable for a mother with rheumatoid arthritis and hypothyroidism, a father with type I diabetes mellitus, and a cousin with mental retardation. Her height is 61 in., weight 116 lb, and BMI 21.9 kg/m^2. Physical and pelvic examinations were normal. Pregnancy test was negative. She was given a progestin challenge test and bled in response to it. Initial prolactin and thyroid studies were normal and basal follicle stimulating hormone (FSH) during her withdrawal bleed was 46 mIU/mL.

Introduction

The ovary is one of the most enigmatic organs in the body. It peaks in oocyte quantity even before a female fetus is born, at approximately 20 weeks in utero, with 5–6 million oocytes. Yet even prior to this peak in oocyte number, the majority of

A.R. Cooper (✉)
Department of Obstetrics and Gynecology Division of Reproductive Endocrinology and Infertility, Washington University School of Medicine, St. Louis, MO, USA
e-mail: coopera@wustl.edu

N.F. Santoro and G. Neal-Perry (eds.), *Amenorrhea: A Case-Based, Clinical Guide*, Contemporary Endocrinology, DOI 10.1007/978-1-60327-864-5_5,

oocytes begin to undergo apoptosis. By birth, 80–90% of oocytes are already lost [1]. Most consider the period of infancy through puberty a relatively quiescent time for the ovary, although during this time follicles are growing and oocytes are actively synthesizing mRNA and protein. By the time of puberty, there are less than 500,000 oocytes remaining and most likely 500 or less will ever grow to an optimal size for ovulation. From puberty to the time of menopause (which normally occurs at 51–52 years of age on average), there is a progressive decline in oocyte quantity and, most likely, quality. The last 10–15 years of menstruation are marked by an accelerated rate of oocyte loss, likely when the follicular pool reaches a critical threshold number of oocytes (thought to be around 25,000) [2]. As the follicle pool diminishes, less estradiol and possibly inhibin-B are released, leading to an increase in FSH. More rapid follicular development occurs and menstrual cycle length shortens partially due to early and more rapid recruitment. It may be that the individual age of menopause is related to the size of the established primordial follicle oocyte pool in utero, and, thus, when the functional pool is depleted, menopause will occur. It is also possible that the rate of expenditure of primordial follicles is accelerated above normal in some women. Natural menopause is an irreversible decline in reproductive function driven by primordial follicle quantity (Fig. 5.1) [1].

We prefer the designation of "primary ovarian insufficiency" (POI) as a more scientifically accurate term for what many still refer to as "premature ovarian failure" (POF) or "premature menopause." The terms POF and premature menopause inappropriately suggest a state of complete, irreversible cessation of ovarian function. Fuller Albright originally coined the term POI in the early 1940s to report what is now evident to be a continuum of impaired ovarian function ranging from a mild dysfunction to severe abnormality [3]. Also, a majority of women interpret the term "failure" as stigmatizing and prefer the term POI as a more positive and more accurate description of their condition (unpublished data). Many prefer the term insufficiency because it conveys the message that there still remains some hope of pregnancy, albeit small. Published evidence has demonstrated that patients who feel more stigma related to this condition experience more symptoms of anxiety and depression, so

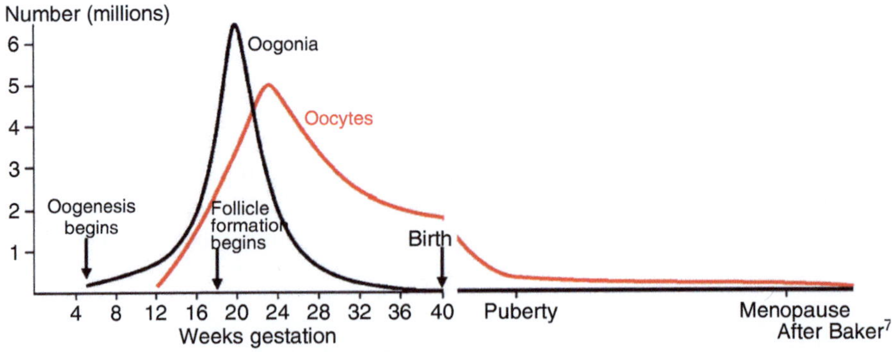

Fig. 5.1 Oocyte quantity (in millions) over the lifespan of a normal female, from in utero through menopause [1]

Table 5.1 POI diagnostic criteria

• <40 years of age
• Absence or irregularity of menstrual cycles ≥4 months
• Menopausal range FSH[a] (defined by individual laboratory criteria)

[a]Menopausal range FSH values need to be repeated and confirmed on two occasions at least 1 month apart

there is good reason to use a term that is both more scientifically accurate and less stigmatizing to patients [4]. A diagnosis of POI comes with significant medical, genetic/heritable, psychologic, and reproductive health concerns. This chapter will describe the condition and provide data to aid the clinician in providing optimal care for women diagnosed with POI. It is our belief that women with POI are best served with a multidisciplinary health care treatment approach in order to address all of their health issues, preventative care, and counseling needs. These issues will be addressed in detail.

POI is defined as absent or irregular periods for 4 months or greater combined with menopausal range FSH in a woman under 40 years of age (Table 5.1). Most have previously defined it as a triad of amenorrhea, hypergonadotropism, and hypogonadism in women younger than 40 years of age. Yet for reasons often unknown to clinicians, 1–2% or more of women develop signs and symptoms of menopause prior to the age of 40 years, an age 2–3 standard deviations outside the normal range [1, 5]. The precise prevalence is difficult to determine, increases with age, and is dependent on the population studied. It may seem natural to call such a process "early menopause" or POF, which implies complete cessation of function of the ovaries and sterility at a significantly earlier age than normal, but these terms are not accurate for young women with this condition as mentioned above. It is well documented that these women have varying and unpredictable menstrual cycles, often periodically ovulate, and still spontaneously conceive 5–10% of the time [6–10].

Menopausal range gonadotropins may not correlate with the degree of ovarian function as they do in a naturally menopausal woman in her sixth decade of life or later. In fact, young women with POF may still ovulate and menstruate while on no therapy despite significantly elevated FSH values (Fig. 5.2) [10, 11]. Furthermore, ultrasound evaluation of these women frequently reveals continued follicular development unlike that in the naturally menopausal woman in her 50s who may have smaller ovaries with little to no basal antral follicles [9, 12]. Such follicular presence or development does not imply normal functionality in these patients. In most cases, the etiology remains a mystery even after thorough evaluation.

The Clinical Spectrum of POI

The presentation and symptoms experienced by women with POI vary depending on the etiology of the condition. Amenorrhea can be a manifestation of numerous underlying medical illnesses. Women who present with primary amenorrhea are less

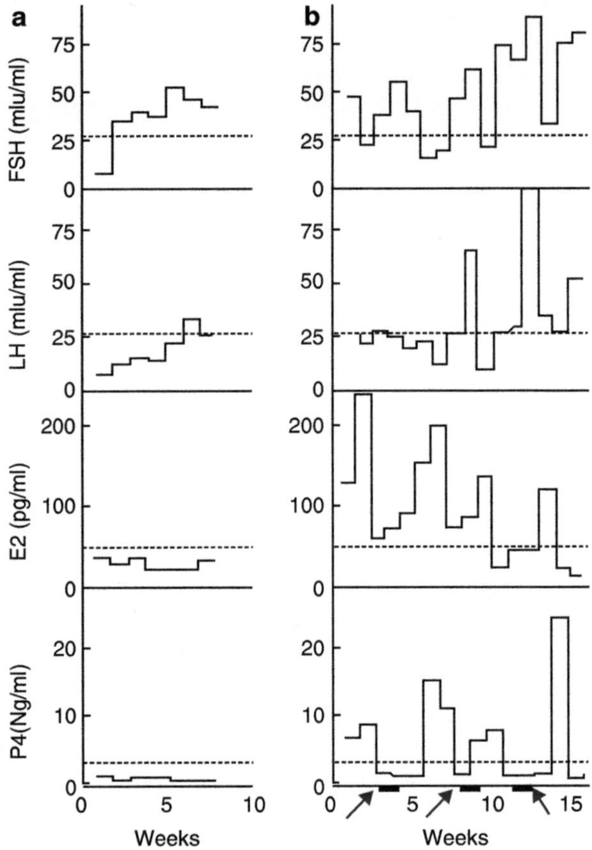

Fig. 5.2 Serial blood samples in an 18-year-old 46,XX patient with spontaneous POI diagnosed at age 14 years. ***Column a*** represents repeated FSH, LH, estradiol (E2), and progesterone (P4) measurements during 4 months of treatment with a GnRH agonist. ***Column B*** demonstrates continued ovulatory cycles and menstrual bleeds (*red arrows* or *solid bars* on the *x*-axis) despite significantly elevated FSH during 4 months of treatment with placebo injections [10, 11]

likely to have developed breasts to Tanner stage 5, less likely to have symptoms of estrogen deficiency, and more likely to have karyotypic abnormalities (50% or more), resulting in conditions such as Turner's syndrome (45,X) [8]. Most adult women who are found to have hypergonadotropic hypogonadism are ultimately given a diagnosis of spontaneous 46,XX POI. Most of these women present with secondary amenorrhea, but many will initially report oligomenorrhea, polymenorrhea, menometrorrhagia, or other dysfunctional uterine bleeding. In women with secondary amenorrhea, estrogen withdrawal symptoms are common and infertility is sometimes part of the history, although for many women the condition precedes any attempt at conception.

Some women who will ultimately meet the criteria for a diagnosis of POI will be completely asymptomatic. Others may only present to subspecialists due to infertility or irregular menstrual cycles. Often while taking a detailed patient history, some clues may surface leading a physician to suspect POI, but this is not always the case. Regardless, it is often a random, or more commonly a basal (drawn on day 2–4 of the menstrual cycle), FSH value abnormality that directs the physician toward uncovering the earliest stage of POI, occult POI.

One way to differentiate between degrees of ovarian insufficiency is to categorize the clinical and laboratory findings, more specifically, to quantify their ovarian function based on their menstrual regularity, fertility, and FSH values. Using this sub-categorization of findings, clinicians can develop a spectrum, referring to women as normal, or as being in the occult, biochemical, or overt stages in the continuum of ovarian function associated with POI (Table 5.2) [6, 13].

With the advent and rapid progression of assisted reproductive technologies (ART) in the last several decades, clinicians have been able to distinguish women who have a poor response to gonadotropin stimulation, significantly less oocytes recovered during in vitro fertilization (IVF), poorer quality embryos, and lower pregnancy rates from women with a similar age and infertility diagnosis. Many have suggested that these women demonstrate "early ovarian aging," have ovaries "older than their chronological age," or exaggerated FSH values during the follicular phase or during clomiphene citrate challenge tests [14, 15]. Terms such as "diminished ovarian reserve (DOR)" and "premature ovarian aging (POA)," and sometimes unexplained infertility, have been used to refer to women who have such a response but do not meet the criteria for POI [16–20]. It is difficult to determine if these patients are representing varying time points on a similar clinical spectrum of disease or whether they are entirely different patient populations. It is important to point out that impaired ovarian function as represented by POI is not a stable state. Therefore, it is best not to consider this condition as representing an irreversible decline in ovarian function, but rather an intermittent and unpredictable ovarian function that can undergo temporary remission. In other words, depending upon when in the course of her condition and to whom a woman presents for diagnosis, she might receive an ostensibly different diagnosis from each of three different clinicians. Thus, while it is worth noting that the relationship between DOR and POA and patients with POI warrants further investigation, the remainder of this chapter will focus specifically on women with overt POI, meaning loss of regular menstruation and the presence of menopausal level gonadotropins.

Table 5.2 Clinical states of POI [6, 13]

Clinical State	Serum FSH Level	Fertility	Menses
Normal	Normal	Normal	Regular
Occult	Normal	Reduced	Regular
Biochemical	Elevated	Reduced	Regular
Overt	Elevated	Reduced	Irregular or absent

Etiologies

At the present time, most cases of POI remain without an etiologic diagnosis. Germ cell proliferation and depletion, follicular development, and the key cellular and molecular processes involved in normal ovarian function, let alone POI, are still in need of significantly more research. When a causal factor has been associated with the clinical phenotype, a sub-classification can be made in several ways. One way to create a framework for classification is by distinguishing the mechanism by which ovarian function diminishes: (1) A decrease in the initial primordial pool established in utero, (2) increased apoptosis/atresia of the follicles, or (3) failed follicular response or dysfunction [6, 10, 13]. The two major mechanisms are follicle depletion and follicle dysfunction, and several examples of each are listed in Table 5.3 [6]. Further discussion in this text will focus on the most common known or suspected causal factors of POI.

Idiopathic

As discussed, most women with a diagnosis of POI will be in this category. This often leaves women as well as their clinicians frustrated and in pursuit of a significant number of screening and diagnostic studies to attempt to uncover any abnormal findings. In reality, some of these patients may have multifactorial causes, undiscovered iatrogenic, genetic, or environmental causes, or have some combination or partial findings of the rest of the etiologic sub-classifications identified in the following discussion.

Genetic

X Chromosome Abnormalities

As the genomics, proteomics, and similar related fields continue to expand, so does the understanding of the individual sex chromosomes, epigenetic modifications associated with reproduction, and the interactions between autosomes and sex chromosomes. Yet, we are likely only viewing the tip of the iceberg in our current state of knowledge. Although presently we can only identify a genetic cause in a minority of women, many women with POI may have underlying genetic and/or epigenetic etiologies of POI that are yet to be identified. For many years, testing was limited to karyotypes and identification of large chromosomal defects such as absence or partial absence of the X chromosome. We can now identify polymorphisms in the genome down to the single nucleotide with single nucleotide polymorphism (SNP) microarray analyses and associated genome wide association studies (GWAS), thanks to efforts like the Human Genome Project in 2003 and the International HapMap Project in 2005. Thus, there is great potential to accrue more diagnostic accuracy regarding the role of the X chromosome in the etiology of POI.

Table 5.3 Causes of spontaneous POI classified by two major mechanisms [6]

Mechanism and cause	Comments
Ovarian follicle dysfunction	
Signal defect	Presence of ovarian follicles confirmed by biopsy; founder effect; rare disorder outside of Finland
FSH-receptor mutation	Ovarian follicles present on ultrasound examination; rare disorder
G-protein mutation	Secondary amenorrhea, elevated gonadotropin levels, and hypoestrogenemia that responded to gonadotropin therapy developed in patient with pseudohypoparathyroidism [11]; rare disorder
Enzyme deficiency	
Isolated 17,20-lyase deficiency	Ovarian follicles present on biopsy, "moderate ovarian enlargement" due to block in estradiol synthesis; rare disorder
Aromatase deficiency	Ovarian enlargement or hyperstimulation due to inability of the ovary to aromatize androstenedione to estradiol; rare disorder
Autoimmunity	
Autoimmune lymphocytic oophoritis	Antral follicles with lymphocytic infiltration into theca, primordial follicles spared, multifollicular ovaries; accounts for 4% of cases of 46,XX primary ovarian insufficiency; associated with evidence of adrenal autoimmunity
Insufficient follicle number	
Luteinized graafian follicles	Antral follicles imaged by ultrasonography in 40% of patients with idiopathic spontaneous 46,XX primary ovarian insufficiency; on the basis of histologic findings, at least 60% of antral follicles imaged in these patients are luteinized, a major mechanism of follicle dysfunction in these women [7]
Ovarian follicle depletion	
Insufficient initial follicle number	
Blepharophimosis, ptosis, epicanthus inversus syndrome	Mutation in *FOXL2* is a mechanism of familial primary ovarian insufficiency, and disruption of the mouse gene causes a pervasive block in primordial follicle development; rare disorder
Spontaneous accelerated follicle loss	
Turner's syndrome	Although a normal complement of primordial follicles is established in the ovary during fetal development, follicle loss through apoptosis is accelerated so that the store of primordial follicles is typically depleted before puberty; in oocytes, both X chromosomes must be present and remain active to prevent accelerated follicular atresia; the individual genes responsible for this ovarian syndrome have not been identified
Environmental-toxin-induced follicle loss	
Industrial exposure to 2-bromopropane	Exposure to cleaning solvent associated with primary ovarian insufficiency in 16 Korean women [12]

Abnormalities in the X chromosome have been one of the more well-researched areas in POI. It is clear that two copies of the X chromosome are required for normal ovarian function [21]. Women with classic Turner's syndrome (45,X) nearly always have POI prior to the natural age of menarche. Women who present with secondary amenorrhea may actually be found to have mosaicism (usually 45,X/46,XX) on more detailed inspection. While this may seem counterintuitive due to the recognized phenomenon of X chromosome inactivation, many genes on the X chromosome actually escape inactivation and are thought to be critical to normal oocyte/ovarian function, especially for meiosis and folliculogenesis early in development. Both X chromosomes are active at the onset of meiosis in oocytes, during which time a reduced dosage of a particular gene product may have untoward effects. Furthermore, a careful study of X chromosome inactivation and its thorough sequencing has led to the concept that 20% or more of X-linked genes are expressed continuously from both X chromosomes [22–24]. Trisomy X (47,XXX), sometimes present in mosaic form, has also been associated with POI, although whether or not an X trisomy is related to a decrease in fertility and/or ovarian function is still debated [25, 26].

Submicroscopic gene deletions, duplications, translocations, and other mutations within the X chromosome have also been found at a much higher rate in women with POI [27–29]. The degree of haploinsufficiency for particular regions of the X, specifically Xp or Xq, may be responsible for variation in the age or symptomatic presentation of POI [13, 21, 30–32]. Some genes in what has been called the "critical region" of the long arm of X, Xq, may be affected by their relocation in the genome, as with a translocation. Whether this is due to dysfunction at the breakpoint or epigenetic mechanisms, such as chromatin structuring or promoter locations, has yet to be validated. Some of the genes in this region (often cited as Xq13-q21 or beyond) are POF1B, DIAPH2, and others [26, 33–37].

Two of the best characterized X-linked genes associated with POI are the fragile X mental retardation 1 (FMR1) and bone morphogenetic protein-15 (BMP-15) genes. Physicians and geneticists are particularly concerned with the associations between FMR1 and POI due to the constellation of phenotypes associated with abnormalities in the triple-repeat sequence in this gene. Severe expansion of the repeat sequence CGG in the FMR1 gene (in region Xq27) is responsible for one of the most prevalent genetic causes of mental retardation, fragile X syndrome. This full mutation occurs when over 200 CGG repeats are present in the 5′ untranslated region of the gene, causing hypermethylation and failure to transcribe the FMR protein. The normal number of repeats is less than 45 (and some consider 45–54 a gray zone of undetermined significance). The concern regarding POI lies in the premutation range, defined as 55–200 repeats. As the number of repeats increases, transcription and translation are altered. Transcription actually increases but effective translation of the protein diminishes [38]. It appears that excess mutated mRNA, which is unable to be translated, is what is toxic to the cell and this is maximized at a value of approximately 80 repeats. After 100 repeats, the risk of POI or associated FMR1 disorders may plateau or decrease [24, 39–42]. Premutations have been associated with psychologic and/or neurologic diagnoses such as autism, anxiety, hyperactivity, parkinsonian-like disorders, late onset tremor/ataxia in males, and other conditions [39, 43–45]. Concerns with the premutation also apply to future generations. Not only could a premutation expand to a full mutation during meiosis or subsequent development, but also offspring who carry a premutation are at risk for POI and, subsequently, an inability to reproduce [40, 41]. A thorough family history looking for mental retardation, dementia, tremor-ataxia, and other intellectual and psychologic disorders may suggest an increased risk of FMR1 premutation in a woman with POI, though testing should be offered regardless. Anywhere from 2 to 15% of women with POI could carry the FMR1 premutation, depending on the family history, resulting in a situation where the reproductive consequences could be significant if the patient is not made aware of the testing and implication of its results [6, 41, 44]. BMP-15 is a growth factor that appears to have a critical regulatory role in oocyte and follicular development. Its mutations are associated with or may predispose at least certain racial/ethnic subgroups of women to POI, but at present the clinical implications of this finding are unclear [46, 47].

Autosomal Gene Abnormalities

One of the classic genetic disorders associated with POI is galactosemia. The most common and severe form is the homozygous state where there is a complete lack of the enzyme galactose 1-phosphate uridyl transferase (GALT) and an inability to convert galactose to glucose. An affected individual presents in the first few days of life with significant morbidity and mortality if the condition is not recognized. Without the necessary enzyme, toxic precursors accumulate in large quantities and do significant damage to numerous cells, including those within the ovary [13, 48, 49]. There are several other enzymatic mutations and variants of disease severity that create more mild but significant forms of galactosemia. Galactosemia has been associated with an abundant number of mutations in the GALT gene and is inherited in an autosomal recessive fashion [50, 51]. Frustrating is the fact that homo- or heterozygosity for a particular allelic combination does not seem to predict phenotype sufficiently, including ovarian insufficiency timing and/or severity [52]. Women with classic galactosemia need close monitoring and follow-up with a specialized multidisciplinary team, including those with expertise in inborn errors of metabolism, dieticians, and endocrinologists. Most women with the classic form go on to develop ovarian failure, and some, like those with galcotokinase (GALK) mutation, do not have an increased risk. Yet, many women with other variants, and even those who have good dietary compliance, develop POI and it is difficult to predict future outcomes for individual patients [51, 52].

A second commonly cited autosomal abnormality is found on chromosome 3 within the FOXL2 gene. The FOXL2 gene is primarily expressed in the eyelids and granulosa cells in humans. The syndrome that results from a mutation in FOXL2 has been termed blepharophimosis, ptosis, epicanthus inversus syndrome (BPES) and is linked with POI, primarily in type 1 BPES. The precise mechanism by which a FOXL2 mutation causes POI is still under investigation. One proposed process, based on animal models, is that a dysfunctional or truncated FOXL2 transcription factor causes a failure in the early stage pregranulosa cell's ability to develop around and nourish a normal-sized primordial oocyte pool, which is likely reliant on FOXL2 expression in the female gonad [13, 53–55].

Numerous other genetic mutations have been implicated in POI. Among them are FSH receptor (FSHR) and inhibin alpha (INHA) [56, 57]. Anything that somehow affects gonadotropin regulation and action has subsequent consequences on ovarian function. Mutations in the actual subunits of FSH and luteinizing hormone (LH) have also been reported, although some would argue that these causes do not fit the definition of "primary" ovarian insufficiency at the level of the ovary [13]. The ataxia telangiectasia mutated (ATM) gene is a particular gene that has been implicated in causing oocytes to stall out in meiosis prophase I and then undergo apoptosis, due to a deficiency in the gene product [58, 59]. The BLM (Bloom syndrome) gene is somewhat similar, as it is a DNA repair gene that controls progression through the cell cycle and in a mutated form causes genomic instability [60]. This mutation has been linked with POI as well. Werner's syndrome (WRN) gene may be another. Next is a family of eukaryotic initiation factor 2B (EIF2B) genes that were found to be mutated in eight patients with POI and leukodystrophy and related central nervous system abnormalities [61]. Other genes that have been reported include PMM2 (phosphomannomutase), AIRE (gene that causes autoimmune polyglandular syndrome (APGS) type I discussed further below), GDF9, NOBOX, and LDX8, among many others [6, 21, 32].

Other Gene Abnormalities

The oocyte is quite dependent on its mitochondrial energy production. Therefore, any mitochondrial dysfunction could be detrimental to oocyte health and predispose a woman to POI. One particular disorder, progressive external ophthalmoplegia, is linked with a mitochondrial DNA polymerase gamma (POLG) mutation, and it segregates with POI in certain families of women [62, 63]. More mitochondrial abnormalities may be uncovered in the future as the biology of this field moves forward. It is likely that further research will uncover mitochondrial defects linked to POI, as the oocyte has more mitochondria than most cells in the body.

Certain steroidogenic enzyme defects result from other genetic mutations. Steroid acute regulatory protein (STAR) is required for mitochondrial membrane transport of cholesterol to start the production of steroids within the cell. A mutation within the STAR gene can result in a severe phenotype. Deficiencies such as 17α-hydroxylase or 17, 20-lyase deficiency and 20, 22-desmolase deficiency have also been associated with POI. Whether the steroidogenic similarities between the ovary and adrenal gland underlie the associated phenotypes remains unclear but is worthy of further research. Aromatase deficiency can also cause a block in the production of estradiol, although in this disorder, the ovaries enlarge due to continued follicular development [6, 13, 32].

Autoimmune Dysfunction

A portion of patients with POI appear to have an autoimmune-associated etiology [34, 64, 65]. There is a higher prevalence of autoimmune disease in women compared to men, and, more importantly, the association of POI with autoimmune dysfunction has been found in several studies to be significantly higher in women with autoimmune disease than that in the general population [66]. That said, the study of autoimmune conditions remains a very complex one, due to the non-Mendelian inheritance patterns and intricate multigenetic loci and environmental interactions. POI has been most commonly linked to autoimmune conditions within the thyroid and adrenal glands. Yet, it has also been associated with conditions such as dry eye syndrome, rheumatoid arthritis, hypoparathyroidism, diabetes mellitus, myasthenia gravis, and pernicious anemia [6, 13, 67]. A subset of such women may present with a polyglandular or syndromic disorder. Yet, women with isolated POI may still be at risk for future autoimmune conditions. Whether or not this implies an autoimmune oophoritis pathogenic process within the ovary, increased lymphocyte activation, or some other complex multifactorial process still needs further investigation. Potential autoantigen targets in the ovary are also a possibility that is a topic of current investigation.

Syndromic POI has been associated with APGS, of which there are four types (I–IV). Type I, due to a mutation in the AIRE gene, is referred to as autoimmune polyendocrinopathy-candidiasis-ectodermal dystrophy (APECED), and the majority of patients with this mutation develop POI and adrenal insufficiency among other disorders [64, 68]. The AIRE gene is predominantly expressed in immune tissues such as the thymus. Such mutations may affect self-tolerance. While mutations in the AIRE gene may still be important in the pathophysiology of autoimmune dysfunction, some investigators have reported that the HLA subtype (especially class II) may be even more significantly associated with the phenotype than the AIRE mutation, or a combination of the two may be more detrimental [69].

For the remainder of women with POI, who do not have mutations in the AIRE gene or who are not HLA class II, an association between POI and other, more isolated autoimmune disorders appears to occur in a proportion higher than that can be accounted for by chance. Specifically, 2–10% of patients with POI have been found to have anti-adrenal antibodies, or more concerning, unrecognized adrenal insufficiency [64, 65, 67, 70, 71]. Due to the fact that POI can precede adrenal insufficiency, and the insidious, often asymptomatic course patients take before an adrenal crisis occurs, many physicians feel that screening for adrenal dysfunction is worthwhile in the POI population [65, 70, 72]. Thyroid autoimmunity is present in about 20% of women with spontaneous POI [6, 13, 64].

To many patients with POI as well as to clinicians, the discovery of an autoimmune etiology or an associated autoimmune disorder implies that the POI may be treatable or reversible by immune modulating therapies. Unfortunately, this is not the case. Most patients with POI, regardless of whether or not they have an associated autoimmune condition, will neither have biopsy-proven oophoritis, nor should they undergo such testing, and the risks of the various, immunomodulating therapies are often too significant to warrant therapy [10, 73, 74].

Iatrogenic/Environmental

Iatrogenic and environmental factors have been associated with POI. Cytotoxic therapies used in a variety of malignant and autoimmune conditions are one of the most prevalent causes. Alkylating agents have been the most ovarian-damaging chemotherapy agents in selected treatment regimens, and bone marrow transplant therapy is nearly 100% toxic to ovarian function [75, 76]. Hopefully, referral practices and public awareness are such that most young reproductive-aged patients are referred for consultations with reproductive endocrinologists prior to the administration of ovary-toxic therapies. Ionizing radiation, used to treat a number of cancers in the abdomen/pelvis, has also been demonstrated to cause ovarian dysfunction and/or failure. Surgical or procedure injury, such as a significant reduction of ovarian tissue or damage to the blood supply (i.e., unilateral oophorectomy, hysterectomy, and uterine artery embolization), is also a potential iatrogenic cause of POI [77, 78].

Numerous environmental factors have been implicated in the search for etiologic factors associated with POI. Tobacco smoke, stress, viral infection, and certain chemicals (2-bromopropane, 1, 3-butadiene, 4-vinylcyclohexane, and polycyclic aromatic hydrocarbons) are among those reported, some of which potentially mediate their effects through a Bax transcription pathway [79–83]. Finally, infiltrative or destructive conditions may also diminish ovarian function, such as with severe endometriosis [84].

Evaluation of Hypergonadotropic Amenorrhea

As discussed above, there is a myriad of ways a woman can present with POI. Disturbances in the menstrual cycle, especially amenorrhea or oligomenorrhea for 3–4 months, warrants an evaluation in nearly all women (with basic diagnostic testing including a pregnancy test, and if negative, FSH, thyroid stimulating hormone (TSH), and prolactin). Once a diagnosis of hypergonadotropic amenorrhea is made, the clinician should perform a basic evaluation, develop a treatment plan, and consider a referral as appropriate.

History

Most women with POI will have had normal puberty and menarche, a period of irregularities in their menstrual cycle, and ultimately a diagnosis of spontaneous POI.

A small portion will present with primary amenorrhea. A very thorough personal and family history is very important for these women. Any symptoms that suggest estrogen deficiency (decreased libido, hot flashes, insomnia, vaginal dryness, etc.), environmental or iatrogenic insults to the ovary, or other related medical conditions should be sought after. A family history is very important and should include questions about other family members with POI, autoimmune conditions, and any neurologic and/or mental delay that could be related to the FMR1 gene or fragile X syndrome as discussed above. A percentage of women with autoimmune or FMR1 premutation etiologies of POI will reveal a significantly associated family history if asked the proper questions. When the potential exists for a genetic diagnosis for the POI, referral to a genetic counselor should be strongly considered. This will help establish a full pedigree and assures that the patient understands all of the implications of genetic testing for such conditions, especially FMR1. A social history that includes details about smoking, drinking, stress, and potential significant changes in weight or associated eating disorders are also important, although not necessarily associated with hypergonadotropic amenorrhea. Early (less than 45 years of age) or premature (less than 40 years of age) menopause in women relatives is a clue to genetic etiologies for POI.

Physical Examination

On physical examination, vital signs and general appearance of the woman should be assessed. Is there a subtle increase in skin pigmentation or vitiligo, or could there be orthostatic hypotension associated with asymptomatic adrenal insufficiency? Is there a neck goiter, lid lag, or fine tremor associated with thyroid disease? Does she have short stature, shield chest, or other suggestions of Turner's syndrome? On the speculum and/or pelvic examination, vaginal atrophy could be noted visually or microscopically, and enlarged ovarian size as may occur in autoimmune oophoritis may be appreciated on bimanual examination [71].

Laboratory Evaluation

Laboratory examinations should always start with a pregnancy test, prolactin, and TSH in the evaluation of amenorrhea. In women with overt POI, the FSH values will generally be in the menopausal range, but should be confirmed with more than 1 month between testing. Since this disorder is associated with intermittent ovarian function, patients with a clear history suggesting hypergonadotropic hypogonadism may still have FSH values transiently in the normal range. In such cases, follow-up is needed to clarify the situation. It is not surprising to see FSH values wax and wane [10, 11]. Estradiol measurements are generally less than 50 pg/mL due to lack of follicular development, but could also vary with the course of the disorder.

The utility of LH values remains controversial. Some would argue that assessment of follicular function may be better served with a transvaginal ultrasound. Others value the FSH:LH ratio in the diagnostic evaluation [7]. Of less controversy is the progestin withdrawal test. Most evidence would support that there is little gained by performing this test in the setting of a suspected diagnosis of POI. This is because the amount of estrogen priming needed to cause a positive progestin withdrawal may well be present in a woman with intermittent or early stage POI, and thus the false reassurance of a positive withdrawal may delay the diagnosis of significant hypogonadism. Over half of women with POI will have a withdrawal bleed [3, 5]. Therefore, the clinical utility of doing this is limited and potentially harmful in terms of ongoing bone loss related to estrogen deficiency [85].

Most expert opinions support obtaining a karyotype in women with POI. Over half of girls who present with primary amenorrhea, and approximately 15% of women with secondary amenorrhea due to POI have karyotypic abnormalities [8]. The reasons for obtaining a karyotype are several: (1) to determine if there is Y chromosome material present, which is associated with potential future malignancy; (2) to evaluate for loss or gain of an X chromosome, which may require further diagnostic studies and have health implications; and (3) to determine if significant levels of mosaicism exist. Further genetic studies should include testing for the FMR1 premutation due to the significant familial and reproductive impact of a potential expansion in the triple-repeat sequence as discussed above. Further molecular testing, to determine if there are submicroscopic or cryptic X chromosome mutations, translocations, deletions, or other abnormalities, is still limited in availability and their clinical usefulness is uncertain at the present time [4, 28].

Other laboratory testing includes an evaluation for potential associated autoimmune conditions. Up to 30–50% of women with POI may have some associated autoimmune disease [86]. Given that thyroid and adrenal disorders are fairly prevalent in women with POI and that there are effective therapies to treat them, they both merit evaluation. Initial work-up of amenorrhea should have included thyroid function studies, but if these have not been done, serum TSH and possibly free thyroxine (T4) should be ordered. Thyroid stimulating and thyroid peroxidase antibodies are also useful. Up to 20–30% of women with POI may have preexisting or will develop thyroid disease, most commonly hypothyroidism [70].

Testing for adrenal insufficiency or the potential to develop such a condition is important. While there are various ways to test for adrenal insufficiency, some may cause false positive or false negative rates. Testing for adrenal antibodies improves the pretest probability of other testing regimens (i.e., ACTH stimulation test, morning cortisol, aldosterone, and plasma renin activity) and, thus, should be performed first, followed by the other testing when clinically indicated [65, 87]. Approximately 5% of patients with POI who are asymptomatic for any adrenal disorder will end up testing positive for adrenal antibodies and approximately 3% will have unrecognized adrenal insufficiency. Detection of these women can ultimately be life-saving if discovered prior to a crisis, which can be precipitated during an elective surgery or trauma [65, 70]. Adrenal cortex and 21-hydroxylase antibodies are the assays most reliable for testing. Predictive models have been made to determine the 5-year probability of developing autoimmune Addison's disease based on age, gender, adrenal function, antibody titers, and co-existing disease [88]. Such a predictive model may help guide physicians regarding the difficult decisions for determining monitoring intervals and follow-up.

Finally, testing for diabetes-related illnesses may be useful due to the risks of untreated disease and minimal cost, although only a small number of women will test positive (2%). Using either a fasting glucose or a 2-h glucose tolerance test is acceptable, although rarely a 2-h test will identify those with intolerance who have a normal fasting value. Testing for pernicious anemia or hyperparathyroidism, with either a vitamin B12 or calcium level, respectively, may not be useful in asymptomatic women [70]. Testing for ovarian antibodies is generally not justified due to their nonspecific nature and need for more research. A number of other, more obscure conditions that have been reported in association with POI can be excluded by performing a serum chemistry profile and CBC with indices [70].

Initial imaging considerations include a pelvic ultrasound to evaluate both the uterus and ovaries, and a bone density test. A significant number of women with POI are found to be osteopenic, and possibly even osteoporotic at the time of diagnosis, and have reduced bone mineral density compared to controls [6, 8, 85, 89]. Such findings not only guide calcium (1,200 mg elemental calcium/day), vitamin D (800 IU/day), exercise, and smoking cessation counseling but also highlight the need for hormone replacement therapies unless contraindications exist.

Emotional Assessment

POI affects a woman's physical health and wellness, yet often the most difficult and profound aspect for women and their caregivers is dealing with the emotional response to the diagnosis and treatment of this chronic condition. The diagnosis usually comes as a shock, as it is often unexpected and unanticipated when undergoing medical evaluation. Living with the condition can be life-changing, as a woman's view of her place in the world is irrevocably altered by this tremendous threat to her self-concept of her femininity and its ties to her fertility potential [90]. Frequently, the most devastating realization for women is impaired fertility and other health issues may be minimized. As a consequence, care must focus on both the physical and emotional needs of women with POI. This aspect of care begins with the diagnosis itself.

Delivering the Diagnosis

How the diagnosis of POI is communicated can influence a woman's emotional response to her health, perception of self, treatment compliance, quality of life, and overall satisfaction with care. One study found that almost half the women interviewed received the diagnosis from their physician over the telephone or by message, and three-quarters reported their doctor spending 15 min or less in communicating the information. The result was that over 70% felt unsatisfied or very unsatisfied with this communication and 89% described feeling emotionally traumatized after hearing the diagnosis. Patients were most satisfied when they felt prepared to hear the diagnosis, perceived the clinician as knowledgeable, felt the clinician spent sufficient time with them, and that the physician was sensitive to their emotional needs [91].

When delivering the diagnosis, steps need to be taken to ensure that the patient is able to hear the news in a non-traumatizing way and know that she will be assisted in getting appropriate help and support in dealing with POI. Buckman has written a six-step protocol for breaking bad news to patients which recommends the following [92]:

- Get started with a private physical setting to talk
- Find out how much the patient knows
- Find out how much the patient wants to know
- Share the information using an agenda developed before you sit down with the patient, so that you have the relevant information at hand
- Respond to the patient's feelings, "Could you tell me a little more about how you're feeling?"
- Plan and follow through by outlining an explicit step-by-step approach that can be carried out

From this perspective, it is ideal to meet physically with a patient, in a private place, and with sufficient time to talk when going over the diagnosis. Physicians need to be able to acknowledge patients' emotions and respond with patience and empathy. In addition, it is helpful to have written materials and resource information about POI available to give, so that the patient does not go home "empty-handed." There is a need to develop evidence-based approaches to provide emotional support and guidance to women experiencing the emotional sequelae associated with POI.

Psychologic Impact

While learning the diagnosis can be traumatic, living with POI can cause women significant, long-term distress and suffering. Using language that can be interpreted as judgmental, such as POF or "premature menopause," may reinforce a sense of stigma and defectiveness, and negatively affect body image. Women with POI describe feeling old, unfeminine, less healthy, empty, and worthless [91]. Over time, patients with POI have been shown to have reduced self-esteem, increased shyness, diminished perception of social supports, increased social anxiety, and more symptoms of depression and anxiety compared with control women [4, 93, 94]. The emotional suffering felt by women with POI is often experienced in isolation, as they may have difficulty in identifying people who they believe can truly understand their feelings or may feel such shame, embarrassment, and/or sense of defectiveness that they are unable to reach out to others. Thus, their sense of self and relationships with others can be profoundly negatively affected. Care should, therefore, include referrals for psychologic assistance, including counseling for women, their partners, and families. There is a need for evidence-based interventions to help these women cope with the emotional sequelae of this disorder. Not all women find the existing lay-led support groups beneficial, and some describe them as harmful.

The awareness of impaired fertility is often the most painful aspect of learning about POI. It is well documented in the literature that infertility is a major life crisis, generating significant sadness, distress, and grief [95]. The losses associated with infertility are multifaceted and, yet, uniquely personal to each woman as they reflect her dreams and hopes for the future: a wish for child/family, status in the community, health, passing on of genes and knowledge, and the experience of pregnancy, among others [96]. Grief is the emotional response to the loss of a significant relationship and often includes such feelings as shock, disbelief, anger, sadness, depression, guilt, shame, blame, and hopefully, eventually, acceptance. When the loss is invisible or intangible to others, as in the desired child, it is even more difficult to grieve [97]. It is helpful for the physician to "name" the sequelae of emotions as "grief," thereby communicating the emotional response as normal and giving permission to grieve and mourn as one is allowed to do with other more tangible losses [98].

Patients often feel urgency in trying to achieve a pregnancy when diagnosed with POI. Because a small percentage of women will become pregnant spontaneously, patients may find themselves in an ambiguous position of "Am I infertile or not?" Thus, they may embark on a journey to find ways to become pregnant quickly, a journey that often leads to the high-tech world of ART. As their life plans are altered, family building, in their view, must now become deliberate, determined, and costly in terms of finances, time, and emotional energy. Patients are often willing to undergo painful, expensive, and, as yet, unproven treatments in the hopes of restoring ovarian function and achieving pregnancy. These therapies carry a risk of interfering with spontaneous conception that can occur, and patients need to be advised about the overall ineffectiveness of these often expensive, unproven interventions [98].

It is important to keep in mind that not all individuals desire to get married or raise children. For those who have this desire, family-building options include egg or embryo donation, adoption, or the hosting of foster children. The passage of time can be important in helping patients arrive at these options, as it allows them the opportunity to grieve and come to terms with the loss of a hoped-for biologic child. When physicians offer donor egg or adoption precipitously after giving the POI diagnosis, it can circumvent grief and potentially cause problems later. Thus, patients avoid doing the emotional work necessary to heal the losses of infertility. Alternative family building does not cure the feelings of infertility, although it does fill the space of the longed-for child. Discussion with patients about choices must go beyond biologic parenthood and alternative family building, and include the achievement of other life goals and purposes, such as career, hobbies/interests, and spirituality [4].

Sexual Impact

The impact of POI on a woman's sexual identity, sexual functioning, and sexual relationship is another aspect of her emotional health that needs to be addressed by caregivers. The earlier in age the POI is identified, the more complex is the impact on all dimensions of sexuality [99]. Sexual identity is especially vulnerable when POI disrupts the normal process of development in an adolescent girl, affecting attachment needs and the ability to achieve autonomy [100]. Even before receiving the diagnosis, symptoms related to POI, such as hot flushes, night sweats, irritability, vaginal dryness, and mood disturbance, may have challenged a woman's sense of stability and affect her sexual functioning. After learning about POI, the loss of the potential to reproduce may impair motivation and desire for sexual activity, as she may feel "What's the use?" The susceptibility to psychosexual distress from POI is greater in women who wish for children and lower in those focused on their professional and social achievements [99].

As in all sexual dysfunction, sexual difficulties for women with POI need to be identified by the physician as a disorder of sexual interest or desire; the ability to be aroused; difficulty in achieving orgasm; and/or sexual pain. Treatment methods for sexual dysfunction, as well as to general health-related matters in POI, should take a multidisciplinary approach and may include a gynecologist (HR treatment), urologist (male partner's sexual dysfunction), psychiatrist (psychopharmacologic treatment of affect disorders), sex therapist (behavioral treatment), couple's therapist (relationship issues), individual psychotherapist (personal issues), and/or physical therapist (pelvic floor issues) [99]. Hormone therapy (HT) may be helpful in arousal and desire disorders. Psychosexual behavioral treatments and couple's and/or individual therapy are useful in many areas. Women and their partners need to understand how POI can affect feelings and functioning (sexually and otherwise), and be given appropriate medical therapies and referrals for psychosocial resources.

Treatment

Genetic Counseling

Genetic counseling is an important part of the diagnostic and treatment strategies for women with POI. This is especially critical when women are found to have karyotypic abnormalities and/or FMR1 premutations. Patients need to be informed about the implications of an abnormal karyotype so as to give informed consent for the testing. In situations with high pre-test probability of a positive test, it is best to offer genetic counseling before actually performing the tests. Such findings have significant implications for each individual woman's reproductive, genetic, and family health.

Family Planning

While much discussion centers on infertility, it is important to note that POI can be transient, and spontaneous remission and/or conception can occur. Therefore, if pregnancy is not desired, appropriate contraception must be discussed. Furthermore, case reports exist of women with POI ovulating and conceiving on oral contraceptive pills [101]. Oral contraceptives have not been proven effective in this specific population of women. This concern, combined with the fact that these women have menopausal FSH levels that may not be adequately suppressed by oral contraceptives, makes it prudent for women with this condition to use a barrier method or intrauterine device.

As discussed, while a diagnosis of POI implies a significant decrease in ovarian reproductive and endocrine function, it does not always imply cessation of function, and 5–10% of women with POI may still spontaneously conceive. General preconceptual health and individual medical and genetic counseling should take place prior to conception, as with any woman hoping to conceive. Regardless of the possibility of spontaneous conception, most realize that the chance of non-assisted conception is low and many, but not all, seek out ART. It should be remembered that many women have cultural or religious objections to ART. However, as discussed in the emotional health section, many do feel a need to attempt aggressive therapies such as IVF with or without egg or embryo donation to make every attempt at conceiving a biologic child.

Finally, as genetic and diagnostic technologies as well as medical treatments and interventions continue to advance, so may the abilities to predict the onset of POI and those who may be at significant risk for such a diagnosis in the future. We are already at a time when we can predict the possibility of POI after systemic cytotoxic therapies in certain cancers and autoimmune diseases. Thus, the research and advances in fertility preservation have been at the forefront of many discussions surrounding ovarian function and/or reserve. Cryopreservation of sperm has successfully been established for decades, especially with the advancement of intracytoplasmic sperm injection, allowing the utilization of as little as a single sperm to achieve a pregnancy. In the same regard, cryopreservation of embryos has also been fairly well accepted as a standard option for fertility preservation, with a success rate surrounding 30% per frozen embryo transfer cycle, although many factors must be considered. The issue for most women with POI is that they may not be married or have a partner to consider embryo freezing. While they may use donor sperm, this option is often not acceptable to some women.

More recently, efforts have been directed toward improving oocyte and ovarian tissue cryopreservation [102]. Although these technologies are improving, they are still considered experimental at most institutions, since very few pregnancies have resulted from thawing of ovarian tissue and oocytes. Moreover, they have not been tested or have been found to be of little use in women who already have a severely compromised oocyte supply. Thus, for most women with POI, regardless of stage, these treatments are not an option at the present time.

Significant controversy still involves the potential success rates and the best mechanisms for freezing, thawing, and re-implanting ovarian tissue, whether it is cortical strips or portions of the whole ovary [103–109]. Even more rare is the very few reports of ovarian transplantation in monozygotic twins discordant for ovarian failure [110]. Thus, physicians are often left with an ethical dilemma when counseling and encouraging patients regarding fertility preservation in many situations. The most important thing is honest and informative counseling, so patients can weigh all of their options. Technology could significantly improve in the future and if the ability to foresee future POI becomes possible, along with fertility preservation improvements, this may become an established and routine option for young women facing the development of iatrogenic POI.

Medical Therapy

Although level I evidence regarding the effectiveness of HT in women with POI is lacking, nearly all expert opinions support the use of HT until at least the natural age of menopause in these women, unless significant contraindications exist [111, 112]. Beyond symptom control, long-term bone and cardiovascular health are at the top of the list of concerns that physicians have when determining whether and how much HT to administer. There have been a handful of research studies that demonstrate significant increased morbidity and mortality in women with early menopause [6, 113–115], which has led to a concern that hormones are warranted in this younger age group of women. A physiologic replacement dose of estradiol in combination with a cyclic progestin is preferred [6]. A dose of 100 μg/day, delivered by skin patch, achieves physiologic, mid-follicular phase estradiol levels in these women. Medroxyprogesterone acetate 10 mg/day for 12 days each month should be taken to induce monthly withdrawal bleeds and to transform the endometrium fully to a secretory phase when given in conjunction with a full replacement dose of estrogen [116, 117]. If a menses does not occur, a pregnancy test should be obtained, and the hormones stopped if positive. Monthly progestin administration reduces the risk of endometrial hyperplasia, and with long-term administration, the development of endometrial carcinoma. The endometrial effects of oral micronized progesterone have not been adequately evaluated at the dose of estrogen recommended as replacement for these young women [118].

Decisions regarding androgen replacement therapies are even more difficult, and there is a need for more research before such treatment can be recommended. Similar to treatment with estrogen and progestin, specific studies on younger patients with POI are lacking, and applying findings from older patients with a natural, rather than pathologic, cessation in ovarian function has problems [119–125]. All such therapies deserve special consideration and collaboration with specialists when appropriate.

Preventative Therapy

The dominant issue of infertility can preclude adequate focus on all the important potential long-term adverse health consequences of diminished ovarian function. Yet, the ovary is important as an endocrine organ as well as a reproductive organ. A 59-year-old woman with natural menopause and a 19-year-old woman with POI are different patients, although both have important health considerations. General health counseling may partially be the same: exercise, good nutrition, smoking cessation, calcium and vitamin D supplementation, and good control of concomitant medical illnesses. A bone density screening test is just as important in the young woman with POI as it is in the older naturally occurring menopausal patient due to the prevalence of osteopenia and, occasionally, osteoporosis [85, 89]. Whenever the ovary ceases or significantly diminishes production of estrogen, progesterone, and androgens, there is associated bone loss over time [10, 98, 126].

Since the advent of the Women's Health Initiative and subsequent studies, there has been great reluctance to utilize HT for preventative health. What is often unrecognized by patients is that nearly all studies on estrogen and progestin (and androgen replacement) therapy have been performed on women who are significantly older (often much older than even 50 years of age), and naturally or surgically menopausal. The applicability of these studies to women with POI is unknown. Fear in young women with POI regarding enhanced cardiovascular risk, cancer, or thrombosis with the use of HT may be completely irrelevant as women with normal ovarian function in their 20s, 30s, and even 40s have hormones being produced endogenously, and non-orally administered HT is simply replacing what would otherwise be present. HT after the natural age of menopause, in considerably higher dosages, and in the presence of concomitant thrombotic or significant medical conditions, warrants individual and more specific consultation with medical providers.

Finally, women with POI are at risk for developing other autoimmune and endocrine disorders [6, 13, 64, 70, 127] and, therefore, merit surveillance. Most commonly, POI-associated thyroid and adrenal disorders will emerge over time. The current literature supports periodic screening for some autoimmune-associated conditions as discussed above. Decisions about when to repeat testing if normal at baseline as well as follow-up of slightly abnormal testing or antibodies predicting future disorders are more complicated and need further research.

Back to the Vignette

The woman in the vignette illustrates one possible presentation of a woman with POI. This particular patient scenario was chosen to highlight the vague and unanticipated symptoms in an otherwise healthy young woman. Many clinicians and often the patient herself might attribute her secondary amenorrhea to stress or weight loss, or might only search for thyroid- or prolactin-associated disorders. Such a patient could have previously been to several physicians who disregarded some of her non-specific complaints and ignored the changes in her menstrual cycle. Her progestin challenge test yields minimal to no information useful for diagnosis, and may in fact delay her diagnosis. Once the diagnosis of POI is confirmed by a second menopausal FSH test 1 month later, significant counseling must be undertaken regarding all of the issues addressed in this chapter. She has a significant family history for various autoimmune conditions and warrants a thorough evaluation for any associated autoimmune disorders. Her smoking is a well-established environmental factor that could further diminish her reproductive years, so counseling regarding cessation of smoking is important. Genetic counseling with FMR1 testing and a karyotype is indicated, due to her POI diagnosis, family history of mental retardation, and her small stature. Counseling regarding her family plans should include an assessment of the overall likelihood of a spontaneous conception (5–10%). She may elect to avoid advanced techniques of reproduction for personal reasons and search out other solutions for becoming a parent, or she may request immediate ART. The clinician should help guide her through these decisions with appropriate outcome information and avoid being judgmental. Her desire for fertility and psychologic needs (sexual health, infertility, and the emotional impact of the diagnosis) are extremely important, and require time, a sensitive physician, and a multidisciplinary approach.

Having guided the patient through the initial diagnosis and work-up, the physician has a responsibility to consider long-term health implications of a diagnosis of POI. All of these things warrant time, patience, discussion, and will likely take place over numerous office visits. Appropriate referrals to subspecialists should be considered as issues are identified. Hopefully, as awareness and treatment options (such as genetic, immunoassay, fertility preservation, and medical therapies) continue to improve, patients, such as the one described here, will find their search for answers more easily navigated and the likelihood of fertility more promising.

References

1. Speroff L, Fritz MA (2005) The ovary-embryology and development. In: Speroff L, Fritz MA (eds) Clinical gynecologic endocrinology and infertility. Lippincott Williams & Wilkins, Philadelphia, pp 97–111
2. Faddy MJ, Gosden RG, Gougeon A, Richardson SJ, Nelson JF (1992) Accelerated disappearance of ovarian follicles in mid-life: implications for forecasting menopause. Hum Reprod 7:1342–1346
3. Albright F, Smith P, Fraser R (1942) A syndrome characterized by primary ovarian insufficiency and decreased stature. Am J Med Sci 204:625–648
4. Davis M, Ventura JL, Wieners M, Covington SN, Vanderhoof VH, Ryan ME et al (2009) The psychosocial transition associated with spontaneous 46,XX primary ovarian insufficiency: illness uncertainty, stigma, goal flexibility, and purpose in life as factors in emotional health. Fertil Steril 93(7):2321–2329

5. Luborsky JL, Meyer P, Sowers MF, Gold EB, Santoro N (2003) Premature menopause in a multi-ethnic population study of the menopause transition. Hum Reprod 18:199–206
6. Nelson LM (2009) Clinical practice. Primary ovarian insufficiency. N Engl J Med 360:606–614
7. Rebar RW (2009) Premature ovarian failure. Obstet Gynecol 113:1355–1363
8. Rebar RW, Connolly HV (1990) Clinical features of young women with hypergonadotropic amenorrhea. Fertil Steril 53:804–810
9. Nelson LM, Anasti JN, Kimzey LM, Defensor RA, Lipetz KJ, White BJ et al (1994) Development of luteinized graafian follicles in patients with karyotypically normal spontaneous premature ovarian failure. J Clin Endocrinol Metab 79:1470–1475
10. Nelson LM, Anasti JN, Kimzey LM et al (1996) Premature ovarian failure. In: Adashi EY, Rock JA, Rosenwaks Z (eds) Reproductive endocrinology, surgery, and technology. Lippincott-Raven, Philadelphia, pp 1393–1410
11. Nelson LM, Kimzey LM, White BJ, Merriam GR (1992) Gonadotropin suppression for the treatment of karyotypically normal spontaneous premature ovarian failure: a controlled trial. Fertil Steril 57:50–55
12. Kalantaridou SN, Nelson LM (2000) Premature ovarian failure is not premature menopause. Ann NY Acad Sci 900:393–402
13. Welt CK (2008) Primary ovarian insufficiency: a more accurate term for premature ovarian failure. Clin Endocrinol (Oxf) 68:499–509
14. Navot D, Rosenwaks Z, Margalioth EJ (1987) Prognostic assessment of female fecundity. Lancet 2:645–647
15. Nikolaou D, Gilling-Smith C (2004) Early ovarian ageing: are women with polycystic ovaries protected? Hum Reprod 19:2175–2179
16. Meden-Vrtovec H (2004) Ovarian aging and infertility. Clin Exp Obstet Gynecol 31:5–8
17. Scott RT, Toner JP, Muasher SJ, Oehninger S, Robinson S, Rosenwaks Z (1989) Follicle-stimulating hormone levels on cycle day 3 are predictive of in vitro fertilization outcome. Fertil Steril 51:651–654
18. Levi AJ, Raynault MF, Bergh PA, Drews MR, Miller BT, Scott RT Jr (2001) Reproductive outcome in patients with diminished ovarian reserve. Fertil Steril 76:666–669
19. Gleicher N, Barad D (2006) Unexplained infertility: does it really exist? Hum Reprod 21:1951–1955
20. Barad DH, Weghofer A, Gleicher N (2007) Age-specific levels for basal follicle-stimulating hormone assessment of ovarian function. Obstet Gynecol 109:1404–1410
21. Simpson JL, Rajkovic A (1999) Ovarian differentiation and gonadal failure. Am J Med Genet 89:186–200
22. Ross MT, Grafham DV, Coffey AJ, Scherer S, McLay K, Muzny D et al (2005) The DNA sequence of the human X chromosome. Nature 434:325–337
23. Carrel L, Willard HF (2005) X-inactivation profile reveals extensive variability in X-linked gene expression in females. Nature 434:400–404
24. Toniolo D, Rizzolio F (2007) X chromosome and ovarian failure. Semin Reprod Med 25:264–271
25. Villanueva AL, Rebar RW (1983) Triple-X syndrome and premature ovarian failure. Obstet Gynecol 62:70s–73s
26. Schlessinger D, Herrera L, Crisponi L, Mumm S, Percesepe A, Pellegrini M et al (2002) Genes and translocations involved in POF. Am J Med Genet 111:328–333
27. Krauss CM, Turksoy RN, Atkins L, McLaughlin C, Brown LG, Page DC (1987) Familial premature ovarian failure due to an interstitial deletion of the long arm of the X chromosome. N Engl J Med 317:125–131
28. Bachelot A, Rouxel A, Massin N, Dulon J, Courtillot C, Matuchansky C et al (2009) Phenotyping and genetic studies of 357 consecutive patients presenting with premature ovarian failure. Eur J Endocrinol 161:179–187
29. Portnoi MF, Aboura A, Tachdjian G, Bouchard P, Dewailly D, Bourcigaux N et al (2006) Molecular cytogenetic studies of Xq critical regions in premature ovarian failure patients. Hum Reprod 21:2329–2334

30. Lachlan KL, Youings S, Costa T, Jacobs PA, Thomas NS (2006) A clinical and molecular study of 26 females with Xp deletions with special emphasis on inherited deletions. Hum Genet 118:640–651
31. Toniolo D (2006) X-linked premature ovarian failure: a complex disease. Curr Opin Genet Dev 16:293–300
32. Simpson JL (2008) Genetic and phenotypic heterogeneity in ovarian failure: overview of selected candidate genes. Ann NY Acad Sci 1135:146–154
33. Rizzolio F, Sala C, Alboresi S, Bione S, Gilli S, Goegan M et al (2007) Epigenetic control of the critical region for premature ovarian failure on autosomal genes translocated to the X chromosome: a hypothesis. Hum Genet 121:441–450
34. Persani L, Rossetti R, Cacciatore C, Bonomi M (2009) Primary ovarian insufficiency: X chromosome defects and autoimmunity. J Autoimmun 33:35–41
35. Rizzolio F, Bione S, Sala C, Goegan M, Gentile M, Gregato G et al (2006) Chromosomal rearrangements in Xq and premature ovarian failure: mapping of 25 new cases and review of the literature. Hum Reprod 21:1477–1483
36. Bione S, Sala C, Manzini C, Arrigo G, Zuffardi O, Banfi S et al (1998) A human homologue of the *Drosophila melanogaster* diaphanous gene is disrupted in a patient with premature ovarian failure: evidence for conserved function in oogenesis and implications for human sterility. Am J Hum Genet 62:533–541
37. Rizzolio F, Pramparo T, Sala C, Zuffardi O, Desantis L, Rabellotti E et al (2008) Epigenetic analysis of the critical region I for premature ovarian failure (POF): demonstration of a highly heterochromatic domain on the long arm of the mammalian X chromosome. J Med Genet 46(9):585–592
38. Feng Y, Zhang F, Lokey LK, Chastain JL, Lakkis L, Eberhart D et al (1995) Translational suppression by trinucleotide repeat expansion at FMR1. Science 268:731–734
39. Hagerman PJ, Hagerman RJ (2004) The fragile-X premutation: a maturing perspective. Am J Hum Genet 74:805–816
40. Conway GS, Payne NN, Webb J, Murray A, Jacobs PA (1998) Fragile X premutation screening in women with premature ovarian failure. Hum Reprod 13:1184–1187
41. Sullivan AK, Marcus M, Epstein MP, Allen EG, Anido AE, Paquin JJ et al (2005) Association of FMR1 repeat size with ovarian dysfunction. Hum Reprod 20:402–412
42. Ennis S, Ward D, Murray A (2006) Nonlinear association between CGG repeat number and age of menopause in FMR1 premutation carriers. Eur J Hum Genet 14:253–255
43. Hagerman PJ, Hagerman RJ (2004) Fragile X-associated tremor/ataxia syndrome (FXTAS). Ment Retard Dev Disabil Res Rev 10:25–30
44. Wittenberger MD, Hagerman RJ, Sherman SL, McConkie-Rosell A, Welt CK, Rebar RW et al (2007) The FMR1 premutation and reproduction. Fertil Steril 87:456–465
45. Coffey SM, Cook K, Tartaglia N, Tassone F, Nguyen DV, Pan R et al (2008) Expanded clinical phenotype of women with the FMR1 premutation. Am J Med Genet A 146A:1009–1016
46. Di Pasquale E, Rossetti R, Marozzi A, Bodega B, Borgato S, Cavallo L et al (2006) Identification of new variants of human BMP15 gene in a large cohort of women with premature ovarian failure. J Clin Endocrinol Metab 91:1976–1979
47. Ledig S, Ropke A, Haeusler G, Hinney B, Wieacker P. BMP15 mutations in XX gonadal dysgenesis and premature ovarian failure. Am J Obstet Gynecol 2008;198:84.e1–e5
48. Kaufman FR, Kogut MD, Donnell GN, Goebelsmann U, March C, Koch R (1981) Hypergonadotropic hypogonadism in female patients with galactosemia. N Engl J Med 304:994–998
49. Levy HL, Driscoll SG, Porensky RS, Wender DF (1984) Ovarian failure in galactosemia. N Engl J Med 310:50
50. Leslie ND, Immerman EB, Flach JE, Florez M, Fridovich-Keil JL, Elsas LJ (1992) The human galactose-1-phosphate uridyltransferase gene. Genomics 14:474–480
51. Kaufman FR, Reichardt JK, Ng WG, Xu YK, Manis FR, McBride-Chang C et al (1994) Correlation of cognitive, neurologic, and ovarian outcome with the Q188R mutation of the galactose-1-phosphate uridyltransferase gene. J Pediatr 125:225–227

52. Waggoner DD, Buist NR, Donnell GN (1990) Long-term prognosis in galactosaemia: results of a survey of 350 cases. J Inherit Metab Dis 13:802–818
53. Uda M, Ottolenghi C, Crisponi L, Garcia JE, Deiana M, Kimber W et al (2004) Foxl2 disruption causes mouse ovarian failure by pervasive blockage of follicle development. Hum Mol Genet 13:1171–1181
54. Uhlenhaut NH, Treier M (2006) Foxl2 function in ovarian development. Mol Genet Metab 88:225–234
55. Ottolenghi C, Uda M, Hamatani T, Crisponi L, Garcia JE, Ko M et al (2004) Aging of oocyte, ovary, and human reproduction. Ann NY Acad Sci 1034:117–131
56. Aittomaki K, Lucena JL, Pakarinen P, Sistonen P, Tapanainen J, Gromoll J et al (1995) Mutation in the follicle-stimulating hormone receptor gene causes hereditary hypergonadotropic ovarian failure. Cell 82:959–968
57. Chand AL, Ooi GT, Harrison CA, Shelling AN, Robertson DM (2007) Functional analysis of the human inhibin alpha subunit variant A257T and its potential role in premature ovarian failure. Hum Reprod 22:3241–3248
58. Barlow C, Liyanage M, Moens PB, Deng CX, Ried T, Wynshaw-Boris A (1997) Partial rescue of the prophase I defects of Atm-deficient mice by p53 and p21 null alleles. Nat Genet 17:462–466
59. Barlow C, Liyanage M, Moens PB, Tarsounas M, Nagashima K, Brown K et al (1998) Atm deficiency results in severe meiotic disruption as early as leptonema of prophase I. Development 125:4007–4017
60. Ellis NA, German J (1996) Molecular genetics of Bloom's syndrome. Hum Mol Genet 5 Spec No:1457–14563
61. Fogli A, Rodriguez D, Eymard-Pierre E, Bouhour F, Labauge P, Meaney BF et al (2003) Ovarian failure related to eukaryotic initiation factor 2B mutations. Am J Hum Genet 72:1544–1550
62. Pagnamenta AT, Taanman JW, Wilson CJ, Anderson NE, Marotta R, Duncan AJ et al (2006) Dominant inheritance of premature ovarian failure associated with mutant mitochondrial DNA polymerase gamma. Hum Reprod 21:2467–2473
63. Luoma P, Melberg A, Rinne JO, Kaukonen JA, Nupponen NN, Chalmers RM et al (2004) Parkinsonism, premature menopause, and mitochondrial DNA polymerase gamma mutations: clinical and molecular genetic study. Lancet 364:875–882
64. Welt CK (2008) Autoimmune oophoritis in the adolescent. Ann NY Acad Sci 1135:118–122
65. Bakalov VK, Vanderhoof VH, Bondy CA, Nelson LM (2002) Adrenal antibodies detect asymptomatic auto-immune adrenal insufficiency in young women with spontaneous premature ovarian failure. Hum Reprod 17:2096–2100
66. Hoek A, van Kasteren Y, de Haan-Meulman M, Hooijkaas H, Schoemaker J, Drexhage HA (1995) Analysis of peripheral blood lymphocyte subsets, NK cells, and delayed type hypersensitivity skin test in patients with premature ovarian failure. Am J Reprod Immunol 33:495–502
67. Hoek A, Schoemaker J, Drexhage HA (1997) Premature ovarian failure and ovarian autoimmunity. Endocr Rev 18:107–134
68. Perheentupa J (2002) APS-I/APECED: the clinical disease and therapy. Endocrinol Metab Clin North Am 31:295–320, vi
69. Halonen M, Eskelin P, Myhre AG, Perheentupa J, Husebye ES, Kampe O et al (2002) AIRE mutations and human leukocyte antigen genotypes as determinants of the autoimmune polyendocrinopathy-candidiasis-ectodermal dystrophy phenotype. J Clin Endocrinol Metab 87:2568–2574
70. Kim TJ, Anasti JN, Flack MR, Kimzey LM, Defensor RA, Nelson LM (1997) Routine endocrine screening for patients with karyotypically normal spontaneous premature ovarian failure. Obstet Gynecol 89:777–779
71. Bakalov VK, Anasti JN, Calis KA, Vanderhoof VH, Premkumar A, Chen S et al (2005) Autoimmune oophoritis as a mechanism of follicular dysfunction in women with 46, XX spontaneous premature ovarian failure. Fertil Steril 84:958–965

72. Bakalov VK, Kalantaridou SN, Godoy H et al (2001) Anti-adrenal antibodies are an effective screening test for autoimmune adrenal insufficiency in young women with premature ovarian failure. In: The Endocrine Society's 82nd Annual Meeting. Toronto, Canada
73. Kalantaridou SN, Nelson LM (1998) Autoimmune premature ovarian failure: of mice and women. J Am Med Womens Assoc 53:18–20
74. Kalantaridou SN, Braddock DT, Patronas NJ, Nelson LM (1999) Treatment of autoimmune premature ovarian failure. Hum Reprod 14:1777–1782
75. Sklar CA, Mertens AC, Mitby P, Whitton J, Stovall M, Kasper C et al (2006) Premature menopause in survivors of childhood cancer: a report from the childhood cancer survivor study. J Natl Cancer Inst 98:890–896
76. Meirow D (2000) Reproduction post-chemotherapy in young cancer patients. Mol Cell Endocrinol 169:123–131
77. Lass A (1999) The fertility potential of women with a single ovary. Hum Reprod Update 5:546–550
78. Hehenkamp WJ, Volkers NA, Broekmans FJ, de Jong FH, Themmen AP, Birnie E et al (2007) Loss of ovarian reserve after uterine artery embolization: a randomized comparison with hysterectomy. Hum Reprod 22:1996–2005
79. Midgette AS, Baron JA (1990) Cigarette smoking and the risk of natural menopause. Epidemiology 1:474–480
80. Matikainen T, Perez GI, Jurisicova A, Pru JK, Schlezinger JJ, Ryu HY et al (2001) Aromatic hydrocarbon receptor-driven Bax gene expression is required for premature ovarian failure caused by biohazardous environmental chemicals. Nat Genet 28:355–360
81. Koh JM, Kim CH, Hong SK, Lee KU, Kim YT, Kim OJ et al (1998) Primary ovarian failure caused by a solvent containing 2-bromopropane. Eur J Endocrinol 138:554–556
82. Kim Y, Jung K, Hwang T, Jung G, Kim H, Park J et al (1996) Hematopoietic and reproductive hazards of Korean electronic workers exposed to solvents containing 2-bromopropane. Scand J Work Environ Health 22:387–391
83. Jick H, Porter J (1977) Relation between smoking and age of natural menopause. Report from the Boston Collaborative Drug Surveillance Program, Boston University Medical Center. Lancet 1:1354–1355
84. Yanushpolsky EH, Best CL, Jackson KV, Clarke RN, Barbieri RL, Hornstein MD (1998) Effects of endometriomas on oocyte quality, embryo quality, and pregnancy rates in in vitro fertilization cycles: a prospective, case-controlled study. J Assist Reprod Genet 15:193–197
85. Popat VB, Calis KA, Vanderhoof VH, Cizza G, Reynolds JC, Sebring N et al (2009) Bone mineral density in estrogen-deficient young women. J Clin Endocrinol Metab 94:2277–2283
86. Alper MM, Garner PR (1985) Premature ovarian failure: its relationship to autoimmune disease. Obstet Gynecol 66:27–30
87. Betterle C, Coco G, Zanchetta R (2005) Adrenal cortex autoantibodies in subjects with normal adrenal function. Best Pract Res Clin Endocrinol Metab 19:85–99
88. Coco G, Dal Pra C, Presotto F, Albergoni MP, Canova C, Pedini B et al (2006) Estimated risk for developing autoimmune Addison's disease in patients with adrenal cortex autoantibodies. J Clin Endocrinol Metab 91:1637–1645
89. Anasti JN, Kalantaridou SN, Kimzey LM, Defensor RA, Nelson LM (1998) Bone loss in young women with karyotypically normal spontaneous premature ovarian failure. Obstet Gynecol 91:12–15
90. Orshan SA, Furniss KK, Forst C, Santoro N (2001) The lived experience of premature ovarian failure. J Obstet Gynecol Neonatal Nurs 30:202–208
91. Groff AA, Covington SN, Halverson LR, Fitzgerald OR, Vanderhoof V, Calis K et al (2005) Assessing the emotional needs of women with spontaneous premature ovarian failure. Fertil Steril 83:1734–1741
92. Buckman R (1992) How to break bad news: a guide for health care professionals. The Johns Hopkins University Press, Baltimore
93. Orshan SA, Ventura JL, Covington SN, Vanderhoof VH, Troendle JF, Nelson LM (2009) Women with spontaneous 46, XX primary ovarian insufficiency (hypergonadotropic hypogonadism) have lower perceived social support than control women. Fertil Steril 92:688–693

94. Schmidt PJ, Cardoso GM, Ross JL, Haq N, Rubinow DR, Bondy CA (2006) Shyness, social anxiety, and impaired self-esteem in Turner syndrome and premature ovarian failure. JAMA 295:1374–1376
95. Greil AL (1997) Infertility and psychological distress: a critical review of the literature. Soc Sci Med 45:1679–1704
96. Mahlstedt PP (1985) The psychological component of infertility. Fertil Steril 43:335–346
97. Burns LH, Covington SN (2006) The psychology of infertility. In: Covington SN, Burns LH (eds) Infertility counseling: a comprehensive handbook for clinicians. Cambridge University Press, New York, pp 1–19
98. Nelson LM (2001) Spontaneous premature ovarian failure: young women, special needs. Menopause Management 10:1–6
99. Graziottin A, Basson R (2004) Sexual dysfunction in women with premature menopause. Menopause 11:766–777
100. Covington SN, Martinez PE, Popat V, Nandagopal R, Ryan M, Nelson LM (2008) The psychology of antecedents to adult reproductive disorders in adolescent girls. Ann NY Acad Sci 1135:155–162
101. Alper MM, Jolly EE, Garner PR (1986) Pregnancies after premature ovarian failure. Obstet Gynecol 67:59S–62S
102. Woodruff TK (2007) The emergence of a new interdiscipline: oncofertility. Cancer Treat Res 138:3–11
103. Meirow D, Levron J, Eldar-Geva T, Hardan I, Fridman E, Zalel Y et al (2005) Pregnancy after transplantation of cryopreserved ovarian tissue in a patient with ovarian failure after chemotherapy. N Engl J Med 353:318–321
104. Donnez J, Dolmans MM, Demylle D, Jadoul P, Pirard C, Squifflet J et al (2004) Livebirth after orthotopic transplantation of cryopreserved ovarian tissue. Lancet 364:1405–1410
105. Gosden RG, Baird DT, Wade JC, Webb R (1994) Restoration of fertility to oophorectomized sheep by ovarian autografts stored at -196 degrees C. Hum Reprod 9:597–603
106. Oktay K, Buyuk E (2004) Fertility preservation in women undergoing cancer treatment. Lancet 363:1830
107. Oktay K, Buyuk E, Veeck L, Zaninovic N, Xu K, Takeuchi T et al (2004) Embryo development after heterotopic transplantation of cryopreserved ovarian tissue. Lancet 363:837–840
108. Oktay K, Sonmezer M (2004) Ovarian tissue banking for cancer patients: fertility preservation, not just ovarian cryopreservation. Hum Reprod 19:477–480
109. Oktay K, Tilly J (2004) Livebirth after cryopreserved ovarian tissue autotransplantation. Lancet 364:2091–2092; author reply 2–3
110. Silber SJ, Lenahan KM, Levine DJ, Pineda JA, Gorman KS, Friez MJ et al (2005) Ovarian transplantation between monozygotic twins discordant for premature ovarian failure. N Engl J Med 353:58–63
111. Pines A, Sturdee DW, Birkhauser MH, Schneider HP, Gambacciani M, Panay N (2007) IMS updated recommendations on postmenopausal hormone therapy. Climacteric 10:181–194
112. Practice Committee of American Society for Reproductive Medicine (2004) Current evaluation of amenorrhea. Fertil Steril 82:S33–S39
113. Jacobsen BK, Knutsen SF, Fraser GE (1999) Age at natural menopause and total mortality and mortality from ischemic heart disease: the Adventist Health Study. J Clin Epidemiol 52:303–307
114. Gallagher JC (2007) Effect of early menopause on bone mineral density and fractures. Menopause 14:567–571
115. Mondul AM, Rodriguez C, Jacobs EJ, Calle EE (2005) Age at natural menopause and cause-specific mortality. Am J Epidemiol 162:1089–1097
116. Gibbons WE, Moyer DL, Lobo RA, Roy S, Mishell DR Jr (1986) Biochemical and histologic effects of sequential estrogen/progestin therapy on the endometrium of postmenopausal women. Am J Obstet Gynecol 154:456–461
117. Bjarnason K, Cerin A, Lindgren R, Weber T (1999) Adverse endometrial effects during long cycle hormone replacement therapy. Scandinavian Long Cycle Study Group. Maturitas 32:161–170

118. Anonymous (1995) Effects of estrogen or estrogen/progestin regimens on heart disease risk factors in postmenopausal women. The Postmenopausal Estrogen/Progestin Interventions (PEPI) Trial. The Writing Group for the PEPI Trial. JAMA 273:199–208
119. Davis SR, McCloud P, Strauss BJ, Burger H (1995) Testosterone enhances estradiol's effects on postmenopausal bone density and sexuality. Maturitas 21:227–236
120. Davis SR, Moreau M, Kroll R, Bouchard C, Panay N, Gass M et al (2008) Testosterone for low libido in postmenopausal women not taking estrogen. N Engl J Med 359:2005–2017
121. Davis SR, van der Mooren MJ, van Lunsen RH, Lopes P, Ribot C, Rees M et al (2006) Efficacy and safety of a testosterone patch for the treatment of hypoactive sexual desire disorder in surgically menopausal women: a randomized, placebo-controlled trial. Menopause 13:387–396
122. Floter A, Nathorst-Boos J, Carlstrom K, von Schoultz B (2002) Addition of testosterone to estrogen replacement therapy in oophorectomized women: effects on sexuality and well-being. Climacteric 5:357–365
123. Lobo RA, Rosen RC, Yang HM, Block B, Van Der Hoop RG (2003) Comparative effects of oral esterified estrogens with and without methyltestosterone on endocrine profiles and dimensions of sexual function in postmenopausal women with hypoactive sexual desire. Fertil Steril 79:1341–1352
124. Myers LS, Dixen J, Morrissette D, Carmichael M, Davidson JM (1990) Effects of estrogen, androgen, and progestin on sexual psychophysiology and behavior in postmenopausal women. J Clin Endocrinol Metab 70:1124–1131
125. Shifren JL, Braunstein GD, Simon JA, Casson PR, Buster JE, Redmond GP et al (2000) Transdermal testosterone treatment in women with impaired sexual function after oophorectomy. N Engl J Med 343:682–688
126. Prior JC, Vigna YM, Schechter MT, Burgess AE (1990) Spinal bone loss and ovulatory disturbances. N Engl J Med 323:1221–1227
127. LaBarbera AR, Miller MM, Ober C, Rebar RW (1988) Autoimmune etiology in premature ovarian failure. Am J Reprod Immunol Microbiol 16:115–122

Chapter 6
Hyperprolactinemia and Pituitary Causes of Amenorrhea

Pouneh Fazeli and Lisa B. Nachtigall

Introduction

Pituitary causes of amenorrhea constitute approximately 18% of cases of secondary amenorrhea but only approximately 7% of cases of primary amenorrhea [1]. The most common pituitary cause of amenorrhea is hyperprolactinemia constituting 80% of all pituitary causes of secondary amenorrhea and approximately 15% of cases of secondary amenorrhea due to any cause [2]. In this chapter, we review the causes, clinical presentation, diagnostic evaluation, and current treatment strategies for amenorrhea due to hyperprolactinemia and other pituitary disorders. We present an illustrative case of secondary amenorrhea due to a pituitary cause.

Case

The patient is a 33-year-old woman with a history of running competitively beginning at the age of 12 years. She had her first menstrual period at the age of 15 years and then was oligoamenorrheic until the age of 18 years when she was started on oral contraceptives. She stopped running competitively after graduating from college but continued to run 7 miles daily, 6 days per week. At the age of 32 years, she stopped the oral contraceptive pill in order to attempt to become pregnant. Three months after discontinuing the oral contraceptive pill, she remained amenorrheic and her gynecologist initiated a work-up and asked that she decrease her activity level. History was notable for no other past medical history, and current medications included only a pre-natal vitamin. Physical examination was notable for a BMI of 20.5 kg/m^2. She appeared non-Cushingoid and non-acromegalic. Visual fields were intact to confrontation. Laboratory studies demonstrated a negative HCG, normal

L.B. Nachtigall (✉)
Neuroendocrine Clinical Center unit, Massachusetts General Hospital
and Harvard Medical School, Boston, MA 02114, USA
e-mail: lnachtigall@partners.org

N.F. Santoro and G. Neal-Perry (eds.), *Amenorrhea: A Case-Based, Clinical Guide*,
Contemporary Endocrinology, DOI 10.1007/978-1-60327-864-5_6,

Table 6.1 Case

History	
33-year-old woman presenting with amenorrhea	
Competitive runner since the age of 12 years	
Menarche at 15 years of age	
Oligoamenorrhea until 18 years old when started oral contraceptives	
Stopped oral contraceptives at age 32 years	
Amenorrhea >3 months after stopping oral contraceptives	
Physical examination	
BMI: 20.5 kg/m^2	
Non-Cushingoid, non-acromegalic appearing	
Visual fields intact to confrontation	
Laboratory studies	
Prolactin: 45 ng/ml (normal range: 0–20 ng/ml)	
Serum HCG: undetectable	
TSH: 1.3 mIU/L (normal range: 0.5–5 mIU/L)	
Free T4: 1.2 ng/dl (normal range: 0.8–1.8 ng/dl)	
LH: 5 U/L	
FSH: 3 U/L	
Estradiol: 30 pg/ml (normal range:	Follicular phase: <20–145 pg/ml Mid-cycle peak: 112–443 pg/ml Luteal phase: <20–241 pg/ml Post-menopausal: <59 pg/ml)

thyroid function studies, a slightly elevated prolactin level, low-normal FSH and LH, and a low estradiol level of 30 pg/ml (Table 6.1).

Causes of Hyperprolactinemia

The most common cause of hyperprolactinemia is a lactotroph-secreting adenoma [2]. There are other causes of an elevated prolactin level which can also lead to the development of the sequelae of hyperprolactinemia. A non-adenomatous cause of hyperprolactinemia will rarely lead to a prolactin level greater than 200–300 ng/ml [3] (Table 6.2). Extremely elevated prolactin levels generally indicate the presence of a lactotroph adenoma.

Physiologic Causes

Pregnancy

Pregnancy is a common physiologic cause of both amenorrhea and hyperprolactinemia. Prolactin levels increase progressively during pregnancy and are the highest at the time of delivery [4]. Prolactin levels have been shown to be as high

Table 6.2 Causes of hyperprolactinemia

Physiologic causes
Pregnancy
Nipple stimulation
Macroprolactinemia
Stress
Medications[a]
Antipsychotics
Haloperidol
Phenothiazines
Risperidone
Olanzapine
Molindone
Gastric motility agents
Metoclopramide
Domperidone
Cimetidine
Antihypertensives
Methyldopa
Verapamil
Reserpine
Pathophysiologic causes
Lactotroph adenoma
Mass effect/stalk interruption
Trauma (chest wall/CNS)
Primary hypothyroidism
Chronic renal failure

[a]This list is a summary of common medications associated with hyperprolactinemia and does not include all medications associated with hyperprolactinemia

as nearly 600 ng/ml at the time of delivery [4]; therefore, women with amenorrhea and hyperprolactinemia should be evaluated for pregnancy prior to any other diagnostic work-up. Within the first 72 h post-partum, the prolactin levels drop precipitously unless a woman is nursing, since the prolactin levels will increase in response to suckling [4].

Nipple Stimulation

Nipple stimulation can cause a rise in serum prolactin levels but usually only during the first 6 weeks of lactation [4]). This is likely due to the fact that estradiol levels fall precipitously in the post-partum period and, therefore, the lactotroph hypertrophy subsides, diminishing the rise in the prolactin level post-suckling. Therefore, in women who choose to breast feed, prolactin levels should not be checked until at least 6 weeks post-partum. In non-lactating women, nipple stimulation has not been shown to lead to significant increases in serum prolactin levels [5].

Macroprolactinemia

Prolactin circulates in multiple forms. The predominant form is a 23-kD form but rare individuals may have other forms of prolactin, with much higher molecular masses, which predominate. These individuals may have elevated levels of a 150-kD form of prolactin, referred to as big prolactin or macroprolactin [6]. This form of prolactin is thought to be a macromolecule consisting of the 23-kD form of prolactin and an immunoglobulin [6], and has been shown to be cleared from the circulation more slowly, which is likely the cause of the elevated prolactin levels [7].

Macroprolactinemia has historically been considered an asymptomatic condition. Individuals with macroprolactinemia may still experience amenorrhea or galactorrhea, although much less frequently compared to individuals with true hyperprolactinemia [8, 9]. A polyethylene glycol (PEG) precipitation test can be used to determine whether an individual's hyperprolactinemia is due to macroprolactinemia [10]. Macroprolactinemia must be considered in the differential diagnosis for hyperprolactinemia in patients with high serum prolactin concentrations who do not exhibit clinical signs of hyperprolactinemia.

Medications

Psychiatric Medications

Antipsychotics

As dopamine suppresses the production of prolactin, any medications that block dopamine receptors may increase prolactin levels. Such medications include antipsychotic medications including haloperidol (a typical antipsychotic) and risperidone (an atypical antipsychotic), as well as many others (see Table 6.2). Antipsychotics have been shown to be associated with higher prolactin levels in women compared to men [11, 12]. Although both acute and chronic therapy with antipsychotic agents has been shown to increase prolactin levels, acute therapy tends to be associated with a greater elevation [11]; therefore, prolactin levels should likely not be checked in the first 4 weeks of treatment. Risperidone, an atypical antipsychotic agent, has been shown to be associated with significantly greater prolactin levels when compared to the typical antipsychotic haloperidol, but generally the newer atypical agents are thought to induce less of an increase in prolactin levels compared to the typical agents [12, 13].

Antidepressants

Selective serotonin reuptake inhibitors (SSRIs), specifically fluoxetine, have been shown to increase prolactin levels only minimally [14], whereas less commonly used antidepressants, such as the tricyclics, have only rarely been associated with hyperprolactinemia [13].

Other Medications

Gastric motility agents that block dopamine receptors, for example, metoclopramide and domperidone, also raise prolactin levels [13]. Antihypertensive drugs that block dopamine synthesis, such as methyldopa, have also been shown to raise prolactin levels as quickly as 2–6 h after oral administration [15]. Verapamil is the only calcium-channel blocker that has been shown to increase prolactin levels [16]; the mechanism is thought to be due to decreased hypothalamic production of dopamine [17].

Pharmacologic doses of estradiol have been shown to increase prolactin secretion [18]. Estradiol is thought to increase prolactin levels by stimulating lactotroph cell proliferation, likely through a mechanism involving the transforming growth *factor-β* isoforms [19]. Supra-physiologic levels of estradiol, as occur during pregnancy or with assisted reproductive technologies such as ovulation induction or in vitro fertilization, may cause lactotroph cell hyperplasia leading to hyperprolactinemia. Yet oral contraceptive pills are not typically thought to cause hyperprolactinemia [13].

Pathophysiologic Causes

Lactotroph Adenoma

Lactotroph adenomas are responsible for 80% of amenorrhea due to a pituitary cause [2]. Lactotroph adenomas are the most common hyper-secreting pituitary adenomas and are almost always benign but very rarely they can be malignant and metastasize extra-cranially [20]. Prolactin secretion is typically proportional to the size of the adenoma in well-differentiated adenomas and can be very high – in fact, levels on the order of 10^4 ng/ml have been measured [21]. Poorly differentiated lactotroph adenomas may be large but secrete less prolactin than expected based on their size.

Mass Effect/Trauma

The pituitary gland is connected to the median eminence of the hypothalamus via a stalk. Dopamine, produced in the hypothalamus, suppresses the production of prolactin in the pituitary gland. Any compression or interference of the stalk, for example, by a mass or trauma, can lead to an interruption of the flow of dopamine into the pituitary gland and subsequent hyperprolactinemia.

Traumatic injury to the chest wall can lead to hyperprolactinemia [22]. The mechanism is thought to be due to neurogenic stimulation as intercostal nerve blockade was found to reduce serum prolactin levels in a patient with elevated prolactin levels after a traumatic burn injury to the chest wall [22]. Traumatic brain injury can also result in hyperprolactinemia [23] even 12 months after the initial trauma [24].

Primary Hypothyroidism

Thyrotropin releasing hormone, secreted by the hypothalamus, can stimulate pituitary lactotroph cells to secrete prolactin in individuals with hypothyroidism [25]. Primary hypothyroidism can also cause enlargement of the pituitary gland due to thyrotroph hyperplasia and possibly lactotroph hyperplasia. Therefore, primary hypothyroidism can be associated with an enlarged pituitary gland, hyperprolactinemia, and all of its sequelae including amenorrhea and evaluation of an individual with hyperprolactinemia should always include a TSH level. Treatment for the hypothyroidism should result in resolution of the pituitary enlargement and hyperprolactinemia [26].

Chronic Renal Failure

Individuals with chronic renal failure, particularly those receiving hemodialysis, may have elevated prolactin levels [27]. The mechanism by which chronic renal failure leads to hyperprolactinemia appears to be one of both decreased responsiveness of the pituitary to dopamine suppression and therefore increased secretion, and decreased clearance [27].

Clinical Findings in Hyperprolactinemia

Reproductive Dysfunction

Hyperprolactinemia can cause hypogonadotropic hypogonadism. Therefore, common clinical findings in women with hyperprolactinemia include menstrual irregularities, typically oligoamenorrhea or amenorrhea [28]. One mechanism by which elevated prolactin levels decrease gonadotropin levels is thought to be mediated by inhibition of gonadotropin releasing hormone (GnRH) secretion from the hypothalamus by corticotrophin releasing factor, the secretion of which is thought to be stimulated by hyperprolactinemia [29].

Women with hyperprolactinemia who have regular ovulatory cycles may still have difficulty achieving a pregnancy. Infertility in the setting of ovulatory cycles may be due to a shortened luteal phase [30, 31]. Any woman with hyperprolactinemia and otherwise unexplained infertility may benefit from a trial of treatment for hyperprolactinemia prior to initiating more aggressive treatments for infertility.

Galactorrhea

Individuals with hyperprolactinemia may experience galactorrhea [28]. The galactorrhea may be spontaneous or may only be expressible in nature [28]. Galactorrhea is less frequently a symptom of hyperprolactinemia compared to oligoamenorrhea or amenorrhea [28], and importantly is a frequent finding in individuals without hyperprolactinemia [3], particularly in parous women.

Bone Loss

Other findings in hyperprolactinemia include bone loss, which has been shown to be primarily due to hypo-estrogenemia [32]. Treatment of hyperprolactinemia has been shown to improve bone mineral densities in women with hyperprolactinemia [32]. Also, individuals with elevated prolactin levels with regular menstrual cycles have been found to have bone mineral densities comparable to those of women with normal prolactin levels and regular menstrual cycles [32].

CNS Disturbances

New visual problems, particularly new peripheral field cuts, are a worrisome sign and may indicate a rapidly expanding tumor or a tumor which is impinging on the optic chiasm. These individuals should be imaged with a pituitary-protocol MRI and have visual field testing immediately. Headaches may also be associated with pituitary adenomas and may be a sign of rapid tumor expansion. Rarely, hyperprolactinemia may cause headaches independently of tumor mass [33]. Dopamine agonist therapy may relieve headaches, especially *migraine-type*, associated with hyperprolactinemia [34].

Treatment of Hyperprolactinmeia

If there is an underlying cause of hyperprolactinemia, such as a medication, the offending agent should be stopped or changed if this is possible without significant risk to the patient. If this is not possible, then treatment is indicated if the individual is symptomatic (reproductive dysfunction or galactorrhea); treatment with a dopamine agonist (cabergoline or bromocriptine) may be initiated if there is no contraindication. If the individual is on a dopamine-blocking agent for psychiatric illness, then a dopamine agonist may exacerbate the underlying psychiatric disorder and in that case dopamine agonists should be avoided. In these cases, oral contraceptives will protect against the harmful consequences of amenorrhea on bone mineral density (Table 6.3).

Microprolactinomas that are not associated with hypogonadism, menstrual irregularity, infertility, or disruptive galactorrhea do not require treatment but should be observed with a pituitary-protocol MRI. Treatment should be initiated if tumor growth occurs. Growing or symptomatic microprolactinomas should be treated with dopamine agonists unless contraindicated or if acute visual field cuts mandate urgent surgical intervention. If compressive symptoms are noted or a dopamine-agonist is contraindicated, such as in the case of an individual with psychiatric illness on dopamine blocking agents, then surgery is the treatment of choice. Surgery may also be indicated in individuals who are intolerant of dopamine agonist therapy or who do not respond to dopamine agonist therapy, such as patients with predominantly cystic tumors.

There are two dopamine agonists currently used in the treatment of hyperprolactinemia: bromocriptine and cabergoline. Cabergoline has been shown to achieve normal prolactin levels and ovulatory cycles or pregnancy more often than bromocriptine and has been associated with fewer side effects than bromocriptine therapy [35]. Yet in women attempting to conceive, bromocriptine therapy is preferred because of greater experience with the use of bromocriptine during pregnancy [36]. Also, there has been recent data demonstrating an increased incidence of cardiac

Table 6.3 Indications for treatment of hyperprolactinemia

Indications for medical therapy
Macroadenoma
Hypogonadism
Reproductive dysfunction
Amenorrhea
Infertility
Acne and/or hirsutism[a]
Bothersome galactorrhea[a]
Headaches (controversial)[a]
Indications for surgical therapy
Optic nerve compression
Intolerance of dopamine agonists
Dopamine agonists ineffective[b]
Predominantly cystic macroadenoma[b]
Apoplexy or hemorrhage within tumor
Patients on psychiatric medications[b]

[a]Relative indication
[b]If tumor mass is a concern

valve regurgitation in individuals taking high doses of cabergoline for the treatment of Parkinson's disease [37, 38]. In patients using cabergoline for hyperprolactinemia, clinically significant valvular disease has not been demonstrated, although an increased incidence of aortic valve calcification has been shown [37], and recent cross-sectional, observational studies and a meta-analysis have demonstrated an increased incidence of clinically insignificant, mild to moderate tricuspid regurgitation [39–41]. Yet a number of studies have also demonstrated no difference in the prevalence of valvular regurgitation when comparing hyperprolactinemic patients treated with cabergoline to controls [42–44]. Although no clinically significant valvular disease has been demonstrated in patients receiving cabergoline for hyperprolactinemia, the potential risk of valvular dysfunction should be discussed with the patient prior to initiating dopamine agonist therapy. Once a pregnancy has been confirmed, we recommend that the dopamine agonist be stopped.

Women with hyperprolactinemia and regular ovulatory cycles may still be infertile due to a luteal phase defect [30, 31]. Administration of bromocriptine in these women may help lengthen the luteal phase and may result in achievement of a pregnancy.

Other Pituitary Causes of Amenorrhea

Non-Lactotroph Adenomas and Sellar Masses

While the most common cause of pituitary-associated amenorrhea is a lactotroph-secreting adenoma, other pituitary adenomas can also cause amenorrhea. Cushing's disease and acromegaly are the result of hyper-functioning pituitary adenomas of the corticotroph and somatotroph cells of the pituitary, respectively. Amenorrhea is a common finding in Cushing's disease, usually due to increased circulating androgens made by the adrenal gland. In acromegaly, amenorrhea may result from hyperprolactinemia, either due to concomitant production of prolactin by the tumor or stalk compression, compression of the pituitary gonadotrophs, or hyperandrogenism. Therefore, Cushing's and acromegaly should be considered in any individual presenting with amenorrhea and clinical evidence of either cortisol or growth hormone excess, respectively. However, in individuals presenting with primary or secondary amenorrhea, these diagnoses are rare. In a series of 252 patients presenting with primary amenorrhea, Cushing's accounted for one case [1]. Similarly, in a series of 262 individuals presenting with secondary amenorrhea, Cushing's accounted for two of those cases [2]. However, it is possible that these small numbers represent under-reporting and/or failure to diagnose these diseases when present.

Any pituitary adenoma, especially those ≥1 cm in size (macroadenomas), can cause amenorrhea due to mass effect on the gonadotrophs or due to stalk compression. Therefore, in individuals with amenorrhea of unknown cause who do not have an elevated serum FSH, a pituitary-protocol MRI should be part of the initial diagnostic work-up. Similarly, any sellar mass, including craniopharyngiomas and meningiomas, can cause amenorrhea through mass effect or interruption of the stalk

Table 6.4 Differential diagnosis for sellar masses

- Adenomas
  - Hyperfunctioning
    - Prolactinomas
    - Corticotroph adenomas (cause of Cushing's disease)
    - Somatotroph adenomas (cause of acromegaly)
    - Somatomammotroph adenomas (adenoma which co-secretes prolactin and growth hormone)
    - Thyrotroph adenomas (excess TSH secretion)
    - Pleurihormonal adenomas (rare)
  - Non-functioning
- Craniopharyngioma
- Chordoma
- Germ cell tumor
- Granular cell tumor
- Metastatic disease
- Meningioma
- Primary lymphoma
- Sarcoma
- Schwannoma
- Vascular tumor/aneurysms/AV fistula of cavernous sinus
- Cysts
  - Rathke's cleft
  - Dermoid
  - Epidermoid
- Infections/Infiltrative disorders
  - Hemochromatosis
  - Hypophysitis
    - Lymphocytic
    - Granulomatous
    - Xanthomatous
  - Langerhans cell histiocytosis
  - Sarcoidosis
  - Giant cell granuloma
  - Infections/abscess

(Table 6.4). Craniopharyngiomas may be associated with diabetes insipidus and, therefore, should be considered in the differential diagnosis of an individual presenting with amenorrhea and diabetes insipidus. In adults with craniopharyngiomas, CT scan of the sellar area usually demonstrates calcifications within the tumor.

Sheehan's Syndrome

The pituitary gland derives its blood supply from both systemic and hypothalamic sources. The inferior hypophyseal arterial branches comprise the systemic circulation, although the predominant supply to the anterior pituitary is from the hypothalamic-portal circulation. The hypothalamic-portal circulation is derived from the superior hypophyseal arteries which branch from the internal carotid arteries. During pregnancy, increased levels of estrogen can potentiate lactotroph cell growth [19]. The increased size of the pituitary can cause compression of the superior hypophyseal artery and can make it very sensitive to sudden changes in blood supply or hypotension [45]. Therefore, cases of massive postpartum hemorrhage requiring multiple transfusions can result in ischemic necrosis of the pituitary gland, causing postpartum hypopituitarism referred to as Sheehan's syndrome. Postpartum hemorrhage is a rare complication of births in the developed world and therefore Sheehan's syndrome is most commonly seen in developing countries [46, 47].

Sheehan's typically presents months to years after delivery and the most common presenting symptoms of Sheehan's syndrome include inability to lactate and failure to resume menses, although an acute presentation with severe pituitary hypo-functioning resulting in death can also occur [45]. Therefore, clinicians must remain alert to this possibility, particularly in women who have had deliveries complicated by >500 ml of blood loss or the requirement for blood transfusions. Treatment for Sheehan's consists of replacing pituitary hormone deficiencies.

Infiltrative and Infectious Causes

Lymphocytic Hypophysitis

Lymphocytic hypophysitis is an inflammatory condition that affects the pituitary gland. It affects predominantly females (8.5:1) and tends to occur during the latter stages of pregnancy or the postpartum period [48]. A case series of 16 histologically proven cases of lymphocytic hypophysitis found that 71% of the cases were associated with pregnancy [48]. Of all patients studied, 63% had anterior pituitary hypo-functioning and 19% had posterior pituitary dysfunction in the form of diabetes insipidus [48]. This cause of hypopituitarism should be high on the differential diagnosis of individuals presenting with both anterior and posterior pituitary dysfunction, who are pregnant or postpartum. These patients commonly present with symptoms of an expanding sellar mass with headaches and visual field defects, although this is not always the case and patients may present with associated autoimmune dysfunction, such as autoimmune thyroid disease [48]. This condition can be lethal if not detected early as 3/16 patients in the case series died as a result of undiagnosed hypopituitarism [48]. Compressive symptoms usually require surgical intervention, and high-dose corticosteroid treatment has been shown to be effective in some patients [49], although its efficacy has not yet been proven.

Hereditary Hemochromatosis

Hereditary hemochromatosis is a cause of gonadal insufficiency in men due to damage caused to either the testes or the pituitary gonadotroph cells by excessive amounts of iron [50]. In women, hypogonadism is rarely seen [50] but must still be kept on the differential diagnosis, particularly in individuals with a family history of hemochromatosis.

Other

Rarer causes of pituitary-associated amenorrhea include sarcoidosis and tuberculosis. In sarcoidosis, granulomas may infiltrate the pituitary gland resulting in amenorrhea due to destruction of pituitary gonadotroph cells, but more commonly sarcoidosis results in granulomatous infiltration of the hypothalamus, resulting in amenorrhea due to decreased synthesis of GnRH by the hypothalamus [51]. Individuals with sarcoidosis and hypopituitarism may also have diabetes insipidus [51] and, therefore, this should be considered in the differential diagnosis of individuals presenting with amenorrhea and diabetes insipidus. Tuberculous meningitis in childhood has also been associated with amenorrhea. A study of 49 patients with a childhood history of tuberculous meningitis found that 10% had pituitary dysfunction in the form of gonadotropin deficiency [52].

Langerhans cell histiocytosis is a disease in which Langerhans cells, a form of dendritic cell, inappropriately proliferate and infiltrate various regions of the body including the hypothalamic-pituitary axis. The most common pituitary dysfunction noted in Langerhans cell histiocytosis is diabetes insipidus but anterior pituitary deficiencies, including gonadal dysfunction, have also been reported [53].

Other infiltrating and infectious diseases may infiltrate the hypothalamic-pituitary axis and cause gonadal dysfunction resulting in amenorrhea. Similarly, metastatic disease can also rarely infiltrate the pituitary gland and result in amenorrhea. Infiltrating disorders are commonly associated with diabetes insipidus and, therefore, these disorders should always be considered in the differential diagnosis of an individual presenting with both amenorrhea and diabetes insipidus.

Iatrogenic and Other Causes of Pituitary-Associated Amenorrhea

Surgery

Surgical treatment of a pituitary adenoma is a rare cause of hypogonadism [54], although most reports in the literature [55] likely reflect the rates of hypopituitarism for individuals undergoing surgery in the hands of a dedicated pituitary surgeon. As the rates of post-surgical complications have been shown to be higher in individuals undergoing pituitary surgery by surgeons with lower surgical volumes [56], the rates of post-surgical hypogonadism may be higher in individuals who have undergone pituitary surgery by a less-experienced surgeon.

Radiation

Pituitary dysfunction resulting in amenorrhea is a well-known complication of radiation therapy directed at the pituitary gland [54]. A series of 35 male patients were followed for a mean of 4.2 years after radiotherapy and 67% developed gonadal dysfunction if they had surgery followed by radiation compared to 50% who were treated with radiation alone [54]. Individuals who have undergone radiotherapy to the pituitary gland should be monitored closely for the development of pituitary dysfunction with long-term serial biochemical testing.

Radiation therapy for non-pituitary brain tumors has also been associated with hypothalamic-pituitary dysfunction, hyperprolactinemia, and gonadotropin deficiency [57]. Hypopituitarism has been shown to be positively correlated with time since the radiation therapy and with the dose of radiation, whereas hyperprolactinemia and hypogonadism are associated only with the dose of radiation therapy [58]. Therefore, both patients who have undergone radiation therapy for pituitary tumors and those who have undergone radiation for non-pituitary brain tumors should be closely followed for subsequent pituitary dysfunction.

Traumatic Brain Injury and Subarachnoid Hemorrhage

Traumatic brain injury and subarachnoid hemorrhage can cause pituitary dysfunction and amenorrhea. Individuals with traumatic brain injury associated with a coma are more likely to be affected by pituitary dysfunction, especially those who are comatose for days to weeks, but even individuals with a mild head injury can develop hypogonadism [59]. Importantly, even if hypopituitarism is not demonstrated immediately after trauma, it has been shown to present even one year after the injury; therefore, patients with a history of traumatic brain injury should be carefully monitored [24].

Genetic Causes

Recently, mutations in transcription factors involved in the cellular proliferation and differentiation of the pituitary gland have been shown to be the cause of anterior pituitary dysfunction and, therefore, should be on the differential diagnosis for primary amenorrhea. Typically mutations in these transcription factors are associated with other clinical findings that will be a clue to the diagnosis. For example, *HESX1* mutations are associated with septo-optic dysplasia as well as pituitary hormone deficiencies and SOX2 mutations may be associated with sensorineural hearing loss, esophageal atresia, and learning difficulties in addition to hypogonadotropic hypogonadism [60]. LHX3 mutations and PROP1 mutations have also been associated with gonadotropin deficiency, and GLI2 and SOX3 mutations have been associated with hypopituitarism [60]. The inheritance pattern of these genes is variable and ranges from recessive, dominant, X-linked to de novo [60].

Diagnostic Evaluation

History

A thorough history of duration of amenorrhea, pregnancy, changes in weight, changes in terminal hair growth, headache, visual changes, increases in shoe size or ring size, galactorrhea, history of renal disease, and medication history should be obtained from each patient. In adolescents and young women, growth curves may be useful, and in patients with primary amenorrhea, a history of pubertal development should be reviewed. Patients with polycystic ovary syndrome (PCOS) are likely to have had normal breast development, whereas patients with genetic hypopituitarism will usually not report a history of spontaneous breast development.

Pregnancy is a common cause of amenorrhea and physiologic hyperprolactinemia. Weight gain and terminal hair growth are common findings in Cushing's disease as well as other causes of amenorrhea including PCOS. Headache and visual changes can be found in individuals with pituitary tumors and may signal tumor growth. Changes in shoe and ring size are common signs of acromegaly. Galactorrhea is a common symptom of hyperprolactinemia, and renal disease and medications (as discussed above) can cause hyperprolactinemia and subsequent menstrual disturbances.

Physical Examination

Physical examination findings that are helpful in determining a pituitary cause of amenorrhea include a Cushingoid or acromegalic body habitus. Individuals with Cushing's may have disproportionate centripetal obesity (obese abdomen and thin extremities due to muscle atrophy), supraclavicular fullness, a posterior cervical hump, and thin skin which often manifests as easy bruising and violaceous striae on the abdomen, flank, axilla, or thighs. Individuals with acromegaly may demonstrate evidence of soft tissue growth including acral changes, large lips and/or nose, frontal skull bossing, widening of the spaces between teeth, and a pronounced jaw and underbite.

In any woman with primary or secondary amenorrhea, we recommend that a prolactin level be checked as part of the work-up. If the value is <50 ng/ml but is elevated above the normal range, we repeat the measurement to ensure that the elevation is chronic and not due to a transient cause, such as nipple stimulation in a lactating woman, stress [61], recent sexual intercourse [62], or carbohydrate intake [63].

In individuals with any degree of prolactin elevation, pituitary-dedicated MRI imaging is indicated. Individuals with even slightly elevated prolactin levels may have large, non-functioning pituitary adenomas that compress the stalk, thereby causing the prolactin elevation, or their prolactin level may be underestimated secondary to the Hook effect. The Hook effect occurs in the setting of large amounts of antigen (in this case prolactin) saturating both antibodies present in the immunoradiometric sandwich assay: the antibody capturing the antigen and the signaling antibody. When both the capturing and signaling antibody are saturated by the high levels of prolactin, they are not able to sandwich together and give a falsely low prolactin value. Thus, women with macroadenomas (adenomas ≥1 cm) and normal or only mildly elevated prolactin levels should have a prolactin level checked after dilution of the serum sample in order to ensure that a large, well-functioning prolactinoma is not being missed.

Case Correlation

The patient had a pituitary-protocol MRI performed which demonstrated a 3-mm hypo-dense lesion on the right side of the pituitary gland, consistent with a pituitary adenoma. The patient was interested in becoming pregnant. She was subsequently started on low dose bromocriptine (1.25 mg po daily). Her menstrual periods resumed within 6 weeks. A follow-up prolactin level was found to be at our goal of mid-normal range in women attempting to achieve a pregnancy. Within 12 weeks of initiating bromocriptine therapy, a pregnancy was confirmed and the bromocriptine was stopped. As microprolactinomas rarely grow during pregnancy [64], typically patients may be observed for any signs or symptoms that might indicate tumor growth during the pregnancy. If she develops symptoms consistent with tumor growth including headache or visual symptoms, a visual field examination and, if necessary, a non-contrast pituitary-protocol MRI can be performed. The incidence of tumor growth during pregnancy is higher in women with macroprolactinoma (≥1 cm) [64] and therefore in this group of patients, baseline visual field testing prior to pregnancy and during each trimester is recommended. In our patient, we will repeat endocrine testing at least 6 weeks after delivery. This patient illustrates the importance of checking a prolactin level and performing pituitary imaging even when many aspects of the initial presentation are suggestive of hypothalamic amenorrhea due to exercise.

References

1. Reindollar RH, Byrd JR, McDonough PG (1981) Delayed sexual development: a study of 252 patients. Am J Obstet Gynecol 140:371–380
2. Reindollar RH, Novak M, Tho SP, McDonough PG (1986) Adult-onset amenorrhea: a study of 262 patients. Am J Obstet Gynecol 155:531–543
3. Kleinberg DL, Noel GL, Frantz AG (1977) Galactorrhea: a study of 235 cases, including 48 with pituitary tumors. N Engl J Med 296:589–600

4. Tyson JE, Hwang P, Guyda H, Friesen HG (1972) Studies of prolactin secretion in human pregnancy. Am J Obstet Gynecol 113:14–20
5. Jarrell J, Franks S, McInnes R, Gemayel K, Guyda H, Arronet GH, Naftolin F (1980) Breast examination does not elevate serum prolactin. Fertil Steril 33:49–51
6. Gibney J, Smith TP, McKenna TJ (2005) Clinical relevance of macroprolactin. Clin Endocrinol (Oxf) 62:633–643
7. Hattori N, Inagaki C (1997) Anti-prolactin (PRL) autoantibodies cause asymptomatic hyperprolactinemia: bioassay and clearance studies of PRL-immunoglobulin G complex. J Clin Endocrinol Metab 82:3107–3110
8. Leslie H, Courtney CH, Bell PM, Hadden DR, McCance DR, Ellis PK, Sheridan B, Atkinson AB (2001) Laboratory and clinical experience in 55 patients with macroprolactinemia identified by a simple polyethylene glycol precipitation method. J Clin Endocrinol Metab 86:2743–2746
9. Vallette-Kasic S, Morange-Ramos I, Selim A, Gunz G, Morange S, Enjalbert A, Martin PM, Jaquet P, Brue T (2002) Macroprolactinemia revisited: a study on 106 patients. J Clin Endocrinol Metab 87:581–588
10. Olukoga AO, Kane JW (1999) Macroprolactinaemia: validation and application of the polyethylene glycol precipitation test and clinical characterization of the condition. Clin Endocrinol (Oxf) 51:119–126
11. Rivera JL, Lal S, Ettigi P, Hontela S, Muller HF, Friesen HG (1976) Effect of acute and chronic neuroleptic therapy on serum prolactin levels in men and women of different age groups. Clin Endocrinol (Oxf) 5:273–282
12. David SR, Taylor CC, Kinon BJ, Breier A (2000) The effects of olanzapine, risperidone, and haloperidol on plasma prolactin levels in patients with schizophrenia. Clin Ther 22:1085–1096
13. Molitch ME (2008) Drugs and prolactin. Pituitary 11:209–218
14. Meltzer H, Bastani B, Jayathilake K, Maes M (1997) Fluoxetine, but not tricyclic antidepressants, potentiates the 5-hydroxytryptophan-mediated increase in plasma cortisol and prolactin secretion in subjects with major depression or with obsessive compulsive disorder. Neuropsychopharmacology 17:1–11
15. Steiner J, Cassar J, Mashiter K, Dawes I, Fraser TR, Breckenridge A (1976) Effects of methyldopa on prolactin and growth hormone. Br Med J 1:1186–1188
16. Fearrington EL, Rand CH Jr, Rose JD (1983) Hyperprolactinemia-galactorrhea induced by verapamil. Am J Cardiol 51:1466–1467
17. Kelley SR, Kamal TJ, Molitch ME (1996) Mechanism of verapamil calcium channel blockade-induced hyperprolactinemia. Am J Physiol 270:E96–E100
18. Yen SS, Ehara Y, Siler TM (1974) Augmentation of prolactin secretion by estrogen in hypogonadal women. J Clin Invest 53:652–655
19. Hentges S, Sarkar DK (2001) Transforming growth factor-beta regulation of estradiol-induced prolactinomas. Front Neuroendocrinol 22:340–363
20. Walker JD, Grossman A, Anderson JV, Ur E, Trainer PJ, Benn J, Lowy C, Sonksen PH, Plowman PN, Lowe DG et al (1993) Malignant prolactinoma with extracranial metastases: a report of three cases. Clin Endocrinol (Oxf) 38:411–419
21. Delgrange E, Trouillas J, Maiter D, Donckier J, Tourniaire J (1997) Sex-related difference in the growth of prolactinomas: a clinical and proliferation marker study. J Clin Endocrinol Metab 82:2102–2107
22. Morley JE, Dawson M, Hodgkinson H, Kalk WJ (1977) Galactorrhea and hyperprolactinemia associated with chest wall injury. J Clin Endocrinol Metab 45:931–935
23. Lieberman SA, Oberoi AL, Gilkison CR, Masel BE, Urban RJ (2001) Prevalence of neuroendocrine dysfunction in patients recovering from traumatic brain injury. J Clin Endocrinol Metab 86:2752–2756
24. Aimaretti G, Ambrosio MR, Di Somma C, Gasperi M, Cannavo S, Scaroni C, Fusco A, Del Monte P, De Menis E, Faustini-Fustini M, Grimaldi F, Logoluso F, Razzore P, Rovere S, Benvenga S, Degli Uberti EC, De Marinis L, Lombardi G, Mantero F, Martino E, Giordano G, Ghigo E (2005) Residual pituitary function after brain injury-induced hypopituitarism: a prospective 12-month study. J Clin Endocrinol Metab 90:6085–6092

25. Snyder PJ, Jacobs LS, Utiger RD, Daughaday WH (1973) Thyroid hormone inhibition of the prolactin response to thyrotropin-releasing hormone. J Clin Invest 52:2324–2329
26. Groff TR, Shulkin BL, Utiger RD, Talbert LM (1984) Amenorrhea-galactorrhea, hyperprolactinemia, and suprasellar pituitary enlargement as presenting features of primary hypothyroidism. Obstet Gynecol 63:86S–89S
27. Sievertsen GD, Lim VS, Nakawatase C, Frohman LA (1980) Metabolic clearance and secretion rates of human prolactin in normal subjects and in patients with chronic renal failure. J Clin Endocrinol Metab 50:846–852
28. Gomez F, Reyes FI, Faiman C (1977) Nonpuerperal galactorrhea and hyperprolactinemia. Clinical findings, endocrine features and therapeutic responses in 56 cases. Am J Med 62:648–660
29. Kooy A, de Greef WJ, Vreeburg JT, Hackeng WH, Ooms MP, Lamberts SW, Weber RF (1990) Evidence for the involvement of corticotropin-releasing factor in the inhibition of gonadotropin release induced by hyperprolactinemia. Neuroendocrinology 51:261–266
30. Corenblum B, Pairaudeau N, Shewchuk AB (1976) Prolactin hypersecretion and short luteal phase defects. Obstet Gynecol 47:486–488
31. Seppala M, Ranta T, Hirvonen E (1976) Hyperprolactinaemia and luteal insufficiency. Lancet 1:229–230
32. Biller BM, Baum HB, Rosenthal DI, Saxe VC, Charpie PM, Klibanski A (1992) Progressive trabecular osteopenia in women with hyperprolactinemic amenorrhea. J Clin Endocrinol Metab 75:692–697
33. Kemmann E, Jones JR (1983) Hyperprolactinemia and headaches. Am J Obstet Gynecol 145:668–671
34. Bosco D, Belfiore A, Fava A, De Rose M, Plastino M, Ceccotti C, Mungari P, Iannacchero R, Lavano A (2008) Relationship between high prolactin levels and migraine attacks in patients with microprolactinoma. J Headache Pain 9:103–107
35. Webster J, Piscitelli G, Polli A, Ferrari CI, Ismail I, Scanlon MF (1994) A comparison of cabergoline and bromocriptine in the treatment of hyperprolactinemic amenorrhea. Cabergoline Comparative Study Group. N Engl J Med 331:904–909
36. Bronstein MD, Salgado LR, de Castro Musolino NR (2002) Medical management of pituitary adenomas: the special case of management of the pregnant woman. Pituitary 5:99–107
37. Schade R, Andersohn F, Suissa S, Haverkamp W, Garbe E (2007) Dopamine agonists and the risk of cardiac-valve regurgitation. N Engl J Med 356:29–38
38. Zanettini R, Antonini A, Gatto G, Gentile R, Tesei S, Pezzoli G (2007) Valvular heart disease and the use of dopamine agonists for Parkinson's disease. N Engl J Med 356:39–46
39. Kars M, Delgado V, Holman ER, Feelders RA, Smit JW, Romijn JA, Bax JJ, Pereira AM (2008) Aortic valve calcification and mild tricuspid regurgitation but no clinical heart disease after 8 years of dopamine agonist therapy for prolactinoma. J Clin Endocrinol Metab 93:3348–3356
40. Colao A, Galderisi M, Di Sarno A, Pardo M, Gaccione M, D'Andrea M, Guerra E, Pivonello R, Lerro G, Lombardi G (2008) Increased prevalence of tricuspid regurgitation in patients with prolactinomas chronically treated with cabergoline. J Clin Endocrinol Metab 93:3777–3784
41. Bogazzi F, Manetti L, Raffaelli V, Lombardi M, Rossi G, Martino E (2008) Cabergoline therapy and the risk of cardiac valve regurgitation in patients with hyperprolactinemia: a meta-analysis from clinical studies. J Endocrinol Invest 31:1119–1123
42. Vallette S, Serri K, Rivera J, Santagata P, Delorme S, Garfield N, Kahtani N, Beauregard H, Aris-Jilwan N, Houde G, Serri O (2008) Long-term cabergoline therapy is not associated with valvular heart disease in patients with prolactinomas. Pituitary 12(3):153–157
43. Devin JK, Lakhani VT, Byrd BF 3rd, Blevins LS Jr (2008) Prevalence of valvular heart disease in a cohort of patients taking cabergoline for management of hyperprolactinemia. Endocr Pract 14:672–677
44. Nachtigall LB, Valassi E, Lo J, McCarty D, Passeri J, Biller BM, Miller KK, Utz A, Grinspoon S, Lawson EA, Klibanski A (2009) Gender effects on cardiac valvular function in hyperprolactinaemic patients receiving cabergoline: a retrospective study. Clin Endocrinol (Oxf) 72(1):53–58
45. Kelestimur F (2003) Sheehan's syndrome. Pituitary 6:181–188

46. Feinberg EC, Molitch ME, Endres LK, Peaceman AM (2005) The incidence of Sheehan's syndrome after obstetric hemorrhage. Fertil Steril 84:975–979
47. Zargar AH, Singh B, Laway BA, Masoodi SR, Wani AI, Bashir MI (2005) Epidemiologic aspects of postpartum pituitary hypofunction (Sheehan's syndrome). Fertil Steril 84:523–528
48. Thodou E, Asa SL, Kontogeorgos G, Kovacs K, Horvath E, Ezzat S (1995) Clinical case seminar: lymphocytic hypophysitis: clinicopathological findings. J Clin Endocrinol Metab 80:2302–2311
49. Kristof RA, Van Roost D, Klingmuller D, Springer W, Schramm J (1999) Lymphocytic hypophysitis: non-invasive diagnosis and treatment by high dose methylprednisolone pulse therapy? J Neurol Neurosurg Psychiatry 67:398–402
50. Kelly TM, Edwards CQ, Meikle AW, Kushner JP (1984) Hypogonadism in hemochromatosis: reversal with iron depletion. Ann Intern Med 101:629–632
51. Stuart CA, Neelon FA, Lebovitz HE (1978) Hypothalamic insufficiency: the cause of hypopituitarism in sarcoidosis. Ann Intern Med 88:589–594
52. Lam KS, Sham MM, Tam SC, Ng MM, Ma HT (1993) Hypopituitarism after tuberculous meningitis in childhood. Ann Intern Med 118:701–706
53. Kaltsas GA, Powles TB, Evanson J, Plowman PN, Drinkwater JE, Jenkins PJ, Monson JP, Besser GM, Grossman AB (2000) Hypothalamo-pituitary abnormalities in adult patients with langerhans cell histiocytosis: clinical, endocrinological, and radiological features and response to treatment. J Clin Endocrinol Metab 85:1370–1376
54. Snyder PJ, Fowble BF, Schatz NJ, Savino PJ, Gennarelli TA (1986) Hypopituitarism following radiation therapy of pituitary adenomas. Am J Med 81:457–462
55. Sudhakar N, Ray A, Vafidis JA (2004) Complications after trans-sphenoidal surgery: our experience and a review of the literature. Br J Neurosurg 18:507–512
56. Barker FG 2nd, Klibanski A, Swearingen B (2003) Transsphenoidal surgery for pituitary tumors in the United States, 1996-2000: mortality, morbidity, and the effects of hospital and surgeon volume. J Clin Endocrinol Metab 88:4709–4719
57. Constine LS, Woolf PD, Cann D, Mick G, McCormick K, Raubertas RF, Rubin P (1993) Hypothalamic-pituitary dysfunction after radiation for brain tumors. N Engl J Med 328:87–94
58. Agha A, Sherlock M, Brennan S, O'Connor SA, O'Sullivan E, Rogers B, Faul C, Rawluk D, Tormey W, Thompson CJ (2005) Hypothalamic-pituitary dysfunction after irradiation of nonpituitary brain tumors in adults. J Clin Endocrinol Metab 90:6355–6360
59. Benvenga S, Campenni A, Ruggeri RM, Trimarchi F (2000) Clinical review 113: hypopituitarism secondary to head trauma. J Clin Endocrinol Metab 85:1353–1361
60. Kelberman D, Dattani MT (2007) Hypopituitarism oddities: congenital causes. Horm Res 68(suppl 5):138–144
61. Sobrinho LG (2003) Prolactin, psychological stress and environment in humans: adaptation and maladaptation. Pituitary 6:35–39
62. Kruger TH, Haake P, Hartmann U, Schedlowski M, Exton MS (2002) Orgasm-induced prolactin secretion: feedback control of sexual drive? Neurosci Biobehav Rev 26:31–44
63. Quigley ME, Ishizuka B, Ropert JF, Yen SS (1982) The food-entrained prolactin and cortisol release in late pregnancy and prolactinoma patients. J Clin Endocrinol Metab 54:1109–1112
64. Molitch ME (1985) Pregnancy and the hyperprolactinemic woman. N Engl J Med 312: 1364–1370

Chapter 7
Amenorrhea Associated With the Female Athlete Triad: Etiology, Diagnosis, and Treatment

M.J. De Souza and R.J. Toombs

Introduction

The Female Athlete Triad [1, 2] is a syndrome of interrelated conditions that involves disordered eating, low bone mass, and amenorrhea in physically active women and female athletes. This condition was first described by the American College of Sports Medicine in 1997 [1] and is associated with significant health risks. The condition is most common in women involved in sports that emphasize leanness, such as cross country running, gymnastics, and figure skating [2, 3]; however, this condition also impacts recreationally physically active women [4]. Inadequate nutrition precedes the clinical sequelae of amenorrhea and low bone mass. Nutritional deficits are typically associated with internal and external pressures on these women to maintain a low body weight, and most often present as disordered eating [5–7]. The etiology of amenorrhea in exercising women is secondary to inadequate caloric intake in the face of high exercise-related energy expenditure, resulting in a net energy deficit. The energy deficit, in turn, stimulates compensatory mechanisms such as weight loss and energy conservation that translate to hypothalamic suppression of ovarian function and amenorrhea [6, 8, 9].

In the past two decades, much has been learned about symptoms, risk factors, causes, and treatment strategies for the Female Athlete Triad, and particularly amenorrhea, although only limited clinical guidelines are available to date [2, 10]. The only clinical recommendation for the prevention and treatment of amenorrhea in physically active women and athletes is to increase caloric intake and/or reduce exercise energy expenditure [10]. No specific dietary guidelines exist to date, and the rationale for reducing training when caloric intake is already high is likely an excessively conservative approach, since exercise per se does not play a causal role

M.J. De Souza (✉)
Women's Health and Exercise Laboratory, Noll Laboratory, Department of Kinesiology, Penn State University, University Park, PA 16802, USA
e-mail: mjd34@psu.edu

N.F. Santoro and G. Neal-Perry (eds.), *Amenorrhea: A Case-Based, Clinical Guide*, Contemporary Endocrinology, DOI 10.1007/978-1-60327-864-5_7,

in the etiology of athletic amenorrhea [8, 11]. This chapter describes the most recent scientific findings about the relationship between energy balance and menstrual regularity, and provides clinicians with a practical approach to the diagnosis and treatment of these problems commonly observed in physically active adolescent and adult women and female athletes.

A New Model

The Female Athlete Triad was first identified over 10 years ago by the American College of Sports Medicine [1]. Recently, the emergence of a new model for understanding the Female Athlete Triad has greatly advanced our understanding of the condition [2]. Originally, the three components of the Triad were presented as clinical endpoints that included disordered eating, low bone mass, and amenorrhea [1]. The components of the Female Athlete Triad are known to be interrelated since energy deficiency associated with disordered eating plays a causal role in the development of menstrual disturbances [9, 11, 12], and both energy deficiency and a low estrogen environment associated with amenorrhea play a causal role in initiating bone loss [13–15]. In the new Triad model [2] described in Fig. 7.1, these interrelationships are reaffirmed; however, each component of the Female Athlete Triad is represented as a continuum of severity from health to disease. At the "healthy" end of the continuum of each Triad component are optimal energy availability, the presence of normal ovulatory menstrual cycles, and optimal bone health [2]. At the "unhealthy" end of the continuum of each Triad component are

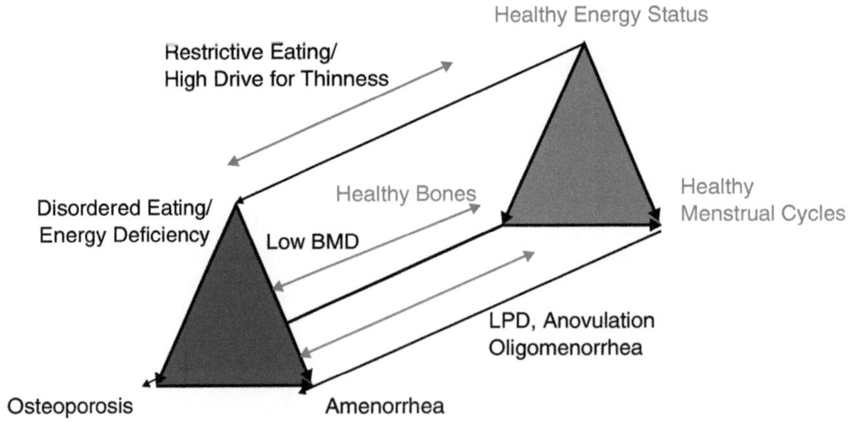

Fig. 7.1 The continuum of the Female Athlete Triad beginning with healthy energy, menstrual, and bone health status at one end of the continuum and the unhealthy outcomes of the Triad at the other end of the Triad continuum, including disordered eating, amenorrhea, and osteoporosis. *BMD* bone mineral density; *LPD* luteal phase defect. Modified and reprinted with permission from Nattiv et al. [2]

the clinical outcomes associated with each, including energy deficiency, with or without disordered eating, abnormal menstrual cycles, functional hypothalamic amenorrhea, and bone loss [2].

Key points that are highlighted by the new model of the Female Athlete Triad are that many athletes may not present with more severe conditions at the extremes of the continuums, but rather may display intermediate, or "subclinical," presentations of one or more of the conditions, and, most importantly, that progression along the three continuums can occur at different rates. For example, an athlete may show signs of restrictive eating but may not meet the clinical criteria for an eating disorder. She may also display subtle menstrual disturbances, such as a change in menstrual cycle length, anovulation, or luteal phase defects, but may not yet have developed amenorrhea. Likewise, she may be losing bone mass but may not yet have dropped below her age-matched normal range for bone mineral density (BMD). While the conditions represented by each continuum can present independent of the other two, it is more likely that, because of the clear associations among the three conditions, an athlete suffering from one element of the Female Athlete Triad is also suffering from the others even if only in a subclinical manner. Thus, it is important to understand that an athlete may present at different stages on each continuum and has the capacity to change stages on each continuum at varying rates. For example, changes can occur daily when considering energy status, monthly when considering the time course necessary for energetic changes to impact menstrual function, and annually when considering the time course necessary for energetic and menstrual changes to impact bone health [2].

The Prevalence of Athletic Amenorrhea

The prevalence of amenorrhea has been reported to range from 6 to 43% in runners [16–21], 1–21% in both high school [22] and collegiate athletes across a wide assortment of sports [3, 23], and as high as 69% in ballet dancers [24]. Of course, the prevalence of amenorrhea in athletes and physically active women grossly exceeds the 2–5% observed in the general population of sedentary college-aged women [25–27].

It is important to note that adolescent athletes are likely to experience a higher prevalence of menstrual cycle disturbances and amenorrhea; Baker et al. [28] demonstrated that adolescent runners experienced a significantly higher prevalence of amenorrhea than their adult counterparts (67% vs. 9%). Primary amenorrhea and delayed menarche have also been reported in many adolescent athletes, particularly gymnasts, ballet dancers, runners, divers, and cheerleaders [3, 29–31]. Primary amenorrhea and delayed menarche in adolescent athletes are often solely attributed to exercise training without appropriate regard for social self-selection factors known to influence the timing of pubertal maturation, particularly in sports like gymnastics and ballet [30, 32].

The Etiology of Athletic Amenorrhea

Primary amenorrhea has recently been defined as the failure to achieve menarche by age 15 in the presence of normal development of secondary sex characteristics [33]. The definition of secondary amenorrhea in the exercise literature has varied, but should be defined conservatively as no menses for 90 days or 3 months, or less than 5 menses in 12 months [6]. Oligomenorrhea is defined as the presence of irregular and inconsistent cycle intervals of 36–90 days [6], although care must be taken to exclude other causes of oligomenorrhea, particularly polycystic ovarian syndrome [34]. Indeed, it is certainly not surprising that many athletes bring their preexisting condition of polycystic ovarian syndrome to the athletic environment.

In athletes, the amenorrhea is hypothalamic in origin, characterized by decreased gonadotropin-releasing hormone (GnRH) pulsatility and, as a result, suppressed levels of circulating gonadotropins and ovarian steroids; however, the responsiveness of the pituitary gland to GnRH remains unaltered [35]. Amenorrhea is associated with an extreme deficiency in estrogen, while less severe perturbations of menstrual function, such as oligomenorrhea and anovulation, have less severe deficits in estrogen, as assessed by daily urinary measurements of ovarian steroids when calculated as an area under the curve [4, 36]. Figure 7.2 demonstrates the examples of the estrogen exposure associated with varying menstrual perturbations in exercising women, contrasted with ovulatory cycles in both sedentary and exercising women when assessed by the daily excretion of urinary estrone and pregnanediol glucuronides.

Physiological Considerations

The significance of energy deficiency as a cause of Female Athlete Triad-related menstrual disturbances and bone loss is now more apparent than ever. Indeed, we have suggested that these menstrual disturbances should be referred to as energy-related menstrual disturbances [37]. Research has well established that one of the primary causes of Triad-related health problems is a chronic energy deficiency [6, 9, 11]. In other words, the amount of calories an athlete or physically active woman consumes is simply not adequate to meet the energetic demands of her daily exercise training energy expenditure, a concept often referred to as low energy availability [2]. When the volume of energy is inadequate to meet energetic demands, the body repartitions energy away from reproduction and growth and toward other more essential energy-consuming processes such as thermoregulation, cell maintenance, and locomotion [38]. The reliance of reproductive function on nutritional factors, such as food availability and energy balance, is also well established in nonwesternized subsistence communities who are impacted by seasonal food availability and high energy expenditures during harvests [39–41]. Energy deficiency in these cases occurs because there is a negative balance between food intake resulting from seasonal availability in food and energy expenditure associated with work in the fields,

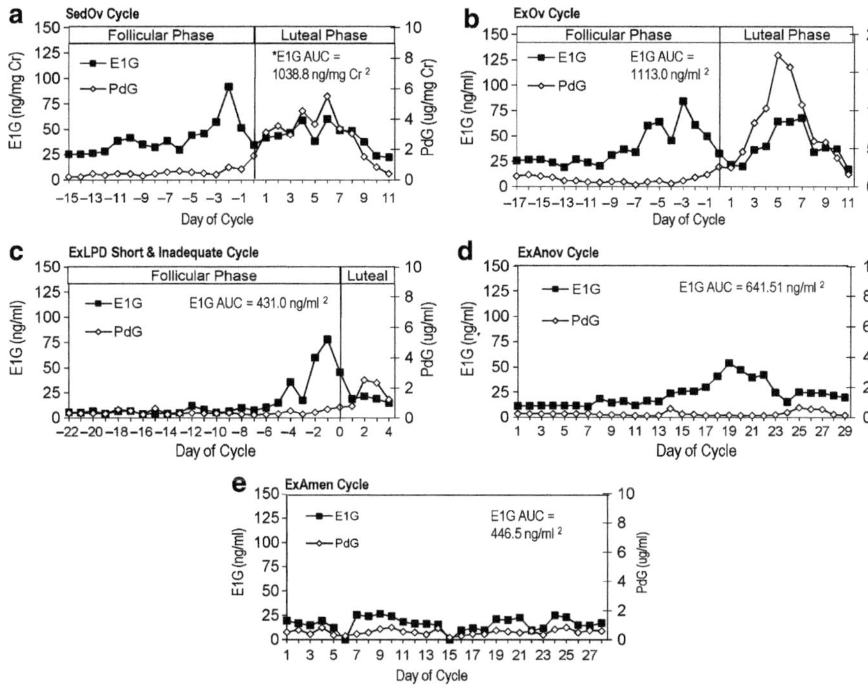

Fig. 7.2 Representative menstrual cycles of exercising women with varying menstrual disturbances and the corresponding estrogen exposure (**c**, **d**, **e**) contrasted to ovulatory cycles and the associated estrogen exposure of both a sedentary woman (**a**) and an exercising woman (**b**). Note the suppressed estrogen exposure associated with anovulatory and amenorrheic menstrual status. *E1G and PdG for SedOv cycle was adjusted based on creatinine excretion; E1G and PdG for all other cycles are corrected for hydration based on specific gravity. *SedOv* Sedentary Ovulatory; *ExOv* Exercising Ovulatory; *ExLPD* Exercising Luteal Phase Deficient; *ExAnov* Exercising Anovulatory; *ExAmen* Exercising Amenorrheic; *E1G* estrone-1-glucoronide; *PdG* pregnanediol glucoronide; *AUC* area under the curve

or travel from one remote location to another [39, 40]. Irrespective of the cause of the energy deficiency, a relative chronic energy drain persists, a concept first published by Michelle Warren in 1980 [42], that results in reproductive suppression. Energy deficiency is often associated with weight loss in a metabolic environment that favors energy conservation. An environment of energy conservation involves a decrease in resting energy expenditure (REE), suppression of total triiodothyronine (TT_3), insulin-like growth factor-1 (IGF-1) and leptin concentrations, and elevated ghrelin and cortisol concentrations [36, 43–46] (see Fig. 7.3). Suppression of REE has been well documented in amenorrheic, exercising women concomitant with the abovementioned alterations in metabolic hormonal profiles consistent with nutritional restriction [13, 36, 47, 48]. Additional evidence for the relationship between energy deficiency and energy-related menstrual disturbances comes from the results of cross-sectional studies of metabolic hormones and substrates in exercising

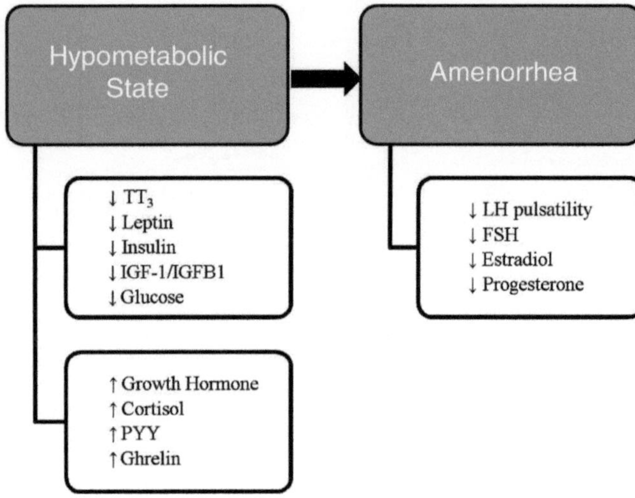

Fig. 7.3 The metabolic and hormonal alterations that are associated with a hypometabolic and amenorrheic environment in exercising women. Metabolic hormones and gut peptides are characteristically altered secondary to an energy deficient environment and gonadotropin and ovarian steroids are characteristically suppressed secondary to an estrogen-deficient environment. TT_3 total triiodothyronine; *IGF-1* insulin-like growth factor-1; *IGFB1* insulin-like growth factor binding protein-1; *PYY* peptide YY; *LH* luteinizing hormone; *FSH* follicle-stimulating hormone

women with subtle menstrual disturbances such as luteal phase defects and anovulation that illustrate similar, but less severe, adaptive changes than those observed in amenorrheic, exercising women [36, 45, 49].

It is noteworthy that a low body weight is not always a reliable indicator of chronic energy deficiency nor is a stable body weight a reliable indicator of energy balance [50]. The metabolic adaptations that act to conserve energy and reduce energy expenditure and body weight can also, in some cases, result in weight stability, albeit at a lower set point that may present as a restoration in energy balance with ongoing chronic alterations indicative of an energy-conserved metabolic and endocrine environment [50]. To forecast the presence of an energy deficiency in our laboratory [12, 13, 36], we have successfully utilized the ratio of REE (as measured in the laboratory) to the Harris–Benedict [51] predicted REE (measured REE/predicted REE). Since the majority of published reports [52–54] of REE in underweight women utilized the Harris–Benedict equation [51] to predict REE, we reasoned that this equation was likely to be useful for our purposes. We further observed that in clinical models of starvation, such as anorexia nervosa [52–54], a reduced ratio of measured REE to predicted REE by the Harris–Benedict equation [51] is often in the range of 60–80%. As such, we operationally defined energy deficiency in exercising women as a ratio of measured REE to predicted REE of less than 90% and energy replete as a ratio of measured REE to predicted REE of greater than 90% [12, 13, 36]. We have successfully utilized this strategy in several published papers to date, and it is consistently corroborated by metabolic hormone (TT_3 and ghrelin concentrations) data, indicative of adaptations to an energy-deficient state [12, 13, 36].

Elegant short-term experiments by Loucks and colleagues [11, 55–57] manipulating both dietary intake and energy expenditure have consistently demonstrated a strong relationship between low energy availability, suppressed metabolic hormones and suppression of the GnRH pulse generator. The design of the Loucks et al. [11] experiments involved having subjects expend 15 kcal/kg lean body mass (LBM) per day during supervised exercise sessions for 5 days at 70% of aerobic capacity while consuming a standardized diet intended to set energy availability at a balanced level of 45 kcal/kg LBM/day or at mild, moderate, and severe levels of energy restriction of 30, 20, 10 kcal/kg LBM/day, respectively [11]. At all levels of restriction, metabolic hormones, including TT_3, IGF-1, insulin, leptin, and cortisol, were altered in an incremental manner with these effects most dramatic at the severe level of energy restriction of 10 kcal/kg LBM/day [11]. Similarly, LH pulsatility was most dramatically impacted at the severe level of energy restriction, but suppression of LH pulsatility was also noted even at mild (30 kcal/kg LBM/day) and modest (20 kcal/kg LBM/day) levels of energy restriction [11].

Convincing evidence for a causal relationship between low energy availability and menstrual cyclicity was provided by the prospective training studies in monkeys elegantly executed by Williams et al. [8, 9]. Williams et al. [8, 9] demonstrated two key relationships, (1) that amenorrhea could be induced in exercising monkeys and that the onset of the amenorrhea was related to the volume of calories restricted during the exercise training, and (2) that the amenorrhea could be reversed by increasing food intake without any moderation of the daily exercise training. The authors point out that the resumption of ovulatory cycles in the amenorrheic monkeys had a dose-dependent relationship with the volume of energy available such that the monkeys that ate the most calories recovered ovulatory function in the shortest time period [9]. It is also noteworthy that in this study, a key marker of energy balance, TT_3, was significantly related to both the induction and reversal of amenorrhea providing additional evidence to support the premise that suppression of reproductive function is linked with adaptive energy conservation when there is an imbalance created by inadequate caloric intake in the face of increased exercise energy expenditure [8, 9].

Psychological Considerations

As previously described, energy deficiency occurs when there is a negative balance between food intake and exercise energy expenditure. Because an athlete's energy supply can be purposely manipulated, it warrants a special comment. It is clear that in many cases of the Female Athlete Triad, there is some form of disordered eating behavior that contributes to the energy deficiency [2, 7, 23, 58]. The disordered eating presents in a variety of ways, but most often as a high drive for thinness (DT) or as a purposeful dietary restriction of caloric intake [2, 7, 23]. The incidence of disordered eating behaviors in physically active women and athletes is reportedly as high as 62%, particularly in esthetic or lean build sports like gymnastics, ballet, and cross country running [59]; whereas, the prevalence of the more severe, clinical eating disorders (anorexia and bulimia) was reportedly ~2–3% in a group of over 400 collegiate athletes [3]. These disordered eating behaviors, of course, can cause a chronic energy deficiency. Women with a high DT demonstrate a preoccupation with body weight and body shape, and a fear of gaining weight [58, 60, 61]. Numerous reports support a strong relationship between disordered eating, DT, and amenorrhea in exercising women [2, 7, 12, 16, 23, 58]. Indeed, in our previous work, we demonstrated that a high DT was associated with energy deficiency as indicated by significant relationships between REE and metabolic hormones such as TT_3 and ghrelin [12]. Figure 7.4 demonstrates the aforementioned relationships. From a physiological standpoint, a high DT promotes the conscious restriction of food intake and/or the excessive participation in exercise; thus, this particular

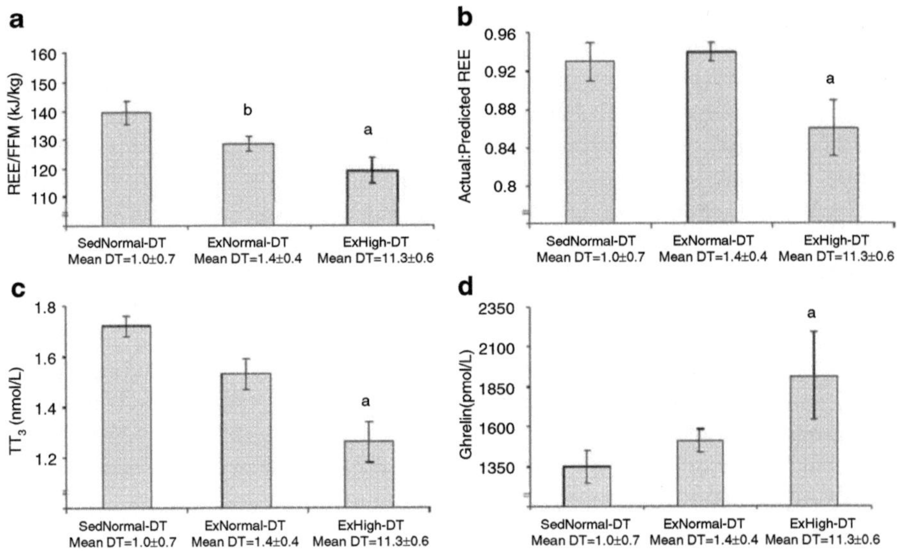

Fig. 7.4 The relationships between drive for thinness (DT) and metabolism in sedentary and exercising women grouped according to DT score on the Eating Disorder Inventory. (**a**) Resting energy expenditure (REE) adjusted for fat-free mass (FFM) among three groups of women categorized by exercise status and DT score to include (1) a sedentary group with a normal DT score, (2) an exercising group with a normal DT score, and (3) an exercising group with a high DT score. (**b**) The ratio of actual REE to predicted REE among the three groups. (**c, d**) The concentrations of total triidothyronine (TT_3) and ghrelin among the three groups. Note the suppressed ratio of measured REE/predicted REE suggestive of an energy deficiency; these data are corroborated by suppressed TT_3 and elevated ghrelin concentrations. [a]$p<0.05$ ExHigh-DT vs. SedNormal-DT and ExNormal-DT. [b]$p<0.05$ ExNormal-DT vs. SedNormal-DT. *SedNormal-DT* Sedentary Normal-DT; *ExNormal-DT* Exercising Normal DT; *ExHigh-DT* Exercising High-DT. Reprinted with permission from De Souza et al. [12]

disordered eating attitude is likely associated with the development of an energy deficit as we have demonstrated in our work [12].

DT is also related to the conscious restriction of food intake, often referred to as cognitive dietary restraint [37]. Cognitive dietary restraint refers to the chronic effort to achieve or maintain a desired body weight by consciously restricting food intake [62]. It has also been associated with compromised reproductive function to include amenorrhea and decreased bone mass [37, 63, 64]. In our own laboratory, we have recently demonstrated that high cognitive dietary restraint scores are associated with reduced lumbar spine and total body BMD in physically active women such that the highest cognitive dietary restraint scores are related to the lowest BMD values and the most severe menstrual disturbances such as amenorrhea [37].

It is also noteworthy to remember that some athletes and physically active women can experience an energy deficiency in the absence of disordered eating; that is, even if they are not consciously restricting their food intake, these individuals may simply not eat enough food to fuel their exercise energy expenditure. A busy class schedule, travel, stress, and other factors can hinder female athletes from maintaining an adequate diet for training. Thus, some athletes who do *not* present with disordered eating symptoms or behaviors are often overlooked in discussions of the Female Athlete Triad. Likewise, it is important to remember that some athletes may present with a clinical eating disorder of anorexia or bulimia nervosa and warrant specialized intervention strategies with trained clinicians.

Bone Health Considerations

Suppression of reproductive function is associated with stress fractures, loss of BMD, the failure to achieve peak bone mass, and osteoporosis [13]. There are numerous reports of significantly lower BMD values on the order of 2–6% at the spine, hip, and total body among amenorrheic athletes when compared to their regularly menstruating counterparts [13, 16, 65–68]. In fact, Christo et al. [68] reported that 38 and 19% of amenorrheic athletes had lumbar and hip BMD Z-scores, respectively, at least one standard deviation below that of an age-matched sedentary population. It is important to note that BMD in exercising women should actually be higher than that observed in a reference population of sedentary women. The current recommendations for appropriate BMD criteria to diagnose low BMD or osteoporosis in athletes utilize the guideline published for premenopausal women by the International Society for Clinical Densitometry [69]. These criteria utilize a Z-score of –2.0 or lower to diagnose low BMD, and when a secondary risk factor is also present, such as hypogonadism or nutritional deficiency, a diagnosis of osteoporosis may be applied [69]. The prevalence of osteopenia in amenorrheic athletes is estimated to range from 1.4 to 50% [16, 65, 70–72]. The prevalence of osteoporosis is lower [16, 72]. Stress fractures are two to four times more common in athletes and physically active women with amenorrhea than their physically active counterparts who are menstruating [2, 73].

A closer look at the negative alterations that occur in the bones of female athletes via peripheral quantitative computed tomography reveals that trabecular BMD as well as cortical thickness are common targets of amenorrhea-associated bone loss in athletes. In a comparison of two samples of elite, retired gymnasts, Ducher et al. [74] observed that those athletes with a history of amenorrhea had significantly reduced trabecular density at the distal radius and tibia and significantly lower bone strength at the distal radius when compared to the eumenorrheic, retired gymnasts. Additionally, cortical thickness was significantly greater and medullary area significantly smaller at the proximal radius of the gymnasts without a history of amenorrhea, providing support for the role of estrogen in endocortical apposition [74]. Moreover, Misra et al. [75, 76] has reported that the low bone mass observed in energy-deficient amenorrheic women may be the consequence of light trabecular and thin cortical bones [75]. In a sample of 34 anorexic adolescents, Misra et al. [75] reported significantly decreased lumbar bone mineral content (BMC) adjusted for bone area (BA) when compared to controls but no significant differences were observed between anorexics and controls in lumbar BA adjusted for height, indicating that the significantly lower BMD of the lumbar spine, composed primarily of trabecular bone, was due to light and undermineralized rather than thin bones. In contrast, no significant differences were reported for whole body BMC adjusted for BA between anorexic women and controls; however, whole body BA adjusted for height was significantly decreased among the anorexic subjects, indicating that at sites of primarily cortical bone, hormonal and nutritional deficiencies lead to thin but poorly mineralized bone [75].

It has generally been accepted that chronic hypoestrogenism is the major cause of bone loss in exercising women. However, the effects of food restriction and energy deficiency on BMD represent an estrogen-independent mechanism for bone loss that involves some of the metabolic-related hormones altered with exercise-associated amenorrhea (see Fig. 7.5). These hormones, i.e., IGF-1 and leptin, play an important role in modulating bone turnover and BMD in these women. Evidence that these factors can impact bone in exercising women with exercise-associated amenorrhea includes several observations that oral contraceptive use in these women and other energy deficient models like anorexia does not unequivocally lead to appropriate recovery of BMD [14, 77, 78]. Therefore, additional factors other than simply estrogen deficiency must be taken into account.

Thus, the mechanism underlying the bone loss observed in amenorrheic athletes is twofold, including both hormonal and nutritional components (see Fig. 7.5) [13, 14]. Bone is an active tissue, undergoing cycles of resorption and formation. In the face of both an estrogen and energy deficiency, an uncoupling of bone turnover occurs, creating the unfavorable environment of increased bone resorption and decreased bone formation, ultimately resulting in bone loss [13]. As demonstrated by Ihle and Loucks [15], the decrease in estrogen that occurs with a reduction in energy availability coincides with an increase in markers of bone resorption, providing support for the role of estrogen in suppressing the bone-resorbing effects of osteoclasts. De Souza et al. [13] also demonstrated that in estrogen-deficient exercising women, urinary C-terminal telopeptide concentrations are elevated. Likewise,

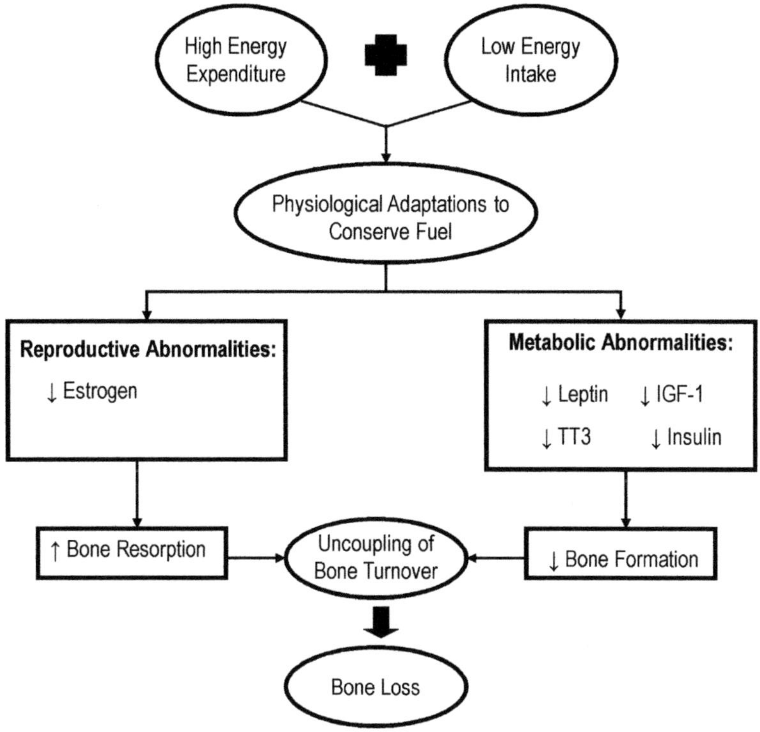

Fig. 7.5 The mechanism for bone loss in exercising amenorrheic women. The combination of a high energy expenditure and a low energy intake suppresses circulating concentrations of certain ovarian steroids and metabolic markers, all of which have an impact on bone metabolism, leading to the uncoupling of bone turnover and subsequent bone loss. TT_3 triiodothyronine; *IGF-1* insulin-like growth factor-1

markers of bone formation appear to be sensitive to alterations in the nutritional and metabolic environment [13, 15]. Ihle and Loucks [15] observed that the decrease in metabolic indicators of nutritional status, namely, insulin, TT_3, and IGF-1, coincided with decreases in bone formation markers. De Souza et al. [13] also reported a significant reduction in osteocalcin and type I procollagen carboxy-terminal propeptide, markers of bone formation, in an environment that was energy deficient but estrogen replete in exercising women.

Recently, the role of leptin, an adipocyte-derived hormone, in modulating the bone loss observed in amenorrheic women has been intensely studied [79]. Several investigators have reported reduced leptin levels in women with amenorrhea, associated with both anorexia and exercise [13, 80, 81], and the absence of the diurnal rhythm of leptin in amenorrheic athletes [82]. In our own laboratory [13], we have demonstrated that leptin was significantly related to markers of bone formation, i.e., osteocalcin and type I procollagen carboxy-terminal propeptide, in exercising women with an energy deficiency. Miller et al. [80] observed significantly reduced leptin in amenorrheic, anorexic women when compared to eumenorrheic, anorexic women, suggesting that leptin exerts a permissive influence on hypothalamic function. Additionally, through central and peripheral mechanisms, leptin exerts both antiosteogenic and osteogenic effects on bone mass [83]. Leptin receptors are present at the level of the hypothalamus; the binding of leptin to these receptors initiates the cascade that results in an increase in cortical bone but a decrease in cancellous bone [83]. Leptin also directly stimulates bone formation at the level of bone cells by stimulating osteoblastic differentiation via leptin receptors present on osteoblasts [83]. However, it has recently been suggested that leptin does not act via the hypothalamus, but rather leptin may regulate bone by inhibiting serotonin synthesis and release in the brainstem, which in turn acts on the hypothalamus via specific serotonin receptors [84].

Diagnosis and Treatment

The optimal occasion to screen for Triad-related disorders, including amenorrhea in athletes, is during the preparticipation physical exam. Recently, the Female Athlete Triad Coalition has published a strategy for the preparticipation exam, and this reference can be located at http://www.femaleathletetriad.org/for-professionals/information-for-physicians/.

Athletes and physically active women presenting with primary or secondary amenorrhea require evaluation, to first rule out pregnancy as well as other underlying endocrinopathies. Since amenorrhea in an athlete is secondary to hypothalamic suppression of the ovarian axis [85], no single blood test or evaluation can confirm such a diagnosis. Indeed the diagnosis of functional hypothalamic amenorrhea secondary to energy deficiency in athletes is a diagnosis of exclusion. An algorithm for the athlete presenting with secondary amenorrhea can be viewed in Fig. 7.6. Endocrinopathies that must be ruled out include (1) pregnancy, (2) pituitary causes such as prolactinomas, (3) adrenal causes such as adult-onset adrenal hyperplasia and Cushing's disease, (4) thyroid disease, (5) ovarian tumors, (6) gonadotropin mutations, (7) hypothalamic causes, (8) premature ovarian failure, and (9) polycystic ovarian syndrome [86]. Other less common causes of amenorrhea exist in a small percentage of cases [86]. The most common causes of amenorrhea are usually identified following a thorough medical history, physical examination, and evaluation of follicle stimulating hormone (FSH), thyroid stimulating hormone (TSH), and prolactin [86]. Readers are referred to the ASRM guidelines [86] for the appropriate algorithms for a more detailed differential diagnosis and interpretation of blood work. If the athlete demonstrates any physical evidence of androgen excess (i.e., hirsutism, acne, androgenic alopecia) or polycystic ovaries, additional laboratory testing that may be useful includes free testosterone and dihydroepiandrosterone sulfate (DHEA-S). A serum estradiol and a progesterone challenge test may be useful to assess the degree of hypoestrogenism [86].

Other diagnostic tests that may be useful for an amenorrheic athlete include a BMD assessment of the anteroposterior spine (L1-L4) and of the total hip, since bone loss or the failure to achieve peak bone mass must be suspected in these

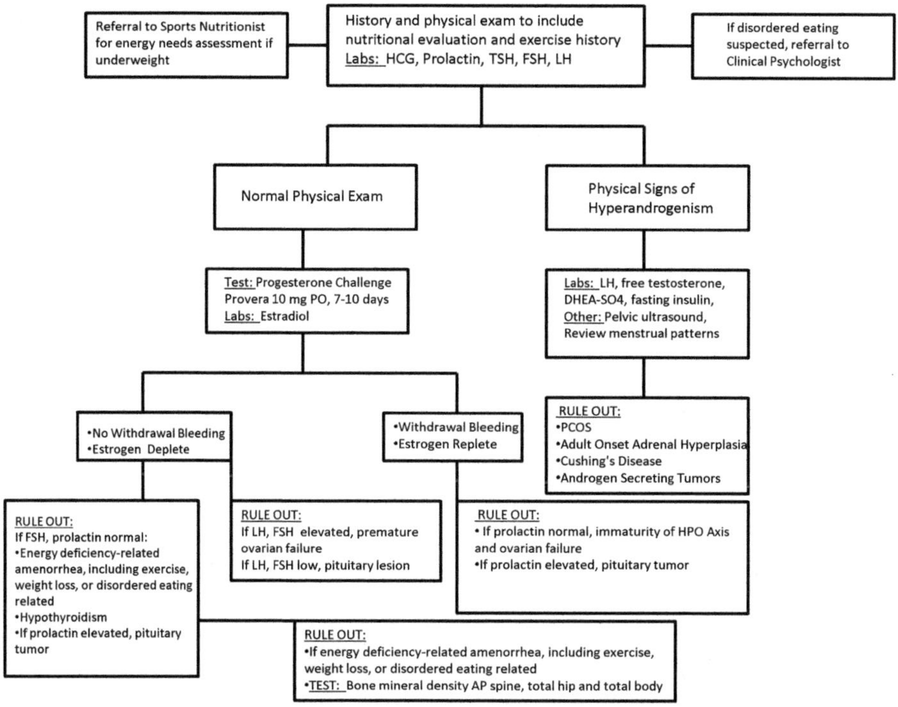

Fig. 7.6 Algorithm for the diagnosis of functional hypothalamic amenorrhea (FHA) among athletes presenting with secondary amenorrhea. A thorough physical exam and evaluation of hormone concentrations are necessary to rule out underlying endocrinopathies. *FSH* follicle-stimulating hormone; *LH* luteinizing hormone; *TSH* thyroid stimulating hormone; *HCG* human chorionic gonadotropin; *DHEA-SO4* dihydroepiandrosterone sulfate; *PCOS* polycystic ovarian syndrome; *AP* anteroposterior

women secondary to energy deficiency and hypoestrogenism [13, 14]. The diagnosis of low BMD in these women should be based on the lowest Z-score observed at these sites [69], and, when athletes are of adolescent age (less than age 20), the diagnosis should be determined from a BMD test of both the total body and the anteroposterior spine. It is most helpful to obtain age-matched controls, particularly in younger women.

Due to the multifaceted nature of exercise-associated amenorrhea, clinicians utilize various treatment strategies, each aimed at addressing an underlying cause or a consequence of the hypothalamic amenorrhea. Few treatment guidelines for amenorrheic athletes are published, but the overwhelming approach recommended is increased food intake and weight restoration, which are likely the best strategies for the resumption of menses and improved bone health [10, 87, 88]. Clinicians must be patient when using this strategy [89–91] and may find it beneficial to enlist the assistance of a registered dietician with demonstrated expertise in the determination of exercise energy expenditure needs. It is important to recall that in monkey studies conducted by Williams et al. [8, 9], the resumption of menses occurred the fastest in the monkeys that ate the most calories during the refeeding paradigm. The assessment of exercise energy expenditure is an essential component of an appropriate refeeding strategy in these exercising women and must be maintained until the goal of resumption of menses has been achieved. In our own laboratory, we are conducting an ongoing 12-month randomized controlled trial to determine the effectiveness of increased energy intake to reverse amenorrhea as well as improve energy and bone marker status in women with exercise-associated amenorrhea; this project is referred to as REFUEL. Preliminary data in five exercising women with amenorrhea demonstrate that an energy prescription of 20–40% above energy expenditure needs averaged 536 calories/day and resulted in the resumption of menses in 3/5 subjects within 4 months and 4/5 subjects within 6 months [92]. Interestingly, we also observed significant changes in metabolic markers that promoted a pro- bone health environment to include decreased ghrelin and increased concentrations of markers of bone formation [92]. Small studies [93–95] of the effects of weight gain on the resumption of menses are reported in the literature, and these results are displayed in Table 7.1. Athletes should also be required to meet the dietary guidelines of 1,000–1,500 mg calcium and 400–800 IU Vitamin D3 intake, either in their daily diet or with supplementation, particularly those athletes who reside at northern latitude and have limited exposure to sunlight.

In some cases, of course, athletes may be noncompliant, particularly those involved in sports which emphasize leanness and in competitive athletes; in these women, it may be necessary to decrease the duration or intensity of training. It may also be helpful, in some cases, to involve a clinical psychologist to help the athlete cope with body image issues or disordered eating behaviors when present. Indeed, cognitive behavioral therapy has been demonstrated to be more beneficial than nutritional counseling alone in some women with hypothalamic amenorrhea with disordered eating behaviors [96] and may likely benefit the athlete struggling with disordered eating behaviors, body image disturbances, and the prescription of increased energy intake.

Because the etiology of bone loss among amenorrheic women is founded upon both a nutritional and hormonal deficiency, weight gain and subsequent resumption of menses have provided hopeful results for the recovery of at least some bone mass. There are a few case studies [97, 98] and small sample size studies [93–95] examining the BMD outcome in amenorrheic athletes who have increased energy intake for the purpose of restoration of menses and improving BMD. In those reports [93–95, 97–101], BMD is positively impacted by ~1–10%, but to date, reports have demonstrated only limited potential to normalize bone mass to that of eumenorrheic, physically active controls. Table 7.1 summarizes these data.

Similar studies have been performed in the anorexic population; among those studies that have included both weight gain and the resumption of menses, increases in BMD have been reported of similar magnitude (1–10%) in those who have recovered menses; whereas, continual decreases in BMD were observed in those who did not recover menses [75, 80, 102]. Weight gain independent of the resumption of menses has shown to have a positive effect on BMD as well as restore the coupling of bone formation and resorption [75, 103–106]. It appears that BMD can be

Table 7.1 Effects of weight gain and resumption of menses on bone mineral density (BMD) among women with exercise-associated amenorrhea

Study	Duration	Weight gain	Menses resumed (# of subjects)	BMD % change	
				Resumed	Did not resume
Observational					
Drinkwater et al. [94]	15.5 months	↑1.9 kg	7 of 9	6.3% (spine)	–3.4% (spine)
Keen and Drinkwater [93]	8.1 years	None	8 of 11	No change	
Warren et al. [95]	2 years	Not reported	7 of 19	17.5% (spine)	4.0% (spine)
Case					
Zanker et al. [97]	12 years	8.1 kg	OC and hormone therapy	16.9% (proximal femur)	
Fredericson and Kent, [98]	8 years	↑BMI 5.5 kg/m^2	OC therapy	25.5% (spine)19.5% (hip)	

increased if both mechanisms that underlie bone loss – hormonal and metabolic – are addressed. However, it is essential to understand that despite some recovery of bone, normalization of BMD is unlikely. It is very interesting to note the recent evidence that increased caloric intake leading to weight gain and the resumption of menses was associated with an increase in BMC adjusted for BA at the spine and, at the level of the whole body, an increase in BA adjusted for height was noted, indicating that both nutritional and hormonal recovery may improve the mineralization of trabecular bone and the growth of cortical bone [75].

For many clinicians, the administration of sex steroids has been a convenient alternative to the recommendation of changes in energy intake or expenditure, but the outcomes, particularly related to bone health, have been equivocal, at best, and are not recommended as the first line of therapeutic options (see Table 7.2). Clearly, an oral contraceptive strategy does nothing to restore fertility in these women. Due to estrogen's role in preserving bone [107] and the hypoestrogenic nature of amenorrhea, oral contraceptive or estrogen therapy has, however, been perceived as a logical strategy to reverse amenorrheic-associated bone loss. The primary problem with this line of thinking is that the bone loss is primarily secondary to energy deficiency, that when exacerbated, results in hypoestrogenism [13]. Thus, oral contraceptive therapy fails to address the root cause of the problem; that is, energy deficiency. As displayed in Table 7.2, the results of several hormonal interventions in exercising amenorrheic women have been confounding [31, 77, 108–110], indicating that oral contraceptive or estrogen therapy may halt the progression of further bone loss and increase BMD slightly but may not completely restore bone mass to that observed in a young, healthy age-matched population [87]. Although significant increases of ~1–9% in bone mass were observed in some studies [77, 109, 110], these improvements in BMD were often site-specific or minimal. Other investigators have reported nonsignificant improvements or no changes in BMD following the oral contraceptive therapy [31, 108]. Bolton et al. [106] have suggested that one reason for the failure of oral contraceptive therapy to yield more positive results to BMD may be because this therapeutic strategy tends to disproportionally suppress bone formation relative to resorption. Another explanation is that oral contraceptive therapy does nothing to reverse the energy deficient environment of suppressed bone formation and, given the data by Bolton et al. [106], may even exacerbate the problem.

In view of the pivotal role of leptin in the regulation of both reproduction and bone turnover [111], recombinant leptin has been administered as a possible treatment for women with hypothalamic amenorrhea associated with exercise or nutritional deficiency [79]. Welt et al. [79] observed an increase in follicular size and the initiation of ovulatory cycles (three of eight subjects) as well as increased levels of luteinizing hormone, estradiol, IGF-1, and bone formation markers following 2–3 months of administration. Two key issues of concern with this therapeutic option is that these improvements were observed in the face of a commensurate loss of body weight and body fat as well as a reduction in hunger and food intake, findings clearly undesirable in an already underweight population of women.

The peptide IGF-1 is also an important link between nutritional status and growth; its presence at normal levels not only indicates nutritional stability, but also mediates

Table 7.2 Effects of hormonal therapy on bone mineral density (BMD) among women with exercise-associated amenorrhea

				BMD % change in Tx group			
Study	Sample	Treatment	Duration	TB	LS	Hip	FN
Hergenroeder et al. [77]	$n=15$	• Ethinyl estradiol (0.035 mg) • Norethindrone (0.5–1.0 mg) or Medroxyprogesterone (10 mg)	12-month intervention	2.7%	9.4%	19.0%	
Castelo-Branco et al. [99]	$n=64$	• Ethinyl estradiol (0.02–0.03 mg) • Desogestrel (0.15 mg)	12-month intervention		2.4–2.5%		
Rickenlund et al. [109]	$n=13$	• Ethinyl estradiol (0.03 mg) • Levonorgestrel (0.15 mg)	10-month intervention	1.8%	1.0%		
De Crée et al. [101]	$n=7$	• Ethinyl estradiol (0.05 mg) • Cyproterone acetate (2 mg)	8-month cohort		9.5%		
Cumming [100]	$n=8$	• Conjugated estrogen (0.0625 mg) or • Transdermal estradiol (0.05 mg)	24-month retrospective observational		8.0%		4.1%
Gibson et al. [108]	$n=34$	• Estriol (1 mg) and Estradiol (2 mg) 12 days • Estriol (1 mg), Estradiol (2 mg), and Norethisterone acetate (1 mg) 10 days • Estriol (0.5 mg) and Estradiol (1 mg) 6 days	9.3-month intervention		No change	No change	No change
Warren et al. [31]	$n=55$	• Premarin (0.625) • Provera (10 mg)	24-month intervention		5.6%		
Warren et al. [110]	$n=27$	• Ethinyl estradiol (0.035 ng) • Norgestimate (0.180–0.250 mg)	10-month intervention		1.5%	No change	

TB total body; *LS* lumbar spine; *FN* femoral neck

anabolic effects on bone [112]. IGF-1 levels are often reduced in amenorrheic athletes [46, 113] and anorexic women [114–116]. Grinspoon et al. [114, 115] administered recombinant human IGF-1 (rhIGF-1) combined with either a placebo or an oral contraceptive to osteopenic, anorexic women. Based on the results of this study [114, 115], it was concluded that a combined treatment of both an anabolic agent such as rhIGF-1 and an antiresorptive agent such as oral contraceptives, but not either treatment alone, may promote an increase in BMD of ~2% among women with anorexia-associated amenorrhea and perhaps also among women with exercise-associated amenorrhea, although not tested to date. As such, this strategy offers only limited potential and requires further investigation as a long-term therapeutic option.

Limited available data suggest that current clinician practices for the treatment of amenorrhea among athletes are changing. Based on a survey administered to 159 physicians of the American Medical Society for Sports Medicine in 1995 [117], 92% reported that they administered sex steroids to treat amenorrheic athletes. Interestingly, calcium supplementation closely followed sex steroid supplementation with up to 87% of the respondents indicating this therapy was also a recommended treatment strategy [117]. Only about 50% of the respondents utilized therapies targeted to the root of the problem, such as increased caloric intake (64%), decreased exercise (57%), and weight gain (43%). More recently, in 2007, Carlson et al. [118] administered a similar survey to 126 clinicians, reporting once again that calcium supplementation seemed to be the preferred method of treatment with 69% of respondents recommending this therapy to more than 75% of patients with athletic amenorrhea. In contrast, however, the administration of sex steroid therapy appeared to decline in use with only 14% of respondents primarily prescribing this therapy [118]. Instead, when compared to the percentage of clinicians in this study who preferentially prescribed sex steroids, a greater percentage of clinicians recommended increased caloric intake (48%), increased body weight (37%), or a reduction in exercise energy expenditure (28%) to greater than 75% of amenorrheic athletes [118]. Thus, this more recent report suggests that clinicians' preferences for treatment have evolved to prefer strategies that involve increased caloric intake and weight gain rather than sacrificing some components of the athlete's exercise training or masking the problem with hormone therapy. Physical therapists and athletic trainers often approach the problem from an educational perspective, offering information regarding changes in diet and training and, when necessary, providing referrals to physicians or dieticians [119].

Conclusions

The Female Athlete Triad is a serious medical condition that signals the presence of an energy deficiency that may be secondary to disordered eating, and is associated with menstrual disturbances and either premature bone loss or the failure to achieve peak bone mass. The etiology of menstrual disturbances associated with the Triad is causally linked to energy deficiency, and as such, there is no justification to fear that exercise itself is unhealthy for women. Indeed, physically active women and athletes have much to gain from physical activity and exercise but must be careful to meet their energetic requirements and include this issue in their training regime. As such, undernutrition plays a key role in triggering Triad-related problems; on the other hand, this means good nutrition is key to preventing the condition. While the conditions represented by each continuum can present independent of the other two conditions, it is more likely that, because of the clear associations among the three conditions, an athlete suffering from one element of the Female Athlete Triad is also suffering from the others, even if only in a subclinical manner. Thus, it is important to understand that an athlete may present at different stages on each continuum and has the capacity to change stages on each continuum at varying rates. For example, changes can occur daily when considering energy status, monthly when considering the time course necessary for energetic changes to impact menstrual function, and annually when considering the time course necessary for energetic and menstrual changes to impact bone health [2].

The nutritional etiology of the Triad warrants emphasis, and treatment strategies should be focused on improving nutritional status in these physically active women and athletes. The best approach recommended is increased food intake and weight restoration, which are likely the best strategies for the resumption of menses and improved bone health [10, 87, 88]. Clinicians must be patient when using this strategy [89–91] and may find it beneficial to enlist the assistance of a registered dietician with demonstrated expertise in the determination of exercise energy expenditure needs. For good reason then, as described in the text of this chapter, most educational efforts aimed at preventing Female Athlete Triad-related problems and amenorrhea in athletes should focus on nutrition and eating behaviors.

References

1. Otis CL, Drinkwater B, Johnson M, Loucks A, Wilmore J (1997) American College of Sports Medicine position stand. The Female Athlete Triad. Med Sci Sports Exerc 29:i–ix
2. Nattiv A, Loucks AB, Manore MM, Sanborn CF, Sundgot-Borgen J, Warren MP (2007) American College of Sports Medicine position stand. The female athlete triad. Med Sci Sports Exerc 39:1867–1882
3. Beals KA, Manore MM (2002) Disorders of the female athlete triad among collegiate athletes. Int J Sport Nutr Exerc Metab 12:281–293
4. De Souza MJ, Miller BE, Loucks AB, Luciano AA, Pescatello LS, Campbell CG, Lasley BL (1998) High frequency of luteal phase deficiency and anovulation in recreational women runners: blunted elevation in follicle-stimulating hormone observed during luteal-follicular transition. J Clin Endocrinol Metab 83:4220–4232
5. Beals KA, Manore MM (2000) Behavioral, psychological, and physical characteristics of female athletes with subclinical eating disorders. Int J Sport Nutr Exerc Metab 10:128–143
6. De Souza MJ, Williams NI (2004) Physiological aspects and clinical sequelae of energy deficiency and hypoestrogenism in exercising women. Hum Reprod Update 10:433–448
7. Sundgot-Borgen J (1994) Risk and trigger factors for the development of eating disorders in female elite athletes. Med Sci Sports Exerc 26:414–419

8. Williams NI, Helmreich DL, Parfitt DB, Caston-Balderrama A, Cameron JL (2001) Evidence for a causal role of low energy availability in the induction of menstrual cycle disturbances during strenuous exercise training. J Clin Endocrinol Metab 86:5184–5193
9. Williams NI, Caston-Balderrama AL, Helmreich DL, Parfitt DB, Nosbisch C, Cameron JL (2001) Longitudinal changes in reproductive hormones and menstrual cyclicity in cynomolgus monkeys during strenuous exercise training: abrupt transition to exercise-induced amenorrhea. Endocrinology 142:2381–2389
10. AAP (2000) American Academy of Pediatrics. Committee on Sports Medicine and Fitness. Medical concerns in the female athlete. Pediatrics 106:610–613
11. Loucks AB, Thuma JR (2003) Luteinizing hormone pulsatility is disrupted at a threshold of energy availability in regularly menstruating women. J Clin Endocrinol Metab 88:297–311
12. De Souza MJ, Hontscharuk R, Olmsted M, Kerr G, Williams NI (2007) Drive for thinness score is a proxy indicator of energy deficiency in exercising women. Appetite 48(3):359–367
13. De Souza MJ, West SL, Jamal SA, Hawker GA, Gundberg CM, Williams NI (2008) The presence of both an energy deficiency and estrogen deficiency exacerbate alterations of bone metabolism in exercising women. Bone 43:140–148
14. De Souza MJ, Williams NI (2005) Beyond hypoestrogenism in amenorrheic athletes: energy deficiency as a contributing factor for bone loss. Curr Sports Med Rep 4:38–44
15. Ihle R, Loucks AB (2004) Dose-response relationships between energy availability and bone turnover in young exercising women. J Bone Miner Res 19:1231–1240
16. Cobb KL, Bachrach LK, Greendale G, Marcus R, Neer RM, Nieves J, Sowers MF, Brown BW Jr, Gopalakrishnan G, Luetters C, Tanner HK, Ward B, Kelsey JL (2003) Disordered eating, menstrual irregularity, and bone mineral density in female runners. Med Sci Sports Exerc 35:711–719
17. Dale E, Gerlach DH, Wilhite AL (1979) Menstrual dysfunction in distance runners. Obstet Gynecol 54:47–53
18. Feicht CB, Johnson TS, Martin BJ, Sparkes KE, Wagner WW Jr (1978) Secondary amenorrhoea in athletes. Lancet 2:1145–1146
19. Glass AR, Deuster PA, Kyle SB, Yahiro JA, Vigersky RA, Schoomaker EB (1987) Amenorrhea in Olympic marathon runners. Fertil Steril 48:740–745
20. Sanborn CF, Martin BJ, Wagner WW Jr (1982) Is athletic amenorrhea specific to runners? Am J Obstet Gynecol 143:859–861
21. Shangold MM, Levine HS (1982) The effect of marathon training upon menstrual function. Am J Obstet Gynecol 143:862–869
22. Nichols JF, Rauh MJ, Barrack MT, Barkai HS, Pernick Y (2007) Disordered eating and menstrual irregularity in high school athletes in lean-build and nonlean-build sports. Int J Sport Nutr Exerc Metab 17:364–377
23. Beals KA, Hill AK (2006) The prevalence of disordered eating, menstrual dysfunction, and low bone mineral density among US collegiate athletes. Int J Sport Nutr Exerc Metab 16:1–23
24. Abraham SF, Beumont PJ, Fraser IS, Llewellyn-Jones D (1982) Body weight, exercise and menstrual status among ballet dancers in training. Br J Obstet Gynaecol 89:507–510
25. Pettersson F, Fries H, Nillius SJ (1973) Epidemiology of secondary amenorrhea. I. Incidence and prevalence rates. Am J Obstet Gynecol 117:80–86
26. Singh KB (1981) Menstrual disorders in college students. Am J Obstet Gynecol 140:299–302
27. Bachmann GA, Kemmann E (1982) Prevalence of oligomenorrhea and amenorrhea in a college population. Am J Obstet Gynecol 144:98–102
28. Baker ER, Mathur RS, Kirk RF, Williamson HO (1981) Female runners and secondary amenorrhea: correlation with age, parity, mileage, and plasma hormonal and sex-hormone-binding globulin concentrations. Fertil Steril 36:183–187
29. Frisch RE, Wyshak G, Vincent L (1980) Delayed menarche and amenorrhea in ballet dancers. N Engl J Med 303:17–19
30. Malina RM (1994) Physical growth and biological maturation of young athletes. Exerc Sport Sci Rev 22:389–433

31. Warren MP, Brooks-Gunn J, Fox RP, Holderness CC, Hyle EP, Hamilton WG, Hamilton L (2003) Persistent osteopenia in ballet dancers with amenorrhea and delayed menarche despite hormone therapy: a longitudinal study. Fertil Steril 80:398–404
32. Malina RM, Ryan RC, Bonci CM (1994) Age at menarche in athletes and their mothers and sisters. Ann Hum Biol 21:417–422
33. ASRM (2006) Current evaluation of amenorrhea.The Practice Committee of the American Society of Reproductive Medicine. Fertil Steril 86:S148–S155
34. Awdishu S, Williams NI, Laredo S, De Souza MJ (2009) Oligomenorrhea in exercising women: a PCOS phenotype or distinct entity? Sports Med 39(12):1055–1069
35. Veldhuis JD, Evans WS, Demers LM, Thorner MO, Wakat D, Rogol AD (1985) Altered neuroendocrine regulation of gonadotropin secretion in women distance runners. J Clin Endocrinol Metab 61:557–563
36. De Souza MJ, Lee DK, VanHeest JL, Scheid JL, West SL, Williams NI (2007) Severity of energy-related menstrual disturbances increases in proportion to indices of energy conservation in exercising women. Fertil Steril 88:971–975
37. Vescovi JD, Scheid JL, Hontscharuk R, De Souza MJ (2008) Cognitive dietary restraint: impact on bone, menstrual and metabolic status in young women. Physiol Behav 95:48–55
38. Wade GN, Schneider JE, Li HY (1996) Control of fertility by metabolic cues. Am J Physiol 270:E1–E19
39. Jasienska G, Ellison PT (1998) Physical work causes suppression of ovarian function in women. Proc Biol Sci 265:1847–1851
40. Ellison PT (1994) Advances in human reproductive ecology. Annu Rev Anthropol 23:255–275
41. Ellison PT (2003) Energetics and reproductive effort. Am J Hum Biol 15:342–351
42. Warren MP (1980) The effects of exercise on pubertal progression and reproductive function in girls. J Clin Endocrinol Metab 51:1150–1157
43. Danforth E Jr, Burger A (1984) The role of thyroid hormones in the control of energy expenditure. Clin Endocrinol Metab 13:581–595
44. Danforth E Jr, Burger AG (1989) The impact of nutrition on thyroid hormone physiology and action. Annu Rev Nutr 9:201–227
45. De Souza MJ, Leidy HJ, O'Donnell E, Lasley B, Williams NI (2004) Fasting ghrelin levels in physically active women: relationship with menstrual disturbances and metabolic hormones. J Clin Endocrinol Metab 89:3536–3542
46. Laughlin GA, Yen SS (1996) Nutritional and endocrine-metabolic aberrations in amenorrheic athletes. J Clin Endocrinol Metab 81:4301–4309
47. Kaufman BA, Warren MP, Dominguez JE, Wang J, Heymsfield SB, Pierson RN (2002) Bone density and amenorrhea in ballet dancers are related to a decreased resting metabolic rate and lower leptin levels. J Clin Endocrinol Metab 87:2777–2783
48. Myerson M, Gutin B, Warren MP, May MT, Contento I, Lee M, Pi-Sunyer FX, Pierson RN Jr, Brooks-Gunn J (1991) Resting metabolic rate and energy balance in amenorrheic and eumenorrheic runners. Med Sci Sports Exerc 23:15–22
49. De Souza MJ, Van Heest J, Demers LM, Lasley BL (2003) Luteal phase deficiency in recreational runners: evidence for a hypometabolic state. J Clin Endocrinol Metab 88:337–346
50. Leibel RL, Rosenbaum M, Hirsch J (1995) Changes in energy expenditure resulting from altered body weight. N Engl J Med 332:621–628
51. Harris JA, Benedict FG (1919) A biometric study of the basal metabolism in man. Carnegie Institution of Washington, Washington, D.C., Pub No. 279
52. Marra M, Polito A, De Filippo E, Cuzzolaro M, Ciarapica D, Contaldo F, Scalfi L (2002) Are the general equations to predict BMR applicable to patients with anorexia nervosa? Eat Weight Disord 7:53–59
53. Melchior JC, Rigaud D, Rozen R, Malon D, Apfelbaum M (1989) Energy expenditure economy induced by decrease in lean body mass in anorexia nervosa. Eur J Clin Nutr 43:793–799

54. Polito A, Fabbri A, Ferro-Luzzi A, Cuzzolaro M, Censi L, Ciarapica D, Fabbrini E, Giannini D (2000) Basal metabolic rate in anorexia nervosa: relation to body composition and leptin concentrations. Am J Clin Nutr 71:1495–1502
55. Loucks AB, Callister R (1993) Induction and prevention of low-T3 syndrome in exercising women. Am J Physiol 264:R924–R930
56. Loucks AB, Heath EM (1994) Induction of low-T3 syndrome in exercising women occurs at a threshold of energy availability. Am J Physiol 266:R817–R823
57. Loucks AB, Verdun M, Heath EM (1998) Low energy availability, not stress of exercise, alters LH pulsatility in exercising women. J Appl Physiol 84:37–46
58. Sanborn CF, Horea M, Siemers BJ, Dieringer KI (2000) Disordered eating and the female athlete triad. Clin Sports Med 19:199–213
59. Smolak L, Murnen SK, Ruble AE (2000) Female athletes and eating problems: a meta-analysis. Int J Eat Disord 27:371–380
60. Garner D (1991) Eating disorder inventory-2 professional manual. Pshychological Assessment Resources, Odessa, FL
61. Sands R (2000) Reconceptualization of body image and drive for thinness. Int J Eat Disord 28:397–407
62. Herman CP, Polivy J (1980) Restrained eating. In: Stunkard AJ (ed) Obesity. WB Saunders, Philadelphia, PA, pp 208–225
63. Van Loan MD, Keim NL (2000) Influence of cognitive eating restraint on total-body measurements of bone mineral density and bone mineral content in premenopausal women aged 18-45 y: a cross-sectional study. Am J Clin Nutr 72:837–843
64. Barr SI, Prior JC, Vigna YM (1994) Restrained eating and ovulatory disturbances: possible implications for bone health. Am J Clin Nutr 59:92–97
65. Drinkwater BL, Nilson K, Chesnut CH III, Bremner WJ, Shainholtz S, Southworth MB (1984) Bone mineral content of amenorrheic and eumenorrheic athletes. N Engl J Med 311:277–281
66. Marcus R, Cann C, Madvig P, Minkoff J, Goddard M, Bayer M, Martin M, Gaudiani L, Haskell W, Genant H (1985) Menstrual function and bone mass in elite women distance runners. Endocrine and metabolic features. Ann Intern Med 102:158–163
67. Nelson ME, Fisher EC, Catsos PD, Meredith CN, Turksoy RN, Evans WJ (1986) Diet and bone status in amenorrheic runners. Am J Clin Nutr 43:910–916
68. Christo K, Prabhakaran R, Lamparello B, Cord J, Miller KK, Goldstein MA, Gupta N, Herzog DB, Klibanski A, Misra M (2008) Bone metabolism in adolescent athletes with amenorrhea, athletes with eumenorrhea, and control subjects. Pediatrics 121:1127–1136
69. ISCD (2004) Diagnosis of osteoporosis in men, premenopausal women, and children. International Society for Clinical Densitometry Position Development Conference. J Clin Densitom 7:17–26
70. Gremion G, Rizzoli R, Slosman D, Theintz G, Bonjour JP (2001) Oligo-amenorrheic long-distance runners may lose more bone in spine than in femur. Med Sci Sports Exerc 33:15–21
71. Tomten SE, Falch JA, Birkeland KI, Hemmersbach P, Hostmark AT (1998) Bone mineral density and menstrual irregularities. A comparative study on cortical and trabecular bone structures in runners with alleged normal eating behavior. Int J Sports Med 19:92–97
72. Khan KM, Liu-Ambrose T, Sran MM, Ashe MC, Donaldson MG, Wark JD (2002) New criteria for female athlete triad syndrome? As osteoporosis is rare, should osteopenia be among the criteria for defining the female athlete triad syndrome? Br J Sports Med 36:10–13
73. Nattiv A (2000) Stress fractures and bone health in track and field athletes. J Sci Med Sport 3:268–279
74. Ducher G, Eser P, Hill B, Bass S (2009) History of amenorrhoea compromises some of the exercise-induced benefits in cortical and trabecular bone in the peripheral and axial skeleton: a study in retired elite gymnasts. Bone 45:760–767
75. Misra M, Prabhakaran R, Miller KK, Goldstein MA, Mickley D, Clauss L, Lockhart P, Cord J, Herzog DB, Katzman DK, Klibanski A (2008) Weight gain and restoration of menses as

predictors of bone mineral density change in adolescent girls with anorexia nervosa-1. J Clin Endocrinol Metab 93:1231–1237

76. Misra M, Prabhakaran R, Miller KK, Goldstein MA, Mickley D, Clauss L, Lockhart P, Cord J, Herzog DB, Katzman DK, Klibanski A (2008) Prognostic indicators of changes in bone density measures in adolescent girls with anorexia nervosa-II. J Clin Endocrinol Metab 93:1292–1297
77. Hergenroeder AC, Smith EO, Shypailo R, Jones LA, Klish WJ, Ellis K (1997) Bone mineral changes in young women with hypothalamic amenorrhea treated with oral contraceptives, medroxyprogesterone, or placebo over 12 months. Am J Obstet Gynecol 176:1017–1025
78. Zipfel S, Seibel MJ, Lowe B, Beumont PJ, Kasperk C, Herzog W (2001) Osteoporosis in eating disorders: a follow-up study of patients with anorexia and bulimia nervosa. J Clin Endocrinol Metab 86:5227–5233
79. Welt CK, Chan JL, Bullen J, Murphy R, Smith P, DePaoli AM, Karalis A, Mantzoros CS (2004) Recombinant human leptin in women with hypothalamic amenorrhea. N Engl J Med 351:987–997
80. Miller KK, Grinspoon S, Gleysteen S, Grieco KA, Ciampa J, Breu J, Herzog DB, Klibanski A (2004) Preservation of neuroendocrine control of reproductive function despite severe undernutrition. J Clin Endocrinol Metab 89:4434–4438
81. Thong FS, McLean C, Graham TE (2000) Plasma leptin in female athletes: relationship with body fat, reproductive, nutritional, and endocrine factors. J Appl Physiol 88:2037–2044
82. Laughlin GA, Yen SS (1997) Hypoleptinemia in women athletes: absence of a diurnal rhythm with amenorrhea. J Clin Endocrinol Metab 82:318–321
83. Lee NJ, Wong IP, Baldock PA, Herzog H (2008) Leptin as an endocrine signal in bone. Curr Osteoporos Rep 6:62–66
84. Yadav VK, Oury F, Suda N, Liu Z, Gao X, Confavreux C, Klemenhagen KC, Tanaka KF, Gingrich JA, Guo XE, Tecott LH, Mann JJ, Hen R, Horvath TL, Karsenty G (2009) A serotonin-dependent mechanism explains the leptin regulation of bone mass, appetite, and energy expenditure. Cell 138:976–989
85. Loucks AB, Laughlin GA, Mortola JF, Girton L, Nelson JC, Yen SS (1992) Hypothalamic-pituitary-thyroidal function in eumenorrheic and amenorrheic athletes. J Clin Endocrinol Metab 75:514–518
86. ASRM (2004) Current evaluation of amenorrhea. The Practice Committee of the American Society of Reproductive Medicine. Fertil Steril 82(suppl 1):S33–S39
87. Vescovi JD, Jamal SA, De Souza MJ (2008) Strategies to reverse bone loss in women with functional hypothalamic amenorrhea: a systematic review of the literature. Osteoporos Int 19:465–478
88. Warren MP, Chua AT (2008) Exercise-induced amenorrhea and bone health in the adolescent athlete. Ann N Y Acad Sci 1135:244–252
89. Kopp-Woodroffe SA, Manore MM, Dueck CA, Skinner JS, Matt KS (1999) Energy and nutrient status of amenorrheic athletes participating in a diet and exercise training intervention program. Int J Sport Nutr 9:70–88
90. Dueck CA, Manore MM, Matt KS (1996) Role of energy balance in athletic menstrual dysfunction. Int J Sport Nutr 6:165–190
91. Dueck CA, Matt KS, Manore MM, Skinner JS (1996) Treatment of athletic amenorrhea with a diet and training intervention program. Int J Sport Nutr 6:24–40
92. Scheid JL WN, West SL, Awdishu S, De Souza MJ (2008) Increased caloric intake in energy deficient exercising women with functional hypothalamic amenorrhea is associated with decreased ghrelin and increased bone formation: preliminary data from an RCT to reverse exercise-associated menstrual disturbances. J Bone Miner Res 23(S1):S286
93. Keen AD, Drinkwater BL (1997) Irreversible bone loss in former amenorrheic athletes. Osteoporos Int 7:311–315
94. Drinkwater BL, Nilson K, Ott S, Chesnut CH III (1986) Bone mineral density after resumption of menses in amenorrheic athletes. JAMA 256:380–382

95. Warren MP, Brooks-Gunn J, Fox RP, Holderness CC, Hyle EP, Hamilton WG (2002) Osteopenia in exercise-associated amenorrhea using ballet dancers as a model: a longitudinal study. J Clin Endocrinol Metab 87:3162–3168
96. Berga SL, Marcus MD, Loucks TL, Hlastala S, Ringham R, Krohn MA (2003) Recovery of ovarian activity in women with functional hypothalamic amenorrhea who were treated with cognitive behavior therapy. Fertil Steril 80:976–981
97. Zanker CL, Cooke CB, Truscott JG, Oldroyd B, Jacobs HS (2004) Annual changes of bone density over 12 years in an amenorrheic athlete. Med Sci Sports Exerc 36:137–142
98. Fredericson M, Kent K (2005) Normalization of bone density in a previously amenorrheic runner with osteoporosis. Med Sci Sports Exerc 37:1481–1486
99. Castelo-Branco C, Vicente JJ, Pons F, Martinez de Osaba MJ, Casals E, Vanrell JA (2001) Bone mineral density in young, hypothalamic oligoamenorrheic women treated with oral contraceptives. J Reprod Med 46:875–879
100. Cumming DC (1996) Exercise-associated amenorrhea, low bone density, and estrogen replacement therapy. Arch Intern Med 156:2193–2195
101. De Crée C, Lewin R, Ostyn M (1988) Suitability of cyproterone acetate in the treatment of osteoporosis associated with athletic amenorrhea. Int J Sports Med 9:187–192
102. Miller KK, Lee EE, Lawson EA, Misra M, Minihan J, Grinspoon SK, Gleysteen S, Mickley D, Herzog D, Klibanski A (2006) Determinants of skeletal loss and recovery in anorexia nervosa. J Clin Endocrinol Metab 91:2931–2937
103. Heer M, Mika C, Grzella I, Heussen N, Herpertz-Dahlmann B (2004) Bone turnover during inpatient nutritional therapy and outpatient follow-up in patients with anorexia nervosa compared with that in healthy control subjects. Am J Clin Nutr 80:774–781
104. Hotta M, Shibasaki T, Sato K, Demura H (1998) The importance of body weight history in the occurrence and recovery of osteoporosis in patients with anorexia nervosa: evaluation by dual X-ray absorptiometry and bone metabolic markers. Eur J Endocrinol 139:276–283
105. Compston JE, McConachie C, Stott C, Hannon RA, Kaptoge S, Debiram I, Love S, Jaffa A (2006) Changes in bone mineral density, body composition and biochemical markers of bone turnover during weight gain in adolescents with severe anorexia nervosa: a 1-year prospective study. Osteoporos Int 17:77–84
106. Bolton JG, Patel S, Lacey JH, White S (2005) A prospective study of changes in bone turnover and bone density associated with regaining weight in women with anorexia nervosa. Osteoporos Int 16:1955–1962
107. Compston JE (2001) Sex steroids and bone. Physiol Rev 81:419–447
108. Gibson JH, Mitchell A, Reeve J, Harries MG (1999) Treatment of reduced bone mineral density in athletic amenorrhea: a pilot study. Osteoporos Int 10:284–289
109. Rickenlund A, Carlstrom K, Ekblom B, Brismar TB, Von Schoultz B, Hirschberg AL (2004) Effects of oral contraceptives on body composition and physical performance in female athletes. J Clin Endocrinol Metab 89:4364–4370
110. Warren MP, Miller KK, Olson WH, Grinspoon SK, Friedman AJ (2005) Effects of an oral contraceptive (norgestimate/ethinyl estradiol) on bone mineral density in women with hypothalamic amenorrhea and osteopenia: an open-label extension of a double-blind, placebo-controlled study. Contraception 72:206–211
111. Khosla S (2002) Leptin-central or peripheral to the regulation of bone metabolism? Endocrinology 143:4161–4164
112. Jenkins PJ, Ibanez-Santos X, Holly J, Cotterill A, Perry L, Wolman R, Harries M, Grossman A (1993) IGFBP-1: a metabolic signal associated with exercise-induced amenorrhea. Neuroendocrinology 57:600–604
113. Laughlin GA, Dominguez CE, Yen SS (1998) Nutritional and endocrine-metabolic aberrations in women with functional hypothalamic amenorrhea. J Clin Endocrinol Metab 83:25–32
114. Grinspoon S, Miller KK, Herzog DB, Grieco KA, Klibanski A (2004) Effects of estrogen and recombinant human insulin-like growth factor-I on ghrelin secretion in severe undernutrition. J Clin Endocrinol Metab 89:3988–3993

115. Grinspoon S, Miller K, Herzog D, Clemmons D, Klibanski A (2003) Effects of recombinant human insulin-like growth factor (IGF)-I and estrogen administration on IGF-I, IGF binding protein (IGFBP)-2, and IGFBP-3 in anorexia nervosa: a randomized-controlled study. J Clin Endocrinol Metab 88:1142–1149
116. Grinspoon S, Miller K, Coyle C, Krempin J, Armstrong C, Pitts S, Herzog D, Klibanski A (1999) Severity of osteopenia in estrogen-deficient women with anorexia nervosa and hypothalamic amenorrhea. J Clin Endocrinol Metab 84:2049–2055
117. Haberland CA, Seddick D, Marcus R, Bachrach LK (1995) A physician survey of therapy for exercise-associated amenorrhea: a brief report. Clin J Sport Med 5:246–250
118. Carlson JL, Curtis M, Halpern-Felsher B (2007) Clinician practices for the management of amenorrhea in the adolescent and young adult athlete. J Adolesc Health 40:362–365
119. Pantano KJ (2009) Strategies used by physical therapists in the U.S. for treatment and prevention of the female athlete triad. Phys Ther Sport 10:3–11

Chapter 8
The Role of Body Weight in Menstrual Disturbances and Amenorrhea

Alex J. Polotsky and Nanette Santoro

Low Body Weight and Menstrual Disturbances

In normal weight women, a 10–15% reduction from ideal body weight (IBW) is associated with amenorrhea [1, 2]. There is considerable interindividual variation in the menstrual cycle manifestations that may occur in association with low body weight. It is likely that the key element involved in eating disorders or low weight related amenorrhea is stress. It appears that the adaptation to the chronic stress involved in food restriction plays a major role. Additives to the low body weight are excessive exercise and a somewhat "driven" personality style. These attributes lead to chronic activation of the adrenocorticotrophic axis and elevated cortisol and corticotrophin releasing factor (CRF) [3]. The end result is functional hypothalamic amenorrhea (FHA), although less severe conditions appear to exist. For example, women who undergo rapid, intense exercise training, and mild dietary restriction will develop a luteal phase defect cycle phenotype, with lengthening of the menstrual cycle, but eventual folliculogenesis and ovulation (albeit with low levels of luteal progesterone secretion and a shortened luteal phase [4]). In many clinical scenarios, it is impossible to separate the relative contributions of body weight, body fat, perceived stress, and exercise to the amenorrhea or menstrual disturbances. This chapter focuses primarily on body weight and body fat as determinants of normal reproductive function.

Case 1

Your next patient is L.G., a 21-year-old college student, who has not had any menstrual bleeding for the last 6 months. She admits to "issues" with eating in the

A.J. Polotsky (✉)
Department of Obstetrics and Gynecology, University of Colorado Denver School of Medicine, Aurora, CO, USA
e-mail: Alex.Polotsky@ucdenver.edu

N.F. Santoro and G. Neal-Perry (eds.), *Amenorrhea: A Case-Based, Clinical Guide*, Contemporary Endocrinology, DOI 10.1007/978-1-60327-864-5_8,

past but denies any active food restriction or excessive exercise. Her weight is 99 pounds; height is 5 ft. 2 in. A pregnancy test is negative.

Eating Disorders – Definition

Body mass below 15% of IBW is one of the diagnostic criteria for anorexia nervosa as defined by the DSM-IV [5]. While the concept of IBW originally came from actuarial life insurance tables and represents the presumably healthiest body mass for given weight [6], BMI) is the most practical and widely acceptable way to assess the degree of deviation from normal, as it is indexed to height and thus the normal BMI range is the same for adults of any size. BMI is easily calculated as the ratio of the body mass in kilograms and square of height in meters. A voluntary BMI threshold below 17.5 kg/m^2 is one of the defining characteristics of anorexia nervosa based upon the ICD-10 diagnostic criteria [7]. Other mandatory diagnostic criteria include distorted body image, menstrual dysfunction and fear of weight gain (Table 8.1). Whereas, DSM-IV defines two additional eating disorders such as bulimia nervosa and "eating disorder not otherwise specified," anorexia is the only entity that is associated with abnormally low body weight and menstrual dysfunction.

Epidemiology of Eating Disorders and Weight-Related Amenorrhea

It has been estimated that up to 1% of the population suffers from restrictive eating disorders [8]. However, the true prevalence of these conditions is probably underestimated as the data are notoriously fraught with methodological problems related to the changing diagnostic criteria and inherent difficulties of self-report [9]. These disorders can take several forms, and appear to have varying relationships to amenorrhea. Common features of eating disorders include an array of attitudes about food, fear of certain foods (because they are believed to cause fatness), body image distortion, and fear of fatness.

The long-term sequelae of FHA and, more broadly, amenorrhea caused by low body weight are only recently beginning to be recognized. Data from the Women's Ischemia Syndrome Evaluation (WISE) study revealed that women with FHA had a 69% prevalence of coronary heart disease as compared to 29% in those without this condition [10]. This profoundly detrimental impact of menstrual irregularities

Table 8.1 DSM-IV diagnostic criteria for anorexia nervosa

Failure to maintain body weight around a minimally normal age- and height-adjusted weight (i.e., body weight less than 85% of that expected for age and height)
Fear of gaining weight or becoming fat, even if inconsistent with current weight
Distorted body image
Absence of three or more spontaneous consecutive menstrual cycles in postmenarcheal females

Adapted from American Psychiatric Association [5]

on overall health is not well appreciated by patients and practitioners alike. More effort is needed to understand the mechanisms underlying the pathophysiology of this association as well as increasing the public awareness of this entity and some potential remedies designed to reverse the pathological chain of events.

Clinical Presentation

The clinical appearance of women with anorexia nervosa includes the following features: lanugo hair; orange-tinted skin (due to elevated circulating carotenoids), a low resting pulse rate, often in the 50s or even 40s (bpm); brittle nails, thinning hair, and an absence of the patient's concern about her emaciated state. Such patients often come to the office accompanied by a concerned relative, usually a parent, and appear to lack an understanding of the fact that they are a cause of concern. The clinical history typically consists of an initial attempt at voluntary weight loss that has now become uncontrollable. The patient is frequently in denial of her behaviors, but family members will often describe extreme food restriction, with consumption of as little as 400 calories a day. To make matters worse, many such women will exercise compulsively out of a worry that they will become overweight if there are any lapses in their vigilance. If queried about their appearance, women in the throes of anorexia nervosa fail to recognize that they are excessively and even dangerously thin. They will express a belief that their body size is "normal" or even a little bit overweight. More savvy patients, who may wish to avoid confrontation, will sometimes conceal this striking body image distortion.

Hypothalamic–pituitary function in anorexia nervosa is similar to that observed in any state of starvation, involuntary or voluntary. It is helpful to conceptualize it as a reaction to the lack of nutrient availability. Thyroid hormone is typically low, with elevated reverse T3, to reduce the metabolic rate. TSH, however, remains in the normal range. Luteinizing hormone (LH) and follicle-stimulating hormone (FSH) are often abnormally low, although they may be within the normal range, due to their inherent pulsatility. Estradiol is typically undetectable. Unlike patients with panhypopituitarism, the somatotrophic and adrenocorticotrophic axes are constitutively activated in women with anorexia. Dynamic pituitary testing is rarely necessary, as the diagnosis is often obvious based on the constellation of signs, symptoms and behaviors.

Women with bulimia are less likely to be underweight and may manifest some, but not all of the features of anorectics. Additional clinical signs of bulimia include erosion of tooth enamel from self-induced vomiting and esophageal damage.

Pathophysiology

Classically, anovulation associated with abnormally low body mass has been linked with WHO anovulation Class I or hypogonadotropic hypogonadism [11]. The mechanisms for impairment of the hypothalamic discharge of GnRH in these cases have been partially elucidated. Caloric restriction or intensive physical activity that exceeds intake produces a reduction in central neural drive of the GnRH pulse generator [2, 12] that is tightly associated with reductions in circulating plasma glucose [13] and increased R ("reverse")T3 [14]. In animal models, hypoglycemia rapidly induces GnRH inhibition, but this inhibition is much more easily elicited in men than in women [15]. Up to 72 h of starvation in normal weight women has not been shown to induce changes in the hypothalamic GnRH pulse generator, as assessed by the measurement of peripheral LH secretion [16]. However, a recently developed animal model of chronic stress [17] provides insight into the combination of mechanisms that contribute to hypothalamic amenorrhea and suggests that both a combination of stressors and an inherent vulnerability to such stressors are necessary to induce menstrual disturbances. In this model, cynomologus monkeys are subjected to mild caloric restriction that does not result in weight loss but reduces the metabolic rate (20% reduction in daily chow). In addition, to mimic the extra energy expenditure in many women with hypothalamic amenorrhea and anorexia nervosa, the animals are trained to run on treadmills for a specified period of time each day. Finally, to create chronic psychogenic stress, the animals are subjected to frequent changes of their cage location, such that unfamiliar animals often surround them. This latter series of experiments highlights in an elegant fashion that the combination of stressors and the susceptibility of the individual help create the amenorrheic phenotype. In the case of restrictive eating, the primary stress may be low body weight and body fat, but the additional components of psychic stress and further energy drainage through exercise are also often present.

Leptin deficiency has been shown to play an important role in hypothalamic amenorrhea. Welt et al. [18] administered recombinant leptin to women with FHA and was able to restore gonadotropin pulsatility (8/8 women) and menstrual cyclicity (3/8 women) along with restoration of normal free T3 and T4. Thus, the low leptin levels in women with weight-loss associated amenorrhea or menstrual disturbances appear to provide the metabolic communication to the central hypothalamic–pituitary axis that reproduction should be switched off, due to a lack of available nutrients. Although the aforementioned experiment provides great insight into the pathophysiology and mechanisms responsible for hypothalamic amenorrhea, leptin does not constitute a credible treatment for the disorder, as its provision of a satiety signal leads to further weight loss if given over a prolonged period of time.

Diagnostic Workup

Women suspected of restrictive eating disorders should undergo a thorough evaluation to exclude other alternative etiologies that may account for extreme thinness. Hyperthyroidism, malabsorption from ulcerative colitis, Crohn's disease, or celiac disease can be ruled out by clinical history, physical examination, and laboratory testing as appropriate. As prudent for any evaluation of secondary amenorrhea, pregnancy must be excluded.

A major goal of the laboratory evaluation of a woman with anorexia nervosa is to rule out a potentially life-threatening emergency. The tragic case of Terry Schiavo was thrust in the public arena because of her family's end-of-life issues. However, little attention was paid to the fact that the patient had reportedly suffered a cardiac arrest due to hypokalemia that was caused by an eating disorder [19]. This underscores the need to evaluate women with anorexia nervosa for electrolyte imbalances. An individual with a potentially life-threatening eating disorder may present to a primary care doctor for the treatment of menstrual irregularity and be reluctant to disclose her eating habits. Sadly, this appears to be exactly what transpired in Ms. Schiavo's case and subsequently led to a $1 million settlement [20].

Once the diagnosis is established, the evaluation for associated comorbidities should be considered. Specifically, the measurement of bone density with dual X-ray absorptiometry may reveal important clinical information useful for the treatment and counseling [21].

Therapeutic Algorithms

Overcoming restrictive eating disorders should involve an approach directed at behavioral modification (Fig. 8.1). It is not sufficient to correct the sex steroid deficiency, although in some cases it may serve as a temporizing measure [22]. The long-term consequences of continuing to live in a state of chronic stress is likely related to the increased risk of heart disease in women with hypothalamic amenorrhea. Moreover, the bone density losses that such women often display may be related to chronic activation of their HPA axis and may not be amenable to estrogen

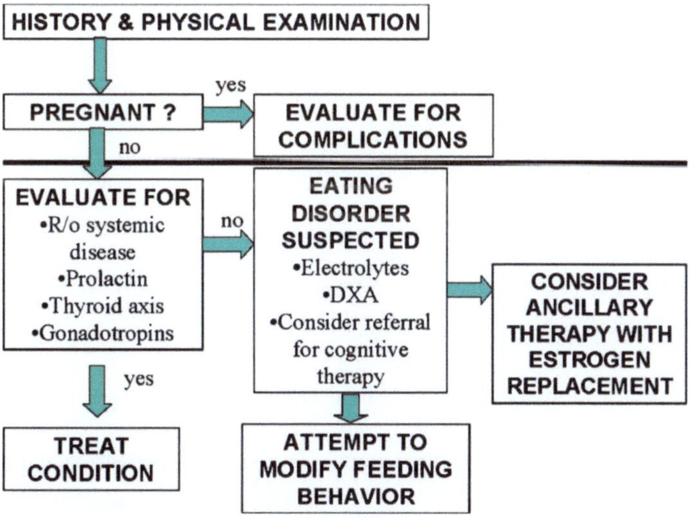

Fig. 8.1 Evaluation of amenorrhea in women with low body mass

replacement alone. Since eating disorders are often initially detected in the teenage years, cognitive behavioral therapy is recommended to lead to permanent change and true healing [23]. Hospitalization may become necessary if out-patient management fails to correct electrolyte imbalance and/or other serious medical or psychiatric complication are present [24]. Among outpatient measures, antidepressants have been found to be more efficacious for patients suffering from bulimia [25]. For anorexia nervosa, American Psychiatric Association recommends antidepressants solely for the prevention of relapse in weight restored patients or psychiatric comorbidities [26].

Obesity and Menstrual Disturbances

Case 2

Your next patient is B.G, a 34-year-old nulligravida, who has been trying to get pregnant for the past 2 years. She does not have any significant past medical or surgical history. Her husband's semen analysis is normal. Hysterosalpingogram reveals bilaterally patent fallopian tubes. Her weight is 205; height is 5 ft. 2 in. She reports infrequent menstrual periods (3–4 per year); menstrual irregularity seems to have started after she gained about 100 pounds in college. She denies any excessive hair growth, has a normal ovarian appearance on ultrasound and does not have any biochemical evidence of hyperandrogenism. A pregnancy test is negative.

Defining Excess Body Mass

The World Health Organization (WHO) categorizes body mass by BMI into the following categories [27]:

- Underweight – less than 18.5 kg/m^2
- Normal weight – 18.5–24.9 kg/m^2
- Overweight – 25.0–29.9 kg/m^2
- Class I obesity – 30.0–34.9 kg/m^2
- Class II obesity – 35.0–39.9 kg/m^2
- Class III obesity – greater than 40 kg/m^2. This category is also sometimes referred to as severe, extreme, or morbid

Epidemiology of Obesity and Menstrual Dysregulation

The obesity epidemic in the United Sates is advancing at an ever-accelerating pace. Currently, 32% of U.S. adults are obese as defined by a BMI of greater than 30 kg/m^2, according to the latest National Health and Nutrition Examination Survey [28].

It is estimated that by 2015, 75% of U.S. adults will be overweight or obese (BMI of greater than 25 kg/m^2) and 41% will be obese [29]. Female adult obesity is associated with a variety of reproductive disturbances, including menstrual cycle irregularities, anovulation and a higher risk of obstetrical complications [30]. Recent data from the Study of Women's Health Across the Nation (SWAN) indicate that increasing high school BMI is consistently and independently associated with reduced lifetime parity [31]. The relative risk of ovulatory infertility is tripled in women with BMI of greater than 27 kg/m^2 compared to women with a normal BMI [32]. When compared with normal weight women, spontaneous abortion rates are higher in obese patients who conceive via either natural or assisted conception [33, 34]. Detrimental effects of obesity on performance in assisted reproductive technology are manifested by higher cycle cancellation, greater requirement for exogenous gonadotropins, and lower birth rates [35, 36]. Menstrual cycle irregularities are significantly more common with increasing body mass, a phenomenon that is often, but not exclusively, ascribed to anovulation [37].

Traditionally, reproductive effects of female adult obesity were attributed to increases in anovulation, amenorrhea, and hyperandrogenism [38]. Most of the existing body of literature concerning obesity and reproduction involves women with polycystic ovary syndrome (PCOS), a condition characterized by hyperandrogenemia and oligomenorrhea and, frequently, accompanying obesity [39–41]. In obese women without PCOS, an influence of adiposity on reproductive outcomes has only recently attracted investigative attention. *Obesity is detrimental to fertility even in women who are ovulatory*. Obesity prolongs the time to pregnancy and is associated with decreased fecundity in women with regular menstrual cycles [42–44]. An increase in waist-hip ratio of as little as 0.1 U was associated with a 30% decrease in the per cycle probability of conception in presumably reproductively normal women undergoing donor sperm insemination [45]. In a cohort of over 3,000 subfertile couples in whom the female partner was confirmed to be ovulatory, the probability of spontaneous conception declined with a BMI over 29 kg/m^2 [46]. Multivariable analysis from the same study indicated that an increase in BMI by 1 unit resulted in a 4% reduction in the likelihood of conception [46].

Clinical Presentation

A typical presentation for obesity-related menstrual irregularity is a woman in her 30s who has been steadily gaining weight since adolescence. It is not uncommon that obesity is the only abnormal finding in an otherwise healthy individual. Prior conceptions and live births may have been attained, depending on the reproductive choice exercised by the patient. While long-standing hirsutism and oligoamenorrhea may be coincident with obesity and suggest the diagnosis of PCOS, the absence of such signs and symptoms may be indicative of so-called simple or non-syndromic obesity [47].

Pathophysiology

Decreased central reproductive drive has been demonstrated in regularly cycling obese women. In the 1970s, when radioimmunoassay became widely available and was used to study day to day reproductive hormone secretion across the human menstrual cycle, obesity was first reported to be associated with long (>14 day) follicular phases and decreased serum gonadotropins and luteal progesterone [48]. In 1986, Grenman et al. examined the reproductive hormonal profile of a group of 25 obese women, and reported lower SHBG, estradiol, androstenedione, and LH in obese compared to normal weight women [49]. Notably, 24 of the 25 obese women reported were cycling regularly. In a large, community-based sample of midlife women from the SWAN study, increasing body size was associated with a greater prevalence of irregular and long menstrual cycles [50]. The latter study, a detailed evaluation of daily hormone patterns from 836 ovulatory cycles, indicated that overweight women (BMI >25 kg/m^2) excreted significantly less urinary LH, FSH, and luteal progesterone metabolites; the association was weight dependent, with women in higher weight centiles excreting progressively less hormone. This relative hypogonadism of obesity may be potentially explained by either central (hypothalamic or pituitary) or peripheral (corpus luteum) defects within the hypothalamic–pituitary–ovarian (HPO) axis. In the studies of ovulatory, morbidly obese women indicate a significant reduction in LH pulse amplitude yet no change in LH pulse frequency compared to normal weight controls [51]. After bariatric surgery induced weight loss, a partial recovery of hypogonadotropic hypogonadism was observed [52].

While there are several potential molecules (reviewed in [53]) that communicate metabolic signals to the HPO axis, leptin has been studied most extensively. Leptin, initially described as a satiety factor [54], conveys an afferent signal to the CNS on the body's fat status – a long-term indicator of nutrient availability. In humans, leptin levels are markedly elevated in obesity [55] and pregnancy [56], and are higher in women than in men [57]. The actions of leptin on the HPO axis are thought to have differential effects on the central and peripheral components of the reproductive system. In the CNS, leptin has been shown to modulate GnRH pulse frequency in vitro [58]. It does not act directly on GnRH neurons, but rather via indirect mechanisms through interneurons secreting hypothalamic neuropeptides, such as neuropeptide Y, galanin-like protein, MSH, and endogenous opioids (reviewed in [59]). In humans, leptin may interrupt normal oocyte maturation [60] and has been correlated with poor implantation potential [61]. The dual low-leptin/high-leptin mechanism has been proposed to take into account the complex nature of leptin-HPG axis interactions [62]. According to this theory, the predominant effect of leptin's action on the HPG axis is determined by its concentration, whereby low leptin exerts a negative influence centrally and elevated leptin yields a negative effect peripherally at the gonadal and/or embryo level.

In 1970, Frisch and Revelle noted a direct relationship between body weight and age at the onset of puberty and concluded that a critical amount of body fat was needed for the onset of puberty [63]. While the original concept was based on the notion that a critical amount of body fatness is needed for menarche, it is not clear whether the degree of fatness causes menarche or whether an increase in body fat is the consequence of the onset of puberty, and the two findings may be coincidentally and independently related to endocrine or genetic factors. The exciting discovery of leptin as an indicator of fat mass gave rise to a speculation that it may represent the missing link in the Frisch hypothesis and thus serve as a trigger of pubertal development.

Leptin administration results in the reversal of pubertal arrest in leptin-deficient mice [64]. When given to normal prepubertal animals, leptin hastens sexual development as manifested by the advancement of vaginal opening [65]. Cheung et al. assessed the temporal sequence of pubertal events in rodents [66, 67] and showed that a rise in serum leptin did not precede pubertal development in rats. Similarly, the expression of leptin mRNA receptor in the hypothalamic of female mouse did not increase with pubertal development. Finally, the administration of leptin to starved animals advanced estrus as compared to food-restricted untreated controls, but first estrus occurred at the same time as mice fed ad libitum. Taken together, these results imply that leptin appears to provide a necessary input of adequacy of energy stores to the brain, and is capable of authorizing but not initiating progression to puberty. Thus, both animal and human data support the notion that leptin is necessary but not sufficient metabolic signal for the reproductive axis.

Diagnostic Workup

It is prudent to exclude other causes for menstrual irregularities before assigning the cause to obesity per se. Evaluation should be targeted to common etiologies, such as premature ovarian insufficiency, PCOS, prolactin, and thyroid abnormalities. Once the diagnosis is confirmed, attention should be paid to proper counseling. It is important to exercise care in avoiding punitive attitudes toward obesity that may discourage the patient and hinder compliance. Patients should be educated on the increased risk obesity poses for congenital anomalies, including neural tube defects and cardiovascular anomalies [68] as well spontaneous abortion [69] and obstetrical complications such as gestational diabetes, cesarean section, preeclampsia, and fetal macrosomia [70].

Therapeutic Algorithms

While exogenous gonadotropins and assisted reproductive technologies are the efficient ways to achieve ovulation and conception in many women, the first line of therapy should be directed at the root of the problem, i.e., large body mass, rather than its consequences (Fig. 8.2). Several investigators have addressed the beneficial effects of weight loss on fertility [71–73]. Few of these studies included long-term follow-up or large numbers of subjects, yet it seems reasonable to support even modest weight reduction in the obese due to the indisputable benefits for overall health.

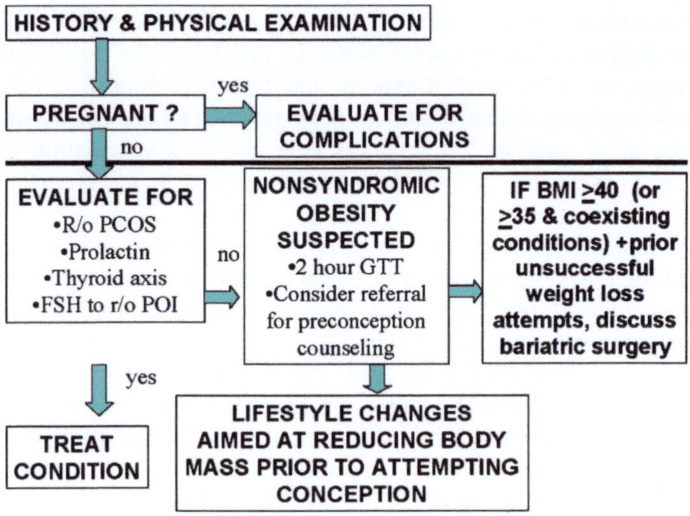

Fig. 8.2 Evaluation of amenorrhea in women with high body mass

The precise amount of the recommended weight loss that may result in the reversal of menstrual irregularities is unknown and is likely subject to wide intrapersonal variance. However, some studies suggest that as little as 5% weight loss may lead to an increased likelihood of conception. One uncontrolled study of a diet and exercise program in infertile women found that approximately 6% weight loss over 36 months resulted in pregnancy in 29 out of 37 subjects [72]. A recent systematic review of pregnancies after bariatric surgery revealed a decrease in prenatal complications and improved neonatal outcomes [74]. While bariatric surgery is understandably limited to the more extreme excesses of body mass, the decreased perinatal morbidity of women who lose weight prior to conception deserves further scientific scrutiny. More research is needed on the effects of modest weight reduction on fertility, as obesity represents one of the few modifiable factors that may be amenable to conservative management.

References

1. Loucks A, Heath E (1994) Dietary restriction reduces luteinizing hormone (LH) pulse frequency during waking hours and increases LH pulse amplitude during sleep in young menstruating women. J Clin Endocrinol Metab 78:910–915
2. Loucks A, Verdun M (1998) Slow restoration of LH pulsatility by refeeding in energetically disrupted women. Am J Physiol 275:R1218–R1226
3. Berga SL, Loucks-Daniels TL, Adler LJ et al (2000) Cerebrospinal fluid levels of corticotropin-releasing hormone in women with functional hypothalamic amenorrhea. Am J Obstet Gynecol 182:776–781, discussion 81–84

4. Loucks AB, Thuma JR (2003) Luteinizing hormone pulsatility is disrupted at a threshold of energy availability in regularly menstruating women. J Clin Endocrinol Metab 88:297–311
5. American Psychiatric Association (1994) Diagnostic and statistical manual of mental disorders, 4th edn. APA, Washington, DC
6. Pai MP, Paloucek FP (2000) The origin of the "ideal" body weight equations. Ann Pharmacother 34:1066–1069
7. McIntosh VVW, Jordan J, Carter FA et al (2004) Strict versus lenient weight criterion in anorexia nervosa. Eur Eat Disord Rev 12:51–60
8. Hoek HW, van Hoeken D (2003) Review of the prevalence and incidence of eating disorders. Int J Eat Disord 34:383–396
9. Wakeling A (1996) Epidemiology of anorexia nervosa. Psychiatry Res 62:3–9
10. Bairey Merz CN, Johnson BD, Sharaf BL et al (2003) Hypoestrogenemia of hypothalamic origin and coronary artery disease in premenopausal women: a report from the NHLBI-sponsored WISE study. J Am Coll Cardiol 41:413–419
11. Anonymous (1973) Agents stimulating gonadal function in the human. Report of a WHO scientific group. World Health Organ Tech Rep Ser 514:1–30
12. Willaims N, Helmreich D, Parfitt D, Caston-Balderrama A, Cameron J (2001) Evidence for a causal role of low energy availability in the induction of menstrual cycle disturbances during strenuous exercise training. J Clin Endocrinol Metab 86:5184–5193
13. Schreihofer D, Amico J, Cameron J (1993) Reversal of fasting-induced suppression of luteinizing hormone (LH) secretion in male rhesus monkeys by intragastric nutrient infusion: evidence for rapid stimulation of LH by nutritional signals. Endocrinology 132:1890–1897
14. Loucks A, Heath E (1994) Induction of low-T3 syndrome in exercising women occurs at a threshold of energy availability. Am J Physiol 266:R817–R823
15. Cameron J (1996) Regulation of reproductive hormone secretion in primates by short-term changes in nutrition. Rev Reprod 1:117–126
16. Berga SL, Loucks T, Cameron J (2001) Endocrine and chronobiological effects of fasting in women. Fertil Steril 75:926–932
17. Williams NI, Berga SL, Cameron JL (2007) Synergism between psychosocial and metabolic stressors: impact on reproductive function in cynomolgus monkeys. Am J Physiol Endocrinol Metab 293:E270–E276
18. Welt CK, Chan JL, Bullen J et al (2004) Recombinant human leptin in women with hypothalamic amenorrhea. N Engl J Med 351:987–997
19. Quill TE (2005) Terri Schiavo – a tragedy compounded. N Engl J Med 352:1630–1633
20. Fine RL (1005) From Quinlan to Schiavo. Proc (Bayl Univ Med Cent) 18:303–310
21. Hotta M, Shibasaki T, Sato K, Demura H (1998) The importance of body weight history in the occurrence and recovery of osteoporosis in patients with anorexia nervosa: evaluation by dual X-ray absorptiometry and bone metabolic markers. Eur J Endocrinol 139:276–283
22. Hergenroeder AC (2001) Risks and benefits of estrogen replacement for eating disorders. AAP News 18:63
23. Berga SL, Loucks TL (2006) Use of cognitive behavior therapy for functional hypothalamic amenorrhea. Ann NY Acad Sci 1092:114–129
24. Golden NH, Katzman DK, Kreipe RE et al (2003) Eating disorders in adolescents: position paper of the Society for Adolescent Medicine. J Adolesc Health 33:496–503
25. Bacaltchuk J, Hay P (2001) Antidepressants versus placebo for people with bulimia nervosa. Cochrane Database Syst Rev CD003391. [see comment] [update in Cochrane Database Syst Rev 2003;(4):CD003391]
26. Anonymous (2000) Practice guideline for the treatment of patients with eating disorders (revision). American Psychiatric Association Work Group on Eating Disorders. Am J Psychiatry 157:1–39
27. Anonymous (2000) Obesity: preventing and managing the global epidemic. Report of a WHO consultation. World Health Organ Tech Rep Ser 894:i–xii
28. Ogden CL, Carroll MD, Curtin LR, McDowell MA, Tabak CJ, Flegal KM (2006) Prevalence of overweight and obesity in the United States, 1999–2004. JAMA 295:1549–1555

29. Wang Y, Beydoun MA (2007) The obesity epidemic in the United States – gender, age, socioeconomic, racial/ethnic, and geographic characteristics: a systematic review and meta-regression analysis. Epidemiol Rev 29:6–28
30. Linne Y (2004) Effect of obesity on women's reproduction and complications during pregnancy. Obesity Rev 5:137–143
31. Polotsky AJ, Hailpern SM, Skurnick JH, Lo JC, Sternfeld B, Santoro N (2009) Association of adolescent obesity and lifetime nulliparity – the Study of Women's Health Across the Nation (SWAN). Fertil Steril 93(6):2004–2011
32. Grodstein F, Goldman MB, Cramer DW, Grodstein F, Goldman MB, Cramer DW (1994) Body mass index and ovulatory infertility. Epidemiology 5:247–250
33. Lashen H, Fear K, Sturdee DW (2004) Obesity is associated with increased risk of first trimester and recurrent miscarriage: matched case-control study. Hum Reprod 19:1644–1646
34. Maheshwari A, Stofberg L, Bhattacharya S (2007) Effect of overweight and obesity on assisted reproductive technology a systematic review. Hum Reprod Update 13:433–444
35. Fedorcsak P, Dale PO, Storeng R et al (2004) Impact of overweight and underweight on assisted reproduction treatment. Hum Reprod 19:2523–2528
36. Spandorfer SD, Kump L, Goldschlag D, Brodkin T, Davis OK, Rosenwaks Z (2004) Obesity and in vitro fertilization: negative influences on outcome. J Reprod Med 49:973–977
37. Windham GC, Elkin E, Fenster L et al (2002) Ovarian hormones in premenopausal women: variation by demographic, reproductive and menstrual cycle characteristics. Epidemiology 13:675–684
38. Rogers J, Mitchell GW (1952) The relation of obesity to menstrual disturbances. N Engl J Med 247:53–55
39. Ehrmann DA, Ehrmann DA (2005) Polycystic ovary syndrome. N Engl J Med 352:1223–1236
40. Pagan YL, Srouji SS, Jimenez Y, Emerson A, Gill S, Hall JE (2006) Inverse relationship between luteinizing hormone and body mass index in polycystic ovarian syndrome: investigation of hypothalamic and pituitary contributions. J Clin Endocrinol Metab 91:1309–1316
41. Holte J, Bergh T, Gennarelli G, Wide L (1994) The independent effects of polycystic ovary syndrome and obesity on serum concentrations of gonadotrophins and sex steroids in premenopausal women. Clin Endocrinol 41:473–481
42. Bolumar F, Olsen J, Rebagliato M, Saez-Lloret I, Bisanti L (2000) Body mass index and delayed conception: a European multicenter study on infertility and subfecundity. Am J Epidemiol 151:1072–1079
43. Gesink Law DC, Maclehose RF, Longnecker MP (2007) Obesity and time to pregnancy. Hum Reprod 22:414–420
44. Jensen TK, Scheike T, Keiding N, Schaumburg I, Grandjean P (1999) Fecundability in relation to body mass and menstrual cycle patterns. Epidemiology 10:422–428
45. Zaadstra BM, Seidell JC, Van Noord PA et al (1993) Fat and female fecundity: prospective study of effect of body fat distribution on conception rates. BMJ 306:484–487
46. van der Steeg JW, Steures P, Eijkemans MJ et al (2008) Obesity affects spontaneous pregnancy chances in subfertile, ovulatory women. Hum Reprod 23:324–328
47. Diamanti-Kandarakis E, Bergiele A (2001) The influence of obesity on hyperandrogenism and infertility in the female. Obes Rev 2:231–238
48. Sherman BM, Korenman SG (1974) Measurement of serum LH, FSH, estradiol and progesterone in disorders of the human menstrual cycle: the inadequate luteal phase. J Clin Endocrinol Metab 39:145–149
49. Grenman S, Ronnemaa T, Irjala K, Kaihola HL, Gronroos M (1986) Sex steroid, gonadotropin, cortisol, and prolactin levels in healthy, massively obese women: correlation with abdominal fat cell size and effect of weight reduction. J Clin Endocrinol Metab 63: 1257–1261
50. Santoro N, Lasley B, McConnell D et al (2004) Body size and ethnicity are associated with menstrual cycle alterations in women in the early menopausal transition: the Study of Women's Health Across the Nation (SWAN) daily hormone study. J Clin Endocrinol Metab 89:2622–2631

51. Jain A, Polotsky AJ, Rochester D et al (2007) Pulsatile luteinizing hormone amplitude and progesterone metabolite excretion are reduced in obese women. J Clin Endocrinol Metab 92:2468–2473
52. Rochester D, Jain A, Polotsky AJ et al (2008) Partial recovery of luteal function after bariatric surgery in obese women. Fertil Steril 92(4):1410–1415
53. Campos DB, Palin MF, Bordignon V, Murphy BD (2008) The 'beneficial' adipokines in reproduction and fertility. Int J Obes 32:223–231
54. Zhang Y, Proenca R, Maffei M, Barone M, Leopold L, Friedman JM (1994) Positional cloning of the mouse obese gene and its human homologue. Nature 372:425–432 [see comment]; [erratum, Nature 1995; 374(6521):479]
55. Considine RV, Sinha MK, Heiman ML et al (1996) Serum immunoreactive-leptin concentrations in normal-weight and obese humans. N Engl J Med 334:292–295
56. Butte NF, Hopkinson JM, Nicolson MA (1997) Leptin in human reproduction: serum leptin levels in pregnant and lactating women. J Clin Endocrinol Metab 82:585–589
57. Kennedy A, Gettys TW, Watson P et al (1997) The metabolic significance of leptin in humans: gender-based differences in relationship to adiposity, insulin sensitivity, and energy expenditure. J Clin Endocrinol Metab 82:1293–1300
58. Lebrethon MC, Vandersmissen E, Gerard A, Parent AS, Junien JL, Bourguignon JP (2000) In vitro stimulation of the prepubertal rat gonadotropin-releasing hormone pulse generator by leptin and neuropeptide Y through distinct mechanisms. Endocrinology 141:1464–1469
59. Moschos S, Chan JL, Mantzoros CS (2002) Leptin and reproduction: a review. Fertil Steril 77:433–444
60. Smith GD, Jackson LM, Foster DL (2002) Leptin regulation of reproductive function and fertility. Theriogenology 57:73–86
61. Cioffi JA, Van Blerkom J, Antczak M, Shafer A, Wittmer S, Snodgrass HR (1997) The expression of leptin and its receptors in pre-ovulatory human follicles. Mol Hum Reprod 3:467–472
62. Caprio M, Fabbrini E, Isidori AM, Aversa A, Fabbri A (2001) Leptin in reproduction. Trends Endocrinol Metab 12:65–72
63. Frisch RE, McArthur JW (1974) Menstrual cycles: fatness as a determinant of minimum weight for height necessary for their maintenance or onset. Science 185:949–951
64. Chehab FF, Lim ME, Lu R (1996) Correction of the sterility defect in homozygous obese female mice by treatment with the human recombinant leptin. Nat Genet 12:318–320
65. Chehab FF, Mounzih K, Lu R, Lim ME (1997) Early onset of reproductive function in normal female mice treated with leptin. Science 275:88–90
66. Cheung CC, Thornton JE, Nurani SD, Clifton DK, Steiner RA (2001) A reassessment of leptin's role in triggering the onset of puberty in the rat and mouse. Neuroendocrinology 74:12–21
67. Cheung CC, Thornton JE, Kuijper JL, Weigle DS, Clifton DK, Steiner RA (1997) Leptin is a metabolic gate for the onset of puberty in the female rat. Endocrinology 138:855–858
68. Stothard KJ, Tennant PW, Bell R, Rankin J (2009) Maternal overweight and obesity and the risk of congenital anomalies: a systematic review and meta-analysis. JAMA 301:636–650
69. Metwally M, Ong KJ, Ledger WL, Li TC (2008) Does high body mass index increase the risk of miscarriage after spontaneous and assisted conception? A meta-analysis of the evidence. Fertil Steril 90:714–726
70. Robinson HE, O'Connell CM, Joseph KS, McLeod NL (2005) Maternal outcomes in pregnancies complicated by obesity. Obstet Gynecol 106:1357–1364
71. Norman RJ, Noakes M, Wu R, Davies MJ, Moran L, Wang JX (2004) Improving reproductive performance in overweight/obese women with effective weight management. Hum Reprod Update 10:267–280
72. Galletly C, Clark A, Tomlinson L, Blaney F (1996) Improved pregnancy rates for obese, infertile women following a group treatment program. An open pilot study. Gen Hosp Psychiatry 18:192–195
73. Clark AM, Ledger W, Galletly C et al (1995) Weight loss results in significant improvement in pregnancy and ovulation rates in anovulatory obese women. Hum Reprod 10:2705–2712
74. Maggard MA, Yermilov I, Li Z et al (2008) Pregnancy and fertility following bariatric surgery: a systematic review. JAMA 300:2286–2296

Chapter 9
Natural and Surgical Menopause

Sara Morelli and Gerson Weiss

Women outnumber men among older adults. In 2002, 33 million women in the US civilian population were aged 55 years and older, with a gender ratio of 81 men per 100 women [1]. By 2030, more than 1.2 billion women in the world will be at least 50 years old [2]. This increasing proportion of the female population will be experiencing the menopausal transition with its accompanying physiology and pathophysiology.

Aging of the female reproductive axis occurs much earlier than aging of other organ systems, generally at a time when a woman is otherwise healthy. Females are born with a fixed number of oocytes (approximately 1–2 million) arrested in prophase I of meiosis. The basis of female reproductive aging is the gradual loss of these oocytes through atresia (beginning in utero and continuing throughout life) and ovulation (during the reproductive years), as well as a diminished sensitivity of the hypothalamic-pituitary axis to estrogen [3]. The median age at onset of irregular menstruation associated with the menopausal transition is 47.5 years, with a median age at final menstrual period (FMP) of 51.3 years [4]. Ethnic differences in the age at menopause have been reported. When compared with Caucasian women, Hispanic and African–American women experience menopause at an earlier age [5, 6], whereas Chinese American and Japanese American women have a later completion of the transition [6]. Lifestyle and social factors play a role in the timing of menopause; cigarette smoking has been shown to advance menopause by as much as 2 years [4, 6], and lower socio-economic status (SES) has been associated with earlier menopause [6].

Defining the Menopausal Transition

Given the wide age range (41–57 years) over which reproductive senescence occurs in normal women [7], and that chronological age is a poor indicator of reproductive aging, defining the menopausal transition has presented a challenge to clinicians as

S. Morelli (✉)
Department of Obstetrics, Gynecology and Women's Health, University of Medicine and Dentistry of New Jersey, Newark, NJ, USA
e-mail: morellsa@umdnj.edu

N.F. Santoro and G. Neal-Perry (eds.), *Amenorrhea: A Case-Based, Clinical Guide*, Contemporary Endocrinology, DOI 10.1007/978-1-60327-864-5_9,

well as the scientific community. The World Health Organization (WHO) presently defines the perimenopause as the "period immediately before the menopause (when the endocrinological, biological, and clinical features of approaching menopause commence) and the first year after menopause" [8]. According to the Massachusetts Women's Health Study, one of the largest longitudinal studies that investigated a method for defining perimenopause based on self-reported data in 1,550 women over 5 years, the two findings that best define the perimenopause are increased menstrual irregularity and 3–11 months of amenorrhea [9].

These definitions still do not clearly define the commencement and natural history of the perimenopause. In 2001, participants of the Stages of Reproductive Aging Workshop (STRAW) convened in order "to address the absence of a relevant staging system for female reproductive aging and to discuss the confusing current nomenclature for the perimenopause" [7]. The workshop's aim was to develop a general staging system for healthy women. The proposed criteria were deemed unsuitable for application in cigarette smokers, women at extremes of body weight (BMI <18 kg/m^2 or >30 kg/m^2), heavy aerobic exercisers (>10 h/week), women with chronic menstrual cycle irregularity, women with previous hysterectomy, or those with abnormal uterine or ovarian anatomy (e.g., fibroids, endometriomas).

As defined by STRAW, reproductive and postreproductive life are divided into seven stages (Fig. 9.1), with the menopausal transition accounting for two of those stages. The stages are anchored around the FMP, defined as the last period preceding 12 months of amenorrhea. They are primarily based on the characteristics of the menstrual cycle and secondarily on follicular phase follicle stimulating hormone (FSH) levels. Stages −5 to −3 span the reproductive years; stages −2 and −1 make up the menopausal transition; and stages +1 and +2 are early and late postmenopause. The age range and duration of each of these stages vary. In fact, not everyone transitions through the described sequence.

There is no clear delineation between the early, peak, and late reproductive stages (stages −5 to −3). An elevated FSH level (defined as an early follicular phase

Final Menstrual Period (FMP)

Stages:	−5	−4	−3	−2	−1	0	+1	+2
Terminology:	Reproductive			Menopausal Transition			Postmenopause	
	Early	Peak	Late	Early	Late*		Early*	Late
				Perimenopasue				
Duration of Stage:	Variable			Variable		(a) 1 yr	(b) 4 yrs	until demise
Menstrual Cycles:	variable to regular	regular		variable cycle length (>7 days different from normal)	≥2 skipped cycles and an interval of amenorrhea (≥60days)	Amen x 12 mos	none	
Endocrine:	normal FSH		↑ FSH	↑ FSH			↑ FSH	

*Stages most likely to be characterized by vasomotor symptoms ↑ = elevated

Fig. 9.1 The STRAW staging system. Reprinted from Soules et al. [7], Fig. 1

level that exceeds 2 SDs of the mean level for a sample of normal women of peak reproductive age [25–30 years], often defined by clinicians as ≥10 mIU/mL) is the first measurable sign of reproductive aging and characterizes stage −3. According to STRAW, a single elevated FSH level is sufficient to categorize a woman as stage −3 and does not require repeating. However, there is significant intercycle variability in early follicular phase FSH levels, and a normal level in a 40- to 45-year-old woman may warrant a second measurement. The early follicular phase serum estradiol (E2) level in the late reproductive stage may be either normal or elevated. Elevated E2 levels may lower FSH levels due to negative feedback at the level of the pituitary; thus, FSH levels cannot be interpreted if E2 is over 80 pg/ml.

The early menopausal transition (stage −2) is characterized by more variable menstrual cycles, whereby the intermenstrual interval changes by seven days or more. The late menopausal transition (stage −1) is characterized by two or more skipped menstrual cycles and at least one intermenstrual interval of at least 60 days in length. Stage 0 is marked by the FMP, followed by 12 months of amenorrhea.

STRAW was the first to recognize that subtle changes in the menstrual cycle are important early markers of the menopausal transition. However, in 2005, Gracia et al. [10] proposed a stricter staging system to distinguish among women with even more subtle changes in cycle length. This system (PENN-5, Penn Ovarian Aging Study) incorporates an additional stage termed the "late premenopause," and redefines the early and late menopausal transition (Table 9.1). The authors used a difference in mean serum reproductive hormone values obtained during the early follicular phase (cycle day 4) to validate their definitions of menopausal status. Significant differences in FSH (8.7 vs. 9.4 mIU/mL, $p=0.04$) and inhibin B (44.9 vs. 39.0 pg/mL, $p=0.003$) were detected between the premenopausal and late premenopausal stages, respectively, as well as between the late premenopausal and early transition stages. Thus, women with only one cycle length change of ≥7 days were distinguished from women with two or more cycle length changes, supporting the notion that early and subtle changes in cycle length reflect significant underlying hormonal changes among women in the earliest phases of the menopausal transition. Of note, differences in

Table 9.1 Menopausal status definitions

STRAW definition		PENN-5 definition	
Premenopause (Stages −5 to −3)	Regular cycles, with no change in cycle length	Premenopause	Regular cycles, with no change in cycle length
Early Transition (Stage −2)	1 cycle length change (≥7 days)	Late Premenopause	1 cycle length change (≥7 days)
		Early Transition	≥2 cycle length changes (≥7 days)
Late Transition (Stage −1)	2–11 months of amenorrhea	Late Transition	3–11 months of amenorrhea
Postmenopause Transition (Stage +1, +2)	≥12 months of amenorrhea	Postmenopause	≥12 months of amenorrhea

Adapted from Gracia et al. [10], Defining menopause status: creation of a new definition to identify the early changes of the menopausal trasition. Menopause 2005.

luteinizing hormone (LH) and E2 levels between the earliest stages did not reach statistical significance. A more in depth review of reproductive hormonal patterns characterizing the menopausal transition will follow later in the chapter.

Ovarian Follicular Depletion is the Primary Driver of the Menopausal Transition

Follicle numbers as well as ovarian volume decrease over the course of reproductive aging. The declining number of primordial follicles over time may be reflected by a decreased size of the antral follicle cohort from which the monthly ovulatory follicle is selected. The number of antral follicles (between 2 and 10 mm on transvaginal ultrasound) has been reported to decrease progressively in women over an age range of 25–46 years [11]. In this study, the antral follicle count measured in the early follicular phase exhibited a mean yearly decline of 4.8% prior to age 37 years, and accelerated to a yearly decline rate of 11.7% thereafter. Additional studies utilizing transvaginal ultrasonography in the early follicular phase confirm the finding of reduced antral follicle counts in older reproductive-aged [12] and menopausal [13] women.

Histologic evidence for accelerated follicular depletion with reproductive aging was provided by a 1987 study by Richardson et al. [14] in which primordial follicle numbers were counted in one ovary obtained from each of 17 healthy women aged 45–55 years undergoing elective total abdominal hysterectomy with salpingo-oophorectomy. Women were divided into three groups: (1) premenopausal (regular menstrual cycles, $n=6$), (2) women undergoing the menopausal transition (defined as the presence of irregular menses with intervals of less than 3 or more than 6 weeks for at least 1 year with or without hot flashes, $n=7$), and (3) postmenopausal (>1 year since last menses, $n=4$). The mean ages of the three groups were similar. The mean number of primordial follicles in premenopausal women was tenfold higher than that in women undergoing the menopausal transition ($1,392 \pm 355$ vs. 142 ± 72, respectively). Follicles were virtually absent in the four postmenopausal ovaries examined; one primordial follicle was identified in one ovary. The data illustrated the dramatic acceleration of follicular depletion which occurs in the last decade of the reproductive years, and "support the view that declining follicular reserve is the immediate cause of both the perimenopausal and menopausal transitions" [14]. However, compelling evidence for independent effects of reproductive aging on the hypothalamic-pituitary-gonadal axis (beyond its release from the negative feedback of ovarian steroids and inhibin due to follicular depletion) exists and will be discussed later in the chapter.

Mullerian inhibiting substance (MIS), also known as anti-mullerian hormone (AMH), is a product of the granulosa cells of primary, secondary, and antral follicles, and is not involved in negative feedback regulation of gonadotropin secretion. It has gained recent attention as a marker of the primordial follicle pool and a predictor for the occurrence of the menopausal transition. The observation that serum

MIS declines detectably over time in younger women still having regular menstrual cycles (prior to the detection of changes in FSH or antral follicle count) illustrates the potential advantage of MIS as an early predictor of declining ovarian reserve [15]. Limitations of its measurement, however, include the inadequate sensitivity of currently available assays to permit accurate assessment of MIS in the years immediately preceding menopause. As women progress to the later stages of the transition, levels of MIS become too low to be detectable [16], and MIS cannot be detected in postmenopausal women [15].

Endocrine Changes in the Menopausal Transition

In 1975, Sherman and Korenman [17] were among the first to describe endocrine changes occurring with advanced reproductive age. The authors collected daily blood samples during several cycles from regularly cycling women (aged 40–41 years, 46–51 years, and a control group aged 18–30 years). The shortest cycle length was observed in the oldest group (mean cycle length 23.5 days in 46- to 51-year olds vs. 30 days in the control group), the shortening being due to a shorter interval between the onset of menses and the LH peak. The authors observed lower serum E2 levels and higher FSH levels throughout the menstrual cycle in the oldest group, "despite the attainment of levels of E2 that might be expected to suppress its secretion, while LH remained indistinguishable from normal" [17]. The finding of a monotropic rise in FSH (but not LH) secretion in the oldest age group led the authors to hypothesize that an ovarian hormone must exist which exerts negative feedback inhibition specifically on FSH secretion by the pituitary, and that this hormone decreases in the late reproductive years due to diminished ovarian follicle number. This hormone was later characterized as inhibin [18].

In the 1980s, Metcalf et al. [19–22] carried out a longitudinal study of weekly hormone secretion in older (median age 42 years) and younger (median age 33 years) women which illustrated the unpredictable hormonal patterns of those undergoing the menopausal transition. In 31 women in the early transition according to STRAW criteria, median cycle length was 29 days (range 18–260 days) with only 52% of cycles being ovulatory. Notably, ovulatory cycles were noted at all stages of the menopausal transition. The authors noted both persistently low and persistently increased urinary estrogen excretion, as well as the sporadic appearance of persistently high FSH and LH levels sometimes associated with high estrogen levels. As stated by the authors, "menstrual cycles in perimenopausal women…are richly varied. Unpredictability is the norm, in marked contrast to the regular succession of ovulatory cycles observed in premenopausal women" [20]. Eight women (aged 44–55 years) were followed during the 6 months following the FMP and exhibited hormonal patterns which were indistinguishable from those observed in the long anovulatory cycles of the menopausal transition. In contrast, older postmenopausal women (aged 57–67 years) exhibited consistently high gonadotropin and low estrogen levels consistent with ovarian failure.

In a similar effort to characterize endocrine features of the perimenopause, Santoro et al. [23] collected daily urinary samples for 12 months on 6 cycling women aged 47 years or older as well as daily samples for a single cycle on 15 women aged 43–47 years. The authors compared menstrual and hormonal patterns in these perimenopausal women to those in midreproductive (aged 19–38 years) and postmenopausal women (aged 54–79 years). Similar to the findings of Sherman and Korenman [17], these authors also demonstrated shorter cycles in perimenopausal women when compared with midreproductive-aged women due to a shortened follicular phase. In contrast, however, overall estrone (E1) conjugate excretion was greater in perimenopausal than in midreproductive-aged women during both follicular and luteal phases. Although others have similarly demonstrated prolonged episodes of unopposed estrogen secretion in women approaching menopause [24], this study was the first to demonstrate significant hyperestrogenemia in ovulatory perimenopausal cycles, a finding that is consistent with the clinical findings of endometrial hyperplasia, enlarging leiomyomata, and dysfunctional bleeding that becomes more prevalent during the perimenopause. These authors also demonstrated elevated gonadotropins (particularly FSH), most pronounced in the early follicular phase, and diminished pregnanediol excretion in the luteal phase of perimenopausal women when compared with that in midreproductive-aged women. Postmenopausal women were found to have tonically elevated LH and FSH and persistently low E1 conjugate excretion. Periods of hypergonadotropic hypoestrogenism were similarly found in some perimenopausal women, becoming more common with proximity to the FMP. In addition to hypergonadotropic hypogonadism, however, perimenopausal cycles can manifest other types of patterns. Elevated gonadotropins with normal estrogen excretion, indicating a failure of negative feedback of estrogen on the hypothalamic-pituitary axis, and failure of estrogen's biphasic, positive feedback on the hypothalamic-pituitary axis have been described [3].

Although the menopausal transition is characterized by menstrual irregularity with interspersed ovulatory and anovulatory cycles, elongated cycles become more frequent and longer in duration as menopause approaches [25]. Miro et al. [26] undertook a study of urinary hormonal profiles during 289 elongated cycles of 34 women undergoing the menopausal transition, STRAW stages −2 to −1. These authors described the concept of estrogen take-off (ETO), a measure of onset of ovarian response to FSH during the follicular phase, defined as time between cycle day 1 and the start of first sustained rise in urinary estrone 3-glucuronide (E1G). The authors demonstrated that elongation of the menstrual cycle is fundamentally the result of a delay in ovarian response (longer ETO), and that this was due to a temporary lack of responsiveness to FSH rather than inadequate FSH stimulus from the pituitary, as they reported an association between longer ETO and higher FSH levels. Similar to the findings of Santoro et al. [23], the authors demonstrated a decline in luteal progesterone synthesis, which correlated with increasing ETO. In the SWAN (Study of Women's Health Across the Nation, a multiethnic observational cohort study of the menopausal transition in 3,302 women aged 42–52 years at seven US sites) study, examination of luteal progesterone excretion over time indicated a progressive decrease [27].

Several studies have investigated ethnic differences in serum FSH and E2 in women undergoing the menopausal transition. A cross-sectional analysis of early follicular serum E2 and FSH concentrations in early perimenopausal patients in the SWAN study reported higher serum FSH levels in African–American and Hispanic women compared with that in Caucasians, but no ethnic differences in E2 levels after adjustment for other factors such as BMI [28]. FSH differences with comparable E2 levels suggest ethnic differences in the pituitary-ovarian relationship during the menopausal transition. A subsequent longitudinal study on SWAN participants evaluated early follicular serum E2 and FSH during three consecutive annual visits [29]. Similar patterns in the decline of E2 and the increase in FSH were found across ethnic groups, but hormone levels differed by race/ethnicity. Consistent with the prior study, African–American women had higher FSH levels but similar E2 levels when compared with Caucasians, whereas Chinese and Japanese women had lower E2 levels but comparable FSH levels. These ethnic differences in E2 and FSH were independent of menopausal status and were indeed suggestive of ethnic differences in the pituitary-ovarian axis.

Markers of ovarian reserve also appear to vary with BMI. A cross-sectional study of 36 women aged 40–52 years found that mean AMH levels (but not FSH, E2, or antral follicle counts) were significantly lower in obese women (BMI $\geq 30\ kg/m^2$) compared with those in normal weight women (BMI $<25\ kg/m^2$) [30]. However, Randolph et al. found in a larger longitudinal cohort study [29] that increasing BMI was associated with increasing E2 and decreasing FSH levels in late perimenopausal and postmenopausal women.

Inhibin and Reproductive Aging

Inhibin is a dimeric glycoprotein composed of an α (alpha)-subunit and a β (beta) A-subunit (inhibin A) or β (beta) B-subunit (inhibin B). During the normal menstrual cycle, inhibin B (a product of antral follicle granulosa cells) is highest in the early to midfollicular phase and decreases in the late follicular phase [31]. Inhibin A is a product of the preovulatory follicle and corpus luteum, and is thus highest in the late follicular and midluteal phases [31]. Production of ovarian inhibin B (and E2) is stimulated by the gonadotropins, and during the follicular phase, inhibin B appears to be the major negative regulator of FSH secretion. The fall in inhibin B in late reproductive age has been shown to trigger the monotropic rise in follicular phase FSH [32].

To evaluate the role of inhibin in reproductive aging, MacNaughton et al. [33] studied serum levels of immunoreactive inhibin in regularly cycling women aged 21–49 years during the early follicular (cycle days 4–7) and midluteal phases (3–12 days prior to menses). Mean follicular phase levels of immunoreactive inhibin were significantly lower in the oldest age group than those in the younger age groups (128 U/l in the 45–49 years age group vs. 239, 235, and 207 U/l in the 20–29, 30–39, and 40–44 years age groups, respectively ($p<0.05$)), while mean FSH levels were significantly higher in the oldest age group. Conversely, the authors found no difference in E2 levels between the oldest and youngest age groups, and LH levels did not differ significantly with age. These results illustrated the concept of differential feedback. The authors postulated that decreasing inhibin levels with age reflected diminished folliculogenesis with approaching menopause.

The availability of assays specific for the inhibin dimers allowed subsequent investigations into the role of each in the endocrinology of the menopausal transition. Klein et al. [34] studied follicular phase secretion of inhibin A and B in older (aged 40–45 years) and younger (aged 20–25 years) ovulatory women and demonstrated that the monotropic rise in FSH seen in older ovulatory women was associated with a decrease in follicular phase levels of inhibin B but not inhibin A. Burger et al. [32] demonstrated similar findings in women undergoing the menopausal transition. These authors studied serum immunoreactive inhibin, inhibin A, inhibin B, FSH, and E2 levels from the follicular phase (or at random in those with >3 months of amenorrhea) of women aged 48–59 years. Women were divided into four menopausal stages (stage 1, premenopausal; stage 2, early perimenopausal [reported change in menstrual cycle frequency in the preceding year with a bleed in the preceding 3 months); stage 3, late perimenopausal [no menses in the preceding 3–11 months]; and stage 4, postmenopausal). FSH rose progressively and immunoreactive inhibin fell progressively with menopausal status, each demonstrating a significant change between early and late perimenopause. The authors demonstrated a significant decline in inhibin B (from 48 to 13.5 ng/l, $p<0.05$) at early perimenopause, which preceded a decline in inhibin A and E2 at late perimenopause (52% and 71% decline from premenopausal levels, $p<0.05$ for both) (Fig. 9.2). Thus, the authors demonstrated that falling inhibin B levels (reflecting a decrease in the size of the primary and early antral follicles) are the important factor in allowing the rise in FSH in older regularly cycling women, whereas inhibin A levels are preserved until late in the menopausal transition. It is important to keep in mind, however, that these hormone measurements have all been made in the early follicular phase of the menstrual cycle, and thus inhibin A levels do not truly reflect maximal secretion of this hormone, as it is primarily a product of the dominant follicle and corpus luteum.

Muttukrishna et al. [35] compared daily serum hormone levels drawn throughout the menstrual cycle in young cycling women (aged 25–32 years) with those of older cycling women (aged 40–50 years) who were subdivided by early follicular phase FSH levels (FSH <8 vs. FSH >8). Young and older women with normal FSH levels exhibited similar patterns of inhibins A and B throughout the cycle. However, older women with elevated basal FSH levels had significantly lower concentrations of inhibin A prior to the LH surge and in the mid-luteal phase, and lower concentrations of inhibin B in the early follicular phase than older women with normal basal FSH levels. The authors concluded that the rise in early follicular phase serum FSH in older women was associated with decreased early follicular phase inhibin B levels, but postulated that lower luteal phase inhibin A levels may also contribute to the rise in early follicular phase FSH levels in women of advanced reproductive age.

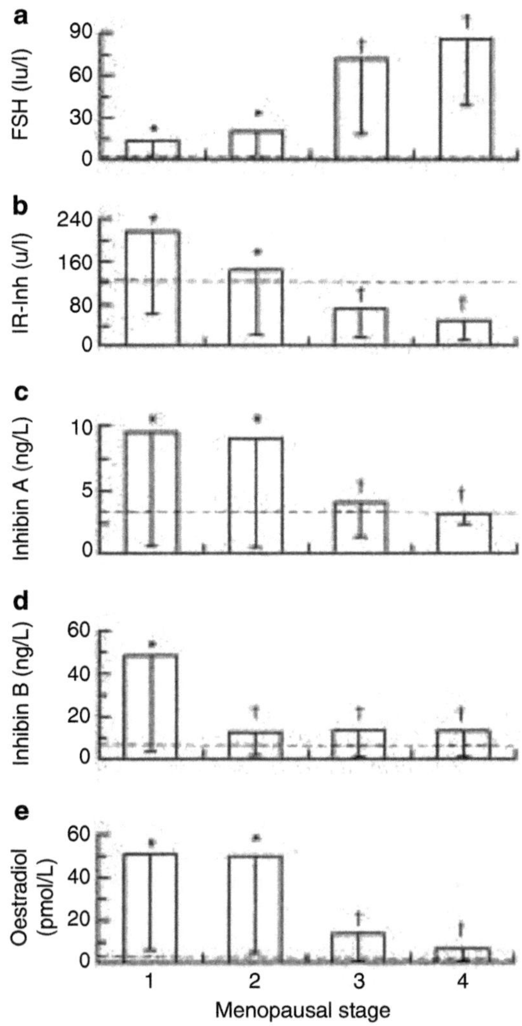

Fig. 9.2 Geometric mean levels (with lower 95% confidence intervals) of (**a**) FSH, (**b**) IR-INH, (**c**) INH-A, (**d**) INH-B, and (**e**) E2 as a function of menopausal status. Menopausal stages as given in text. Values with the same superscript (*asterisk* or *dagger*) are not statistically different; values with differing superscripts are different, $p<0.05$. Reprinted from Burger et al. [32], Fig. 1

Similarly, Santoro et al. [36] and Welt et al. [37] demonstrated lower luteal inhibin A levels in older (aged 43–47 years) vs. younger (aged 19–38 years) cycling women (668 ± 72 vs. 1152 ± 216 total pg, respectively, $p=0.03$) and concluded that lack of negative feedback by both inhibin A and inhibin B may contribute to the FSH rise associated with reproductive aging. These authors and others [38] also demonstrated that activin A levels were significantly elevated throughout the cycle in older women when compared with younger women (21 ± 2 vs. 11 ± 1 total nanogram,

$p < 0.005$), and postulated that activin A may also play an endocrine role in maintaining elevated FSH in older reproductive-aged women. Activin A, a homodimer of the inhibin A β (beta)-subunits, appears capable of direct stimulation of pituitary FSH secretion [39].

Collectively, these studies illustrate that it is primarily a decrease in inhibin B (a reflection of the diminishing ovarian follicular pool) that is the major peptide feedback factor causing a monotropic rise in FSH with advancing reproductive age. However, a decrease in inhibin A after ovulation, manifested later in the menopausal transition, may also be contributory.

Alterations in the Hypothalamic-Pituitary-Ovarian (HPO) Axis with Reproductive Aging

The onset of menopause in humans is related not only to oocyte depletion and ovarian failure, but also to alterations in hypothalamic-pituitary feedback. In 1978, Van Look et al. [40] reported that women of reproductive age with anovulatory dysfunctional uterine bleeding failed to exhibit a normal LH response to an exogenous E2 challenge, supporting the hypothesis that the pathophysiologic defect in these women may be a decrease of hypothalamic sensitivity to positive feedback. The subsequent findings of the Daily Hormone Study (DHS) [3, 41], a substudy of SWAN, supported this notion in its examination of women experiencing anovulatory cycles during the menopausal transition. The authors measured daily urinary LH, FSH, E1 conjugates, and the progesterone urinary metabolite pregnanediol glucuronide (Pdg) over the course of one menstrual cycle ending in bleeding (or up to 50 days in the absence of a menstrual period). In some women, a rise in estrogen followed by an LH surge was observed; however, the absence of ovulation in these cycles (as documented by a lack of threefold increase in Pdg concentrations above a nadir for at least 3 days) indicated a defect at the ovarian level. However, the authors also reported frequent anovulatory cycles in perimenopausal women in which estrogen peaks were equivalent to those that result in LH surges in younger women, yet no LH surges occurred (Fig. 9.3). This finding suggests unresponsiveness of the hypothalamic-pituitary axis to an estrogen peak in older perimenopausal women (failure of "positive feedback"). In other anovulatory cycles, follicular phase estrogen levels similar to those in younger women did not lower LH secretion as occurs in cycles of younger women, indicating decreased negative feedback of estrogen on LH secretion. Collectively, the authors' findings supported the hypothesis that "there is a relative hypothalamic-pituitary insensitivity to estrogen in aging women" [3] with failure of both positive and negative feedback mechanisms.

Although gonadotropins are higher in perimenopausal women than in premenopausal women, levels decline with advancing age after menopause. In contrast, GnRH secretion appears to increase with age in postmenopausal women [42],

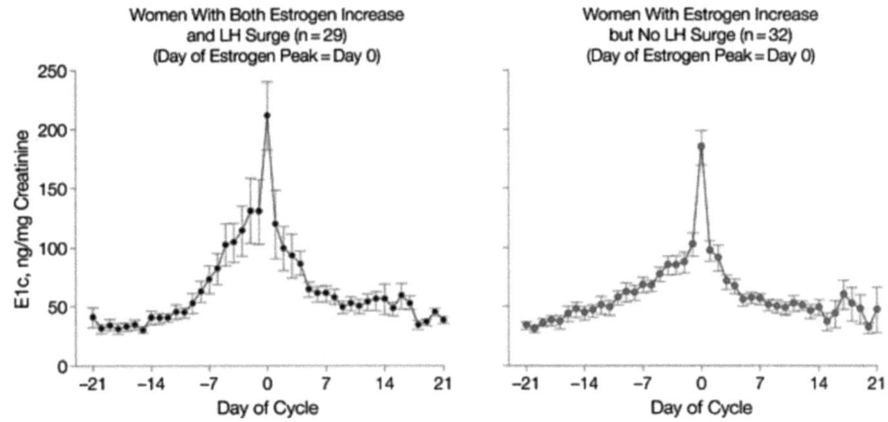

Fig. 9.3 Daily urinary E1c levels in anovulatory older reproductive-age women with estrogen increases. Comparison of E1c levels (estrone conjugates) in women who had an LH surge (*left panel*) vs. those who did not (*right panel*). E1c levels (mean (SEM)) for women with both estrogen increases and LH surges are shown here, where day 0 is the day of maximum E1c. Reprinted from Weiss et al. [3], Fig. 2

which suggests that the pituitary is less responsive to GnRH in older compared with younger postmenopausal women. Gill et al. [42] studied 13 young (aged 45–55 years) and 11 old (70–80 years) postmenopausal women in an effort to investigate the effect of age (and gonadal steroid feedback with administration of exogenous estrogen or estrogen plus progesterone) on GnRH secretion by the hypothalamus in postmenopausal women. At baseline, mean LH and FSH levels were significantly lower in older compared with younger postmenopausal women. Percent inhibition of LH following administration of a fixed, submaximal dose of a GnRH antagonist decreased with age, implying an increase in endogenous GnRH secretion with age. With estrogen and progesterone treatment, mean FSH and LH levels decreased significantly and to a similar degree in both young and old postmenopausal women, implying that responsiveness to gonadal steroid negative feedback at the hypothalamus is maintained with aging. This differs from the previously described findings of the DHS [3] in which a lack of estrogen-negative feedback on LH secretion was seen in a subset of women. This may be explained by the shorter duration of estrogen exposure during the menstrual cycles of women in the DHS compared with that used in the protocol used by Gill et al. [42].

Symptoms of the Menopausal Transition

Whereas some women may experience few or no symptoms during the menopausal transition, many experience a variety of troublesome and sometimes disabling symptoms. These include hot flashes, night sweats, vaginal dryness and painful intercourse, sleep problems, mood and cognitive problems, somatic symptoms, urinary incontinence, bleeding problems, sexual dysfunction, and overall decreased quality of life [43]. Although commonly attributed to menopause, it is a challenge to discern whether these symptoms are truly associated with the hormonal changes of the menopausal transition rather than with aging in general. A 2005 report from the National Institutes of Health highlighted the paucity of scientific data on menopausal symptoms and concluded that although considerable evidence supports the association of vasomotor symptoms, vaginal dryness, and sleep disturbances with menopausal status, there is less information about whether other symptoms such as mood changes, cognitive dysfunction, urinary incontinence, sexual dysfunction, neuromuscular complaints, and overall quality of life are associated with menopausal stage [43].

The Penn Ovarian Aging Study studied 404 women of a mean age of 42.3 years spanning all stages of the menopausal transition over 9 years of follow-up [43]. After adjustment for various risk factors for menopausal symptoms such as age, race, BMI, smoking, and history of depression, the authors found that menopausal stage was significantly associated with hot flashes, aches, joint pain, stiffness, and depressed mood. The risk of hot flashes increased throughout the menopausal transition and was greatest in the postmenopausal group (OR 2.87, 95% CI 1.76–4.87, $p<0.001$). The risk of depression was greatest in the late premenopausal stage (STRAW −3), and depressed mood decreased postmenopause. There was no significant association of menopausal stage with poor sleep, decreased libido, or vaginal dryness. Perceived stress was significantly associated with all menopausal symptoms. Others have found a similar association with perceived stress, as well as an overall increase in symptom reporting in women of low SES [45].

Increased FSH levels, decreased levels of inhibin B, and within-woman fluctuations of E2 (all measured during early follicular phase) were significantly and independently associated with menopausal symptoms.

A follow-up study of the same cohort of women [46] assessed headache, irritability, mood swings, anxiety, and concentration difficulties over the menopausal transition. Of these symptoms, only headache was associated with menopausal stage, and significantly decreased after menopause. Mean FSH levels were inversely associated with mood swings and mean testosterone levels were associated with irritability (p value for both <0.01), indicating a decrease in symptoms as hormone levels increased around menopause. Again, perceived stress independently correlated with all symptoms in the study.

A longitudinal Australian population-based study of 438 women aged 45–55 years followed over 7 years [47] found that the symptoms that were specifically related to hormonal changes during the menopausal transition were vasomotor symptoms, vaginal dryness, and breast tenderness. Hot flashes, night sweats, and vaginal dryness increased and breast tenderness decreased concurrent with the significant drop in E2 levels and rise in FSH levels found in the late menopausal transition. Difficulty in sleeping did not appear to be a direct effect of menopausal hormonal changes, but was predicted by hot flashes and psychosocial factors such as depression.

Hot Flashes

Hot flashes and night sweats (collectively known as vasomotor symptoms) are reported with high frequency (up to 80%) in women during the menopausal transition [43]. They manifest as a transient sensation of heat with or without objective signs of skin vasodilation accompanied by variable degrees of flushing, sweating, palpitations, anxiety, irritability, and even panic [48]. The timing of their appearance in relation to the FMP varies by study; whereas one group reported an acceleration in prevalence of hot flashes during the menopausal transition to peak at about the time of the FMP [4], others have reported the greatest frequency 3 months or more after the FMP [49]. A prospective longitudinal study of 57 Norwegian women undergoing the menopausal transition reported a peak prevalence of hot flashes during the first year following the FMP [50]. Some report that these symptoms generally subside within 1 year [51], whereas others have reported a mean duration of approximately 5 years in both estrogen users and non-users [52].

A number of longitudinal cohort studies including both SWAN [41, 53] and the Penn Ovarian Aging Study [44, 54] have found that African–American women are more likely than white women to report hot flashes. A population-based study of women aged 45–54 years [54] also revealed that African–American women were more likely than Caucasian women to report any hot flashes (RR=2.08), severe hot flashes (RR=2.19), and hot flashes for more than 5 years (RR=1.61). The reasons for this are unknown, but may be due to racial differences in a number of risk factors for hot flashes, including high BMI, current smoking, less than 12 drinks in the past year, and lower estrogen levels [55]. Indeed, obesity and smoking have been reported to increase the risk for hot flashes [56–59].

The physiologic mechanism for the initiation of flashes is not entirely understood. A growing body of evidence supports the hypothesis that flashes result from a physiologic response to a marked narrowing of hypothalamic thermoregulatory set point or neutral zone, which increases the sensation of intense heat in response to internal and environmental triggers (Fig. 9.4). The exact trigger that induces this change in the hypothalamic thermoregulatory set point during menopause is not completely understood.

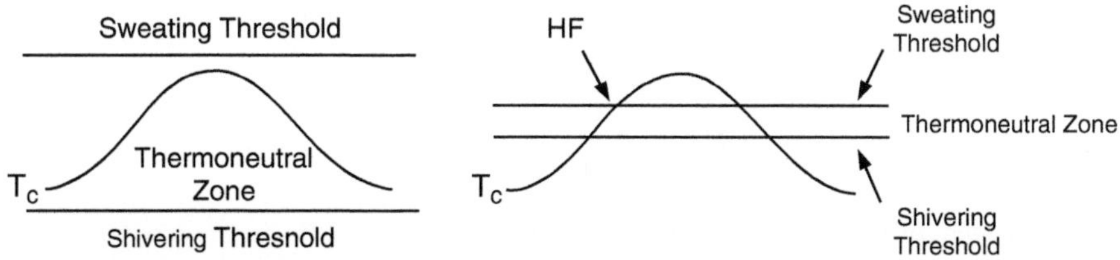

Fig. 9.4 Small core body temperature (Tc) elevations that act within a reduced thermoneutral zone trigger hot flashes in symptomatic postmenopausal women. Reprinted from Freedman [69], Fig. 3

The withdrawal (or decrease in levels) of estrogen, rather than hypoestrogenism per se, appears to precipitate menopausal flashes [47, 49]. However, estrogen withdrawal alone does not explain the cause of vasomotor symptoms, as evidenced by the observation that there is no significant correlation between plasma hormone levels and the occurrence of vasomotor symptoms [60]. Furthermore, 73% of women experience vasomotor symptoms prior to menopause, which may occur during both ovulatory and anovulatory cycles [61]. Data from the SWAN study revealed that most of the premenopausal women experiencing vasomotor symptoms had estrogen secretion that was similar in quantity to or higher than the estrogen secretion of younger women, and revealed no relationship between hot flashes and ambient hormones [61].

A temporal relationship between pulsatile release of LH and initiation of menopausal flashes has been clearly demonstrated [62] (Fig. 9.5). However, it is not LH release by the pituitary itself which directly causes the flashes, as demonstrated by

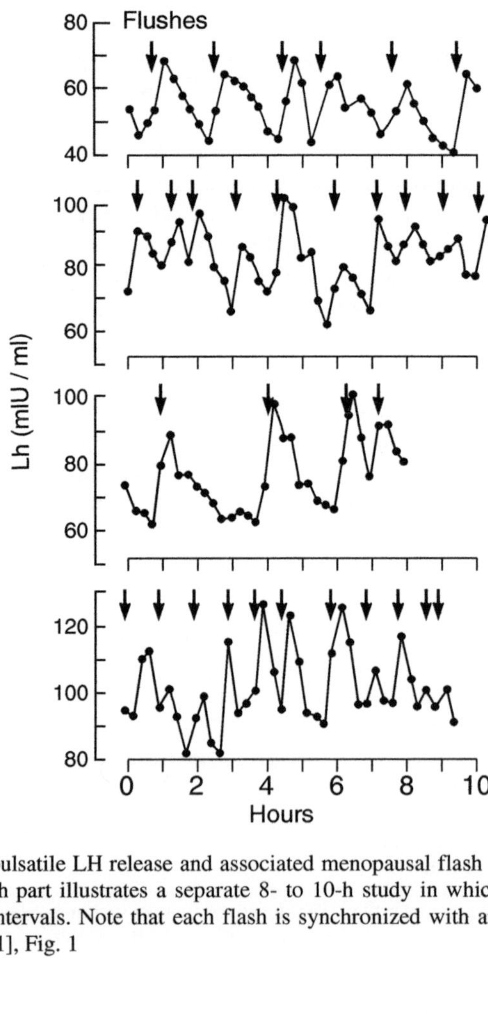

Fig. 9.5 Pattern of pulsatile LH release and associated menopausal flash episodes. *Arrows* indicate flash onset. Each part illustrates a separate 8- to 10-h study in which blood samples were obtained at 15-min intervals. Note that each flash is synchronized with an LH pulse. Reprinted from Casper et al. [61], Fig. 1

the presence of menopausal flashes in hypophysectomized women [63]. Furthermore, studies in which a GnRH agonist was administered to menopausal women with frequent hot flashes demonstrated the complete suppression of LH and FSH pulses, but no changes in frequency or severity of flash episodes [64]. Thus, a hypothalamic mechanism likely initiates both the pulsatile release of LH and flash episodes [62]. A study of serum levels of pituitary hormones during severe menopausal flashes demonstrated a significant rise in growth hormone, LH, and ACTH but not prolactin, TSH, or FSH [65]. Given that norepinephrine is the neurotransmitter believed to be the predominant hypothalamic stimulus of pituitary growth hormone [66], pulsatile LH release [67], and heat dissipation [68], the authors hypothesized that increased hypothalamic norepinephrine activity due to ovarian failure is the "neuroendocrine link between estrogen deficiency and cyclic activation of adjacent thermoregulatory neurons" [65].

Estrogen withdrawal may also be correlated with a decline in circulating levels of serotonin, another neurotransmitter that appears to play a central role in the pathophysiology of hot flashes [69]. This decline may increase the sensitivity of hypothalamic serotonin (5-HT_{2A}) receptors and may also contribute to a narrowing of the thermoregulatory neutral zone [70]. Similarly, animal studies report that increased CNS levels of norepinephrine are associated with a narrowing of the thermoregulatory neutral zone [71]. Thus, instability in both serotonin and norepinephrine levels during menopause (as a result of estrogen withdrawal) appears to contribute to increased risk of hot flashes.

Estrogen, by itself or with progestins, is the most consistently effective therapy for the treatment of vasomotor symptoms [43]. Concerns regarding the use of hormone therapy arose from the findings of the Women's Health Initiative (WHI) [72, 73], a large prospective randomized study designed to evaluate the effect of hormone therapy on the incidence of cardiovascular disease and other adverse outcomes. Although this trial was not designed to evaluate the efficacy of hormone therapy in the treatment of menopausal symptoms, excluded perimenopausal women, and thus was not carried out on a study population representative of most who seek hormone therapy for menopausal symptoms, data from the WHI have been widely interpreted as demonstrating an unfavorable risk-to-benefit ratio for hormone therapy – *regardless of its timing or indication.* This is a most unfortunate outcome of the study, as the presence of menopausal symptoms tips the risk-to-benefit ratio for hormone therapy in a favorable direction for many, if not most women, favoring its short-term use.

Hormone therapy (combined conjugated equine estrogen (CEE) 0.625 mg/day plus medroxyprogesterone acetate (MPA) 2.5 mg/day) was not found to reduce the incidence of cardiovascular disease after 5.2 years of follow-up [73], at which time the estrogen–progestin trial was terminated. Whereas an increased risk of breast cancer was reported with estrogen–progestin therapy (HR 1.24, $p<0.001$) [74], the use of 0.625 mg/day CEE alone in women with previous hysterectomy revealed no increased risk of breast cancer [75]. An increased risk of stroke (12 additional strokes per 10,000 person-years), however, was reported in the estrogen-only arm [75]. Other known risks of hormonal therapy include a twofold to threefold increased risk of venous thromboembolism and an increased risk of gall bladder disease [76].

Absolute contraindications for hormone therapy include undiagnosed vaginal bleeding, active thromboembolic disease, and active breast cancer [76]. The risks of hormone therapy in those without absolute contraindications must be balanced against the benefits, which include excellent control of vasomotor symptoms, treatment of genitourinary atrophy, and preservation of bone health. In assessing the patient for potential hormone therapy vs. nonhormonal options, one must consider factors such as personal history, family history, social history, and current medication use. Thromboembolic risk, cancer (including breast cancer) risk, cardiovascular health (including blood pressure, lipid profile, and tobacco use), bone density, vaginal health, urinary symptoms, and sexual function must all be taken into account.

In women with intact uteri, the use of estrogens with either cyclic or continuous progestins has been shown to relieve vasomotor symptoms and vaginal atrophy [77, 78]. The Postmenopausal Estrogen/Progestin Interventions Trial [77], a randomized, double-blind, placebo-controlled trial conducted in 875 postmenopausal women, evaluated the effect of 0.625 mg CEE alone or in combination with (1) 10 mg MPA given cyclically, (2) 2.5 mg MPA daily, or (3) 200 mg micronized progesterone given cyclically. At both 1 and 3 years of treatment, all treatment groups demonstrated a statistically significant protective effect against vasomotor symptoms compared with placebo. Women with more severe vasomotor symptoms at baseline experienced a greater treatment effect. Breast discomfort was significantly more common in those treated with progestins.

The Women's Health, Osteoporosis, Progestin, Estrogen (HOPE) study, a randomized, double-blind, placebo-controlled trial conducted in 2,673 postmenopausal women, demonstrated that lower doses of CEE with daily MPA (lowest dose 0.3 mg CEE with 1.5 mg MPA) provide significant relief in vasomotor symptoms and vaginal atrophy above placebo and as effectively as commonly prescribed doses (0.625 mg CEE/2.5 mg MPA) [78]. These lower doses also confer endometrial protection comparable to that of standard dose regimens [79], with higher rates of amenorrhea [80] and more favorable changes in lipids, lipoproteins, and hemostatic factors, with minimal changes in carbohydrate metabolism [81] after 1–2 years of therapy.

A randomized, double-blind, placebo-controlled study of the lowest doses of transdermal estrogen available (0.023 mg/day 17β-estradiol and 0.0075 mg/day levonorgestrel or 0.014 mg/day 17β-estradiol alone) revealed a significant reduction in frequency of moderate and severe hot flashes after 12 weeks of treatment [82]. After 2 years of therapy, use of the 0.014 mg/day 17β-estradiol patch alone in women with intact uteri revealed similar rates of endometrial hyperplasia, endometrial proliferation, and vaginal bleeding when compared to placebo [83], with significant increase in bone mineral density (BMD) above placebo [84].

Although not generalizable to short-term treatment of a younger perimenopausal population, the results of the WHI dramatically increased the interest of patients and healthcare practitioners in nonhormonal therapies for menopausal symptoms.

Centrally acting agents that have been studied include the selective serotonin reuptake inhibitors (SSRIs), serotonin-norepinephrine reuptake inhibitors (SNRIs), clonidine, and gabapentin.

A double-blind, randomized, cross-over trial of the SSRI fluoxetine for the treatment of hot flashes evaluated 81 women with a history of, or increased risk of, breast cancer, experiencing at least 14 hot flashes per week [85]. The women were randomized to 20 mg/day of fluoxetine vs. placebo for 4 weeks, followed by a second 4-week period in which the patients were crossed over to the alternative treatment arm. The study demonstrated no significant difference in hot flash scores (frequency × severity) by the end of the first treatment period (50% decrease in score in the fluoxetine arm vs. 36% decrease in the placebo arm), although the cross-over analysis demonstrated a significantly greater improvement in score with fluoxetine ($p=0.02$). However, the study did not adjust for confounding factors such as age or use of tamoxifen during the study period, a medication commonly associated with hot flashes as a side effect.

A randomized, double-blind, placebo-controlled trial evaluated the efficacy of controlled-release paroxetine (12.5 mg/day, 25.0 mg/day, or placebo) in the treatment of menopausal hot flashes in 165 women [86]. After 6 weeks of treatment, median hot flash composite scores (severity × frequency) were reduced by 62.2% in those taking 12.5 mg/day and 64.6% in those taking 25.0 mg/day, compared with 37.8% for those in the placebo group. This treatment difference remained after adjustment for age, breast cancer history, or antiestrogen use. A subsequent randomized, double-blind, placebo-controlled, cross-over trial demonstrated the efficacy of paroxetine (at doses of 10–20 mg) in the treatment of menopausal hot flashes [87] compared with placebo. The variability in results of studies evaluating different SSRIs may be related to the selectivity of different agents in this class for the serotonin vs. the norepinephrine transporter. Paroxetine is the SSRI with the highest activity at the norepinephrine transporter, whereas fluoxetine has a much lower affinity for the norepinephrine transporter [88].

Of the SNRIs, venlafaxine has been the most widely studied, and its efficacy in the management of menopausal hot flashes has been demonstrated in several randomized control trials [89, 90]. A recent randomized, double-blind, placebo-controlled trial [86] randomized 80 postmenopausal women with at least 14 hot flashes per week to receive extended release venlafaxine (37.5 mg/day for one week followed by 75 mg/day for 11 weeks) or placebo. Those receiving venlafaxine experienced a 51% reduction in patient-perceived hot flash scores, compared to a 15% reduction in the placebo group ($p<0.001$). Commonly observed side effects in the treatment group included dry mouth, sleeplessness, and decreased appetite.

Among the centrally acting agents studied for the treatment of vasomotor symptoms, desvenlafaxine, the active metabolite of venlafaxine, has been assessed in the largest randomized controlled trials to date [91]. A recent double-blind, placebo-controlled trial randomized 567 postmenopausal women experiencing at least 50 hot flashes per week to receive desvenlafaxine (100 or 150 mg/day) or placebo [92]. Patients randomized to desvenlafaxine experienced a significantly greater decrease in number of moderate to severe hot flashes after 12 weeks of therapy, despite the large placebo effect observed (60 and 66% decrease in 100 mg and 150 mg groups, respectively, compared with 47% decrease in placebo group, $p \leq 0.002$). This effect persisted at 26 weeks of therapy only in the 150 mg/day group. However, side effects were common (primarily nausea and dizziness), and the discontinuation rate due to side effects was 29%, most commonly during the first week of therapy.

Gabapentin is an anticonvulsant that has demonstrated superior efficacy to placebo in the treatment of vasomotor symptoms in all placebo-controlled trials [91]. Its mechanism of action in the treatment of hot flashes is unclear. A double-blind, placebo-controlled trial randomized 197 postmenopausal women with at least 14 hot flashes per week to receive gabapentin 900 mg/day or placebo for 4 weeks [93]. Hot flash scores decreased by 51% in the gabapentin group compared with 26% in the placebo group ($p < 0.001$). Reported side effects included dizziness, unsteadiness, and drowsiness which decreased to baseline levels by the fourth week. Another randomized placebo-controlled trial assessed gabapentin (titrated to 2,400 mg/day) in comparison with conjugated estrogens (0.625 mg/day) for 12 weeks [94]. Gabapentin and estrogen were similarly effective in reducing hot flash composite score at 12 weeks, and each had a significantly superior treatment effect when compared with placebo.

The α_2-adrenergic receptor agonist clonidine has been used for treatment of hot flashes, but small trials of short duration have demonstrated modest efficacy at best [91]. Doses ranged from 0.5 to 1.5 mg/day, and common side effects such as dizziness and dry mouth make this drug difficult to tolerate and contribute to high discontinuation rates. This option should be reserved only for patients who cannot tolerate other nonhormonal options.

Urogenital Symptoms

Vaginal dryness is reported by many perimenopausal women and becomes increasingly more common throughout the menopausal transition. Symptoms related to vaginal atrophy include itching, discomfort, and painful intercourse. Estimates of the prevalence of vaginal dryness range from 7 to 39% in perimenopause, and from 17 to 30% in postmenopause [43]. In addition, urinary symptoms are reported in as many as 36–39% of menopausal women [43]. If vaginal lubricants do not adequately alleviate mild dryness and dyspareunia, estrogen therapy may be needed. Oral estrogens with or without progestins as well as a variety of vaginal estrogen preparations are beneficial in the treatment of urogenital atrophy. A variety of options for local estrogen therapy are available and include creams, pessaries, tablets, and the E2-releasing ring. A recent meta-analysis of 19 randomized clinical trials comparing the safety and efficacy of different estrogenic preparations revealed significant improvement above placebo in vaginal symptoms in users of the cream (CEE), E2-releasing ring, and E2 tablets [95]. One trial found significant side effects (uterine bleeding, breast pain, and perineal pain) following cream administration when compared to tablets. There were no significant differences between treatment groups in endometrial hyperplasia or increasing endometrial thickness (>5 mm). As a treatment choice, women preferred the E2-releasing vaginal ring for ease of use, comfort of product, and overall satisfaction.

Bone

The rate of bone remodeling is increased in older adults. Osteoporosis occurs when the rate of resorption exceeds the rate of formation, and is defined by a Working Group of the World Health Organization as a BMD (T-score) that is 2.5 SD below the mean peak value in young adults [96]. Common risk factors for osteoporosis in postmenopausal women include thin habitus, physical inactivity, cigarette smoking, alcohol abuse, low calcium intake, little sunlight exposure, early menopause, and first-degree relative with low-trauma fracture [97]. Other risk factors include the use of certain medications (e.g., excessive thyroxine, heparin, phenytoin, and glucocorticoids) as well as endocrinopathies (primary hyperparathyroidism, thyrotoxicosis, and Cushing's syndrome), hematologic diseases (multiple myeloma, lymphoma, and leukemia), and malabsorption syndromes (celiac disease and Crohn's disease) [97].

Treatment of osteoporotic postmenopausal women with antiresorptive therapy increases BMD of the lumbar spine by 5–10% after 2–3 years, after which bone density changes very little. This change is associated with a decrease in the fracture rate of approximately 50% [97]. Although the response to medication is usually evaluated by serial measurements of BMD, the aim of treatment is to prevent fractures, which is the key end point of clinical trials of osteoporosis therapy. There are a number of therapeutic options that prevent further fractures in postmenopausal women with osteoporosis [97].

Trials evaluating calcium and vitamin D supplementation reveal variable efficacy in the prevention of fractures in postmenopausal women. A Dutch study of 1,278 men and women aged 70 years and older who were treated with vitamin D (400 IU/day) or placebo for 3.5 years revealed no difference in rates of hip fracture [98]. However, in a French study of 3,270 institutionalized elderly women (mean age 84 years) who were treated with calcium (1,200 mg/day) and vitamin D (800 IU/day) for 3 years, the risk of hip fractures was 30% lower than the risk in the placebo group [99]. Similarly, in a US study of 389 community-dwelling women and men aged over 65 years who were treated with calcium (500 mg/day) and vitamin D (700 IU/day) for 3 years, the rate of nonvertebral fractures was decreased (RR 0.4, $p=0.03$), despite only a modest increase in BMD, evident primarily after the first year of therapy [100]. Possible explanations for the differences between these studies include differences in the population studied (the French women had lower dietary calcium intakes), dose of vitamin D, and coadministration of calcium.

A number of randomized, controlled trials report that estrogen or estrogen/progestin combinations prevent bone loss; on average, compared with placebo, increases in BMD of between 3 and 10% are observed, depending on the bone measured, the age of the participants, and the duration of therapy [101]. However, randomized, controlled trials of hormone replacement therapy with fracture reduction as the primary outcome are lacking, and information about the effect of estrogen-replacement therapy on risk of fracture in postmenopausal women is thus limited [97]. Due to the lack of antifracture efficacy data from randomized trials, the US Food and Drug Administration has withdrawn CEEs as an approved treatment for osteoporosis [102]. A meta-analysis of 22 randomized trials of HRT with fracture data, which included a number of unpublished studies, reported a 33% reduction in nonvertebral fractures ($p=0.03$) when women started therapy before age 60 years [103]. This effect, however, was reduced to 12% ($p=0.22$) in women starting therapy after 60 years of age. Considering that most women starting therapy for prevention/treatment of osteoporosis (and those at the highest risk of fracture) are older than 60 years, estrogen is no longer considered the first-line therapy for the prevention and treatment of postmenopausal osteoporosis.

Bisphosphonates are a useful treatment option for the treatment of postmenopausal osteoporosis and have been evaluated (both alone and in combination with HRT) for their efficacy in the prevention of bone loss in postmenopausal women with low BMD. Their exact mechanism of action is uncertain, but their net effect is increased osteoclast cell death, thereby decreasing bone resorption. Alendronate is given at a dose of 10 mg/day for the treatment of postmenopausal osteoporosis, or 5 mg/day for the prevention of osteoporosis. A recent meta-analysis of six randomized, placebo-controlled, double-blind trials evaluating the efficacy of alendronate (5–20 mg/day, range 1–4.5 years of therapy) in the prevention of hip fractures in postmenopausal women [104] revealed an overall risk reduction of hip fracture of 45% ($p=0.007$) in patients with a T-score of less than or equal to −2.0 or with a vertebral fracture. In patients with osteoporosis (WHO criteria), the overall risk reduction was 55% ($p=0.0008$).

A randomized, placebo-controlled trial to evaluate the effects of alendronate (10 mg/day) and CEE (0.625 mg/day), in combination and separately, on BMD in hysterectomized postmenopausal osteoporotic women [105] revealed a significantly greater increase in BMD after 2 years of therapy at both the lumbar spine and femoral neck in the combination group above that seen in either the CEE or alendronate group. The effects on BMD of alendronate alone did not differ significantly from those of CEE alone at any site, and a significant increase in BMD at all sites was seen for all treatment groups above that of placebo group. Fracture risk was not assessed in this study. In contrast, a 1 year randomized, placebo-controlled trial evaluating CEE (0.625 mg/day, ±cyclic or daily medroxyprogesterone acetate (up to 5 mg/day) depending on hysterectomy status) alone or in combination with risedronate (5 mg/day) in postmenopausal women [106] revealed significant increases in lumbar spine BMD in both treatment groups, but no difference between treatment groups was seen. Important differences between these two studies include the duration of therapy as well as the patient population studied (the population in the former study had substantially lower BMD and more years since menopause than the population in the latter). Thus, although bisphosphonates alone appear to be effective in increasing BMD and decreasing fracture rate [97], a clear and consistent benefit of combination therapy (bisphosphonates + HRT) above either treatment alone remains to be demonstrated. The optimal duration of bisphosphonate therapy is not known. It should be noted that alendronate has been associated with esophagitis, and should be taken with a glass of water while upright before breakfast in order to maximize absorption while minimizing the risk of esophagitis [93].

Raloxifene is a nonsteroidal selective estrogen receptor modulator (SERM) that has estrogen-agonist effects on bone. It inhibits bone resorption in postmenopausal women without stimulating the breast or endometrium, leading to an increase in BMD and a reduction in markers of bone turnover [107]. The multiple outcomes of raloxifene (MORE) trial [108] studied the effects of raloxifene in 7,705 postmenopausal women with osteoporosis, in which the women were randomized to receive raloxifene 60 or 120 mg/day or placebo, as well as calcium and vitamin D supplementation. After 4 years, the cumulative relative risks for one or more new vertebral fractures were 0.64 (95% CI 0.53–0.76) with the 60 mg dose and 0.57 (95% CI 0.48–0.69) with the 120 mg dose. For both doses, BMD at the lumbar spine and femoral neck was significantly increased over that of placebo after 4 years ($p<0.001$), and decreases in biochemical markers of bone turnover were significantly greater in both raloxifene groups when compared with that in the placebo group ($p<0.001$). Notably, the nonvertebral fracture risk was not significantly reduced. A meta-analysis of seven clinical studies evaluating the anti-vertebral fracture efficacy of raloxifene in postmenopausal women (after 1–3 years of treatment) confirmed the findings of the MORE trial, reporting an overall 40% reduction in vertebral fracture in patients treated with 60 mg/day, and a 49% reduction in vertebral fracture in patients treated with 120 or 150 mg/day [109]. The more recently published raloxifene use for the heart (RUTH) trial [110] also reported a significantly reduced risk of clinical vertebral (but not nonvertebral) fractures in women randomized to 60 mg/day of raloxifene vs. placebo (HR 0.65, 95% CI 0.47–0.89), but these women were not selected on the basis of osteoporosis. Collectively, the data support the use of raloxifene in postmenopausal women with predominantly spinal osteoporosis, but the drug's major limitations are the adverse effects associated with its estrogenic actions. In particular, the MORE trial [108] revealed a significantly increased risk of deep venous thrombosis in women receiving raloxifene compared with placebo (RR 2.76, 95% CI 1.30–5.86).

Surgical Menopause

Approximately 600,000 hysterectomies are performed each year in USA [111], and 50–60% of hysterectomy procedures involve oophorectomy [112]. The theoretical benefits of prophylactic oophorectomy at the time of hysterectomy include the prevention of ovarian cancer and fewer reoperations for ovarian pathology. Common indications for bilateral oophorectomy at the time of hysterectomy include familial breast–ovarian cancer syndromes, severe endometriosis, bilateral tubo-ovarian abscesses, and ovarian, endometrial, or fallopian tube cancers. If a woman has not yet experienced natural menopause, surgical menopause happens immediately upon removal of the ovaries. However, hysterectomy alone is associated with earlier menopause. The mean age of ovarian failure in women who have had hysterectomy is reported to be 45.4±4.0 years, significantly lower than the mean age of 49.5±4.0 years in women without hysterectomy in one series ($p<0.001$) [113]. This may be explained by damage to the ovarian artery at the time of hysterectomy, or misclassification of oophorectomized women as women with intact ovaries.

With bilateral oophorectomy, the decline in circulating E2 is abrupt as opposed to gradual. Accordingly, the prevalence and severity of symptoms differ significantly in women who experience natural vs. surgical menopause [114]. The abrupt decline in E2 after surgical menopause is associated with more frequent and severe symptoms [43, 112]. These symptoms include hot flashes, sexual dysfunction, depression, and vaginal dryness [43, 115]. In one study, moderate to severe hot flashes (defined as episodes that affected a women's capacity to function) were experienced by hysterectomized women 1.7 times more often than their naturally menopausal counterparts [115].

Conflicting data exist as to whether or not the postmenopausal ovary is a major androgen-producing gland. Several reports suggest that the postmenopausal ovaries are an important source of androgens, including studies which demonstrated higher androgen levels in the ovarian veins than peripheral veins of postmenopausal women [116, 117]. The primary estrogen produced after menopause is E1, derived principally from peripheral aromatization of adrenal and ovarian androstenedione, resulting in low circulating levels of estrogen in naturally menopausal women. The reported decline in androgens seen with surgical menopause is sustained throughout the menopausal period, as demonstrated in a study by Laughlin et al. [118] which demonstrated that plasma testosterone levels were 40% lower in oophorectomized women than that in intact postmenopausal women, independent of time since surgery. In contrast, an apparent return to premenopausal testosterone levels was demonstrated in intact women, some evaluated >20 years after natural menopause. In distinct contrast to these studies, Couzinet et al. reported that circulating androgens in postmenopausal women are of adrenal rather than ovarian origin by demonstrating very low plasma androgen levels in postmenopausal women with adrenal insufficiency, and similar levels between oophorectomized and nonoophorectomized postmenopausal women with normal adrenal function [119]. Several studies have also demonstrated absent to low expression of steroidogenic enzymes necessary for androgen biosynthesis (P450cc, 3β-hydroxysteroid dehydrogenase, P450c17) in the postmenopausal ovary [119, 120], supporting the hypothesis that the postmenopausal ovary is not a major androgen-producing gland.

In women who have undergone oophorectomy, some studies report that oral or transdermal testosterone improves sexual function and psychological well-being; however, these studies did not demonstrate any benefit of testosterone in the treatment of vaginal dryness, sleep disturbances, or mood [43, 121]. The consequences of the lower testosterone levels many years after oophorectomy for the health and well-being of aging women remain unknown. Furthermore, high doses (approximately

300 μg/day) are necessary to improve libido and sex drive. This dosage results in elevated circulating levels, which may produce unwanted androgenic side effects such as hirsutism, acne, and weight gain. The decision to institute androgen therapy must be weighed against these potential side effects; additionally, the long-term risks of taking testosterone have not been studied in this population [43]. Hormone therapy (estrogen with or without androgens) should be discussed preoperatively, as the menopausal symptoms associated with acute hypoestrogenism after surgical castration are generally much more severe than those associated with natural menopause.

A number of studies report an association of oophorectomy with an increased risk of cardiovascular disease (CVD) as well as mortality from all causes. In a recent cohort study including 1,274 women who had unilateral oophorectomy and 1,091 women who underwent bilateral oophorectomy with a median follow-up period of 25 years [122], women with bilateral oophorectomy before age 45 years experienced an increased mortality associated with CVD compared with age-matched women without oophorectomy (HR 1.44; 95% CI, 1.01–2.05). Within this age group, mortality was further increased in women who were not treated with estrogen through age 45 years or longer (HR 1.84; 95% CI, 1.27–2.68) but not in women treated with estrogen. Unilateral oophorectomy was not associated with increased cardiovascular mortality. Limitations of this study include its use of a predominantly white cohort as well as lack of data regarding risk factors for CVD (e.g., smoking status, adiposity, cholesterol and blood pressure measurements, and SES) in either the study cohort or control group. A recent meta-analysis [123] revealed that although natural menopause did not influence the rate of CVD (RR 1.14; 95% CI, 0.86–1.51), bilateral oophorectomy even around the age of 50 years increased CVD risk (RR 2.62; 95% CI, 2.05–3.35). Furthermore, bilateral oophorectomy prior to the age of 50 years increased the risk substantially (RR 4.55; 95% CI, 2.56–8.10). Data from the Nurses' Health Study [124] revealed that over 24 years of follow-up, when compared with ovarian conservation, bilateral oophorectomy at the time of hysterectomy (after adjustment for CVD risk factors) was associated with an increased risk of death from CVD (HR 1.28; 95% CI, 1.00–1.64) as well as an increased risk of all-cause mortality (HR 1.12; 95% CI, 1.03–1.21). Those who had never used estrogen therapy and underwent oophorectomy before age 50 years had a higher risk of CVD (HR 1.98, 95% CI 1.18–3.32). Although further studies are necessary, cardiovascular protection linked to ovarian conservation in younger women should prompt reconsideration of routine prophylactic oophorectomy in women not at high risk of developing ovarian cancer.

Summary

Worldwide, an increasing proportion of women are experiencing the menopausal transition. It is thus imperative that providers of women's health care achieve an adequate understanding of the diagnosis of the menopausal transition and proper management of menopause-related health issues. Although not all women will progress through a predicted sequence, use of the recently proposed STRAW criteria may be helpful in counseling the perimenopausal woman regarding her expected course. Measurement of serum FSH levels (with concomitant E2 measurement) is helpful in determining a woman's menopausal status, although normal values may be encountered during advanced reproductive age. Measurements of serum inhibin and possibly AMH may prove clinically useful with further study.

The use of estrogen in the peri- and postmenopausal woman requires careful consideration of her personal history, family history, and comorbidities. This chapter has provided a review of nonhormonal options available for the treatment of vasomotor symptoms as well as postmenopausal osteoporosis. Finally, recent data indicating an association between surgical menopause and increased cardiovascular and all-cause mortality prompt the gynecologist to reconsider routine prophylactic oophorectomy at the time of hysterectomy for benign disease.

References

1. Smith D (2003) The older population in the United States: March 2002. U.S. Census Bureau current population reports (Report No. P20-546). US Census Bureau, Washington, DC
2. World Health Organization (1996) Research on the menopause in the 1990s: Report of a WHO scientific group. WHO Technical Report Series 866. WHO, Geneva
3. Weiss G, Skurnick JH, Goldsmith LT et al (2004) Menopause and hypothalamic-pituitary sensitivity to estrogen. JAMA 292:2991–2996
4. McKinlay SM, Brambilla D, Posner JG (2008) The normal menopause transition. Maturitas 61:4–16
5. Bromberger JT, Matthews KA, Kuller LH et al (1997) Prospective study of the determinants of age at menopause. Am J Epidemiol 145:124–133
6. Gold EB, Bromberger J, Crawford S et al (2001) Factors associated with age at natural menopause in a multiethnic sample of midlife women. Am J Epidemiol 153:865–874
7. Soules MR, Sherman S, Parrott E et al (2001) Executive summary: stages of reproductive aging workshop (STRAW). Fertil Steril 76:874–878
8. WHO Scientific Group (1996) Research on the menopause in the 1990's: a report of the WHO Scientific Group, vol. 866. World Health Organization, Geneva. pp 1–79
9. Brambilla DJ, McKinlay SM, Johannes CB (1994) Defining the perimenopause for application in epidemiologic investigations. Am J Epidemiol 140:1091–1095
10. Gracia CR, Sammel MD, Freeman EW et al (2005) Defining menopause status: creation of a new definition to identify the early changes of the menopausal transition. Menopause 12:128–135
11. Scheffer GJ, Broekmans FJ, Dorland M et al (1999) Antral follicle counts by transvaginal ultrasonography are related to age in women with proven natural fertility. Fertil Steril 72:845–851
12. Santoro N, Isaac B, Neal-Perry G et al (2003) Impaired folliculogenesis and ovulation in older reproductive aged women. J Clin Endocrinol Metab 88:5502–5509
13. Giacobbe M, Mendes Pinto-Neto A et al (2004) The usefulness of ovarian volume, antral follicle count and age as predictors of menopausal status. Climacteric 7:255–260
14. Richardson SJ, Senikas V, Nelson JF (1987) Follicular depletion during the menopausal transition: evidence for accelerated loss and ultimate exhaustion. J Clin Endocrinol Metab 65:1231–1237
15. de Vet A, Laven JS, de Jong FH et al (2002) Antimüllerian hormone serum levels: a putative marker for ovarian aging. Fertil Steril 77:357–362
16. Santoro N (2004) Can a blood test predict the onset of menopause? Menopause 11:585–586

17. Sherman BM, Korenman SG (1975) Hormonal characteristics of the human menstrual cycle throughout reproductive life. J Clin Investig 55:699–706
18. McLachlan RI, Robertson DM, Healy DL (1987) Circulating immunoreactive inhibin levels during the normal human menstrual cycle. J Clin Endocrinol Metab 65:954–961
19. Metcalf MG, Donald RA, Livesy JH (1981) Pituitary-ovarian function in normal women during the menopausal transition. Clin Endocrinol 14:245–255
20. Metcalf MG, Donald RA, Livesey JH (1981) Classification of menstrual cycles in pre- and perimenopausal women. J Endocrinol 91:1–10
21. Metcalf MG, Donald RA, Livesey JH (1982) Pituitary-ovarian function before, during and after the menopause: a longitudinal sudy. Clin Endocrinol 17:489–494
22. Metcalf MG (1988) The approach of menopause: a New Zealand study. N Z Med J 101: 103–106
23. Santoro N, Brown JR, Adel T et al (1996) Characterization of reproductive hormonal dynamics in the perimenopause. J Clin Endocrinol Metab 81:1495–1501
24. O'Connor KA, Ferrell RF, Brindle E et al (2009) Total and unopposed estrogen exposure across stages of the transition to menopause. Cancer Epidemiol Biomarkers Prev 18:828–836
25. Taffe JR, Dennerstein L (2002) Menstrual patterns leading to the final menstrual period. Menopause 9:32–40
26. Miro F, Parker SW, Aspinall LJ et al (2004) Origins and consequences of the elongation of the human menstrual cycle during the menopausal transition: the FREEDOM study. J Clin Endocrinol Metab 89:4910–4915
27. Santoro N, Crawford SL, Lasley WL et al (2008) Factors related to declining luteal function in women during the menopausal transition. J Clin Endocrinol Metab 93:1711–1721
28. Randolph JF Jr, Sowers MF, Gold EB et al (2003) Reproductive hormones in the early menopausal transition: relationship to ethnicity, body size, and menopausal status. J Clin Endocrinol Metab 88:1516–1522
29. Randolph JF Jr, Sowers MF, Bondarenko IV et al (2004) Change in estradiol and follicle-stimulating hormone across the early menopausal transition: effects of ethnicity and age. J Clin Endocrinol Metab 89:1555–1561
30. Su HI, Sammel MD, Freeman EW et al (2008) Body size affects measures of ovarian reserve in late reproductive age women. Menopause 15:857–861
31. Groome NP, Illingworth PG, O'Brien M et al (1996) Measurement of dimeric inhibin B throughout the human menstrual cycle. J Clin Endocrinol Metab 81:1401–1405
32. Burger HG, Cahir N, Robertson DM et al (1998) Serum inhibins A and B fall differentially as FSH rises in perimenopausal women. Clin Endocrinol 48:809–813
33. MacNaughton J, Banah M, McCloud P et al (1992) Age related changes in follicle stimulating hormone, luteinizing hormone, oestradiol and immunoreactive inhibin in women of reproductive age. Clin Endocrinol 36:339–345
34. Klein NA, Illingworth PJ, Groome NP et al (1996) Decreased inhibin B secretion is associated with the monotropic FSH rise in older, ovulatory women: a study of serum and follicular fluid levels of dimeric inhibin A and B in spontaneous menstrual cycles. J Clin Endocrinol Metab 81:2742–2745
35. Muttukrishna S, Child T, Lockwood GM et al (2000) Serum concentrations of dimeric inhibins, activin A, gonadotrophins and ovarian steroids during the menstrual cycle in older women. Hum Reprod 15:546–556
36. Santoro N, Adel T, Skurnick JH (1999) Decreased inhibin tone and increased activin A secretion characterize reproductive aging in women. Fertil Steril 71:658–662
37. Welt CK, McNicholl DJ, Taylor AE et al (1999) Female reproductive aging is marked by decreased secretion of dimeric inhibin. J Clin Endocrinol Metab 84:105–111
38. Ream NE, Wyman TL, Phillips DJ et al (1998) Net increase in stimulatory input resulting from a decrease in inhibin B and an increase in activin A may contribute in part to the rise in follicular phase follicle-stimulating hormone of aging cycling women. J Clin Endocrinol Metab 83:3302–3307

39. Ying SY (1988) Inhibins, activins and follistatins: gonadal proteins modulating the secretion of follicle-stimulating hormone. Endocr Rev 9:267–293
40. Van Look PF, Hunter WM, Fraser IS et al (1995) Impaired estrogen-induced luteinizing hormone release in young women with anovulatory dysfunctional uterine bleeding. J Clin Endocrinol Metab 80:608–613
41. Santoro N, Lasley B, McConnell D et al (2004) Body size and ethnicity are associated with menstrual cycle alterations in women in the early menopausal transition: the Study of Women's Health Across the Nation (SWAN) Daily Hormone Study. J Clin Endocrinol Metab 89:2622–2631
42. Gill S, Sharpless JL, Rado K et al (2002) Evidence that GnRH decreases with gonadal steroid feedback but increases with age in postmenopausal women. J Clin Endocrinol Metab 87:2290–2296
43. National Institutes of Health (2005) National Institutes of Health State-of the Science Conference statement: management of menopause-related symptoms. Ann Intern Med 142:1003–1013
44. Freeman EW, Sammel MD, Lin H et al (2007) Symptoms associated with menopausal transition and reproductive hormones in midlife women. Obstet Gynecol 110:230–240
45. Miller SA, Santoro N, Lo Y et al (2005) Menopause symptoms in HIV-infected and drug-using women. Menopause 12:348–356
46. Freeman EW, Sammel MD, Lin H et al (2008) Symptoms in the menopausal transition: hormone and behavioral correlates. Obstet Gynecol 111:127–136
47. Dennerstein L, Dudley E, Hopper JL et al (2000) A prospective population-based study of menopausal symptoms. Obstet Gynecol 96:351–358
48. Kronenberg F (1994) Hot flashes: phenomenology, quality of life, and search for treatment options. Exp Gerontol 29:319–336
49. Guthrie JR, Dennerstein L, Hopper JL et al (1996) Hot flashes, menstrual status and hormone levels in a population-based sample of midlife women. Obstet Gynecol 88:437–442
50. Overlie I, Moen MH, Holte A et al (2002) Androgens and estrogens in relation to hot flashes during the menopausal transition. Maturitas 41:69–77
51. Rapkin AJ (2007) Vasomotor symptoms in menopause: physiologic condition and central nervous system approaches to treatment. Am J Obstet Gynecol 196:97–106
52. Col NF, Guthrie JR, Politi M et al (2009) Duration of vasomotor symptoms in middle-aged women: a longitudinal study. Menopause 16:453–457
53. Gold EB, Colvin A, Avis N et al (2006) Longitudinal analysis of the association between vasomotor symptoms and race/ethnicity across the menopausal transition: Study of Women's Health Across the Nation. Am J Public Health 96:1226–1235
54. Freeman EW, Sammel MD, Grisso JA et al (2001) Hot flashes in the late reproductive years: risk factors for African American and Caucasian women. J Womens Health Gend Based Med 10:67–76
55. Miller SR, Gallicchio LM, Lewis LM et al (2006) Association between race and hot flashes in midlife women. Maturitas 54:260–269
56. Gold EB, Block G, Crawford S et al (2004) Lifestyle and demographic factors in relation to vasomotor symptoms: baseline results from the study of women's health across the nation. Am J Epidemiol 159:1189–1199
57. Gallicchio L, Miller SR, Visvanathan K et al (2006) Cigarette smoking, estrogen levels, and hot flashes in midlife women. Maturitas 53:133–143
58. Gallicchio L, Visvanathan K, Miller SM et al (2005) Body mass index, estrogen levels, and hot flashes in midlife women. Am J Obstet Gynecol 193:1353–1360
59. Whiteman MK, Staropoli CA, Langenberg PW et al (2003) Smoking, body mass, and hot flashes in midlife women. Obstet Gynecol 101:264–272
60. Hutton JD, Jacobs HS, Murray MS et al (1978) Relation between plasma oestrone and oestradiol and climacteric symptoms. Lancet 1:678–681
61. Skurnick JH, Weiss G, Goldsmith LT et al (2009) Longitudinal changes in hypothalamic and ovarian function in perimenopausal women with anovulatory cycles: relationship with vasomotor symptoms. Fertil Steril 91:1127–1134

62. Casper RF, Yen SSC, Wilkes MM (1979) Menopausal flashes: a neuroendocrine link with pulsatile luetinizing hormone secretion. Science 205:823–825
63. Mulley G, Mitchell JRA, Tattarsall RB (1977) Hot flashes after hypophysectomy. Br Med J 2(6094):1062
64. Casper RF, Yen SSC (1981) Menopausal flashes: effect of pituitary gonadotropin desensitization by a potent luteinizing hormone-releasing factor agonist. J Clin Endocrinol Metab 53:1056–1058
65. Meldrum DR, Defazio JD, Erlik Y et al (1984) Pituitary hormones during the menopausal hot flash. Obstet Gynecol 64:752–756
66. Weiner RJ, Ganong WF (1978) Role of brain monoamines and histamine in regulation of anterior pituitary secretion. Physiol Rev 58:905–976
67. Bhattacharya AN, Dierschke DJ, Yamaji T et al (1972) The pharmacological blockade of the circhoral mode of LH secretion in the ovariectomized rhesus monkey. Endocrinol 90:778–786
68. Cox B, Lomax P (1977) Pharmacologic control of temperature regulation. Ann Rev Pharmacol Toxicol 17:341–353
69. Stearns V, Ullmer L, Lopez JF et al (2002) Hot flashes. Lancet 360:1851–1861
70. Berendsen HH (2000) The role of serotonin in hot flashes. Maturitas 36:155–164
71. Freedman RR (2005) Pathophysiology and treatment of menopausal hot flashes. Semin Reprod Med 23:117–125
72. Rossouw JE, Anderson GL, Prentice RL et al (2002) Risks and benefits of estrogen plus progestin in healthy postmenopausal women: principal results from the Women's Health Initiative randomized controlled trial. JAMA 288:321–333
73. Manson JE, Hsia J, Johnson KC et al (2003) Estrogen plus progestin and the risk of coronary heart disease. N Engl J Med 349:523–534
74. Chlebowski RT, Hendrix SL, Langer RD et al (2003) Influence of estrogen plus progestin on breast cancer and mammography in healthy postmenopausal women: the Women's Health Initiative Randomized Trial. JAMA 289:3243–3253
75. Anderson GL, Limacher M, Assaf AR et al (2004) Effects of conjugated equine estrogen in postmenopausal women with hysterectomy. The Women's Health Initiative randomized control trial. JAMA 291:1701–1712
76. Sikon A, Thacker HL (2004) Treatment options for menopausal hot flashes. Clev Clin J Med 71:578–582
77. Greendale GA, Reboussin BA, Hogan P et al (1998) Symptom relief and side effects of postmenopausal hormones: results from the Postmenopausal Estrogen/Progestin Interventions trial. Obstet Gynecol 92:982–988
78. Utian WH, Shoupe D, Bachmann G et al (2001) Relief of vasomotor symptoms and vaginal atrophy with lower doses of conjugated equine estrogens and medroxyprogesterone acetate. Fertil Steril 75:1065–1079
79. Pickar JH, Yeh IT, Wheeler JE et al (2003) Endometrial effects of lower doses of conjugated equine estrogens and medroxyprogesterone acetate: two-year substudy results. Fertil Steril 80:1234–1240
80. Archer DF, Dorin M, Lewis V et al (2001) Effects of lower doses of conjugated equine estrogens and medroxyprogesterone acetate on endometrial bleeding. Fertil Steril 75:1080–1087
81. Lobo RA, Bush T, Carr BR et al (2001) Effects of lower doses of conjugated equine estrogens and medroxyprogesterone acetate on plasma lipids and lipoproteins, coagulation factors, and carbohydrate metabolism. Fertil Steril 76:13–24
82. Bachmann GA, Schaefers M, Uddin A et al (2007) Lowest effective transdermal 17β (beta)-estradiol dose for relief of hot flashes in postmenopausal women. Obstet Gynecol 110:771–779
83. Johnson SR, Ettinger B, Macer JL et al (2005) Uterine and vaginal effects of unopposed ultralow-dose transdermal estradiol. Obstet Gynecol 105:779–787
84. Ettinger B, Ensrud KE, Wallace R et al (2004) Effects of ultralow-dose transdermal estradiol on bone mineral density: a randomized clinical trial. Obstet Gynecol 104:443–451
85. Loprinzi CL, Sloan JA, Perez EA et al (2002) Phase III evaluation of fluoxetine for treatment of hot flashes. J Clin Oncol 6:1578–1583

86. Stearns V, Beebe KL, Iyengar M et al (2003) Paroxetine controlled release in the treatment of menopausal hot flashes: a randomized control trial. JAMA 289:2827–2834
87. Stearns V, Slack R, Greep N et al (2005) Paroxetine is an effective treatment for hot flashes: results from a prospective randomized clinical trial. J Clin Oncol 28:6919–6930
88. Nemeroff CB, Owens MJ (2004) Pharmacologic differences among the SSRIs: focus on monoamine transporters and the HPA axis. CNS Spectr 9(6 suppl 4):23–31
89. Loprinzi CL, Kugler JW, Sloan JA et al (2000) Venlafaxine in management of hot flashes in survivors of breast cancer: a randomized control trial. Lancet 356:2059–2063
90. Evans ML, Pritts E, Vittinghoff E et al (2005) Management of postmenopausal hot flashes with venlafaxine hydrochloride: a randomized, controlled trial. Obstet Gynecol 105:161–166
91. Jenkins MR, Sikon AL (2008) Update on nonhormonal approaches to menopausal management. Clev Clin J Med 75(suppl 4):S17–S24
92. Archer DF, Dupont CM, Constantine GD et al (2009) Desvenlafaxine for the treatment of vasomotor symptoms associated with menopause: a double-blind, randomized, placebo-controlled trial of efficacy and safety. Am J Obstet Gynecol 200:238e1–238e10
93. Butt DA, Lock M, Lewis JE et al (2008) Gabapentin for the treatment of menopausal hot flashes: a randomized controlled trial. Menopause 15:310–318
94. Reddy SY, Warner H, Guttuso T et al (2006) Gabapentin, estrogen and placebo for treating hot flashes: a randomized controlled trial. Obstet Gynecol 108:41–48
95. Suckling J, Lethaby A, Kennedy R (2006) Local oestrogen for vaginal atrophy in postmenopausal women. Cochrane Database Syst Rev (4):CD001500
96. Kanis JA, Melton LJ III, Christiansen C et al (1994) The diagnosis of osteoporosis. J Bone Miner Res 9:1137–1141
97. Eastell R (1998) Treatment of postmenopausal osteoporosis. N Engl J Med 338:736–746
98. Lips P, Graafmans WC, Ooms ME et al (1996) Vitamin D supplementation and fracture incidence in elderly persons: a randomized, placebo-controlled clinical trial. Ann Intern Med 124:400–406
99. Chapuy MC, Arlot ME, Delmas PD et al (1994) Effect of calcium and cholecalciferol treatment for three years on hip fractures in elderly women. Br Med J 308:1081–1082
100. Dawson-Hughes B, Harris SS, Krall EA et al (1997) Effect of calcium and vitamin D supplementation on bone density in men and women 65 years of age or older. N Engl J Med 337:670–676
101. Greendale GA, Wells B, Marcus R et al (2000) How many women lose bone mineral density while taking hormone replacement therapy? Results from the Postmenopausal Estrogen/Progestin Interventions Trial. Arch Intern Med 160:3065–3071
102. Fitzpatrick LA, Litin SC, Bell MR (2000) The Women's Health Initiative: a heart to HRT conversation. Mayo Clin Proc 75:559–561
103. Torgerson DJ, Bell-Syer SE (2001) Hormone replacement therapy and prevention of nonvertebral fractures: a meta-analysis of randomized trials. JAMA 285:2891–2897
104. Papapoulos SE, Quandt SA, Liberman UA et al (2005) Meta-analysis of the efficacy of alendronate for the prevention of hip fractures in postmenopausal women. Osteoporos Int 16:468–474
105. Bone HG, Greenspan SL, McKeever C et al (2000) Alendronate and estrogen effects in postmenopausal women with low bone mineral density. J Clin Endocrinol Metab 85:720–726
106. Harris ST, Eriksen EF, Davidson M et al (2000) Effect of combined risedronate and hormone replacement therapies on bone mineral density in postmenopausal women. J Clin Endocrinol Metab 86:1890–1897
107. Riggs BL, Hartmann LC (2003) Selective estrogen-receptor modulators-mechanism of action and application to clinical practice. N Engl J Med 348:618–629
108. Delmas PD, Ensrud KE, Adachi JD et al (2002) Efficacy of raloxifene on vertebral fracture risk reduction in postmenopausal women with osteoporosis: four-year results from a randomized clinical trial. J Clin Endocrinol Metab 87:3609–3617
109. Seeman E, Crans GG, Diez-Perez A et al (2006) Anti-vertebral fracture efficacy of raloxifene: a meta-analysis. Osteoporos Int 17:313–316

110. Ensrud KE, Stock JL, Barrett-Connor E et al (2008) Effects of Raloxifene on fracture risk in postmenopausal women: the Raloxifene Use for the Heart Trial. J Bone Miner Res 23:112–120
111. Keshavarz H, Hillis SD, Kieke BA et al (2002) Hysterectomy surveillance: United States, 1994–1999. MMWR CDC Surveill Summ 51(SS-5):1–8
112. Hendrix SL (2005) Bilateral oophorectomy and premature menopause. Am J Med 118:131S–135S
113. Siddle N, Sarrel P, Whitehead M (1987) The effect of hysterectomy on the age at ovarian failure: identification of a subgroup of women with premature loss of ovarian function and literature review. Fertil Steril 47:94–100
114. Bachmann G (2001) Physiologic aspects of natural and surgical menopause. J Reprod Med 46:307–315
115. Oldenhave A, Jaszmann LJ, Everaerd WT et al (1993) Hysterectomized women with ovarian conservation report more severe climacteric complaints than do normal climacteric women of similar age. Am J Obstet Gynecol 168:765–771
116. Judd HL, Judd GE, Lucas WE et al (1974) Endocrine function of the postmenopausal ovary: concentration of androgens and estrogens in ovarian and peripheral vein blood. J Clin Endocrinol Metab 39:1020–1024
117. Fogle RH, Stanczyk FZ, Zhang X et al (2007) Ovarian androgen production in postmenopausal women. J Clin Endocrinol Metab 92:3040–3043
118. Laughlin GA, Barrett-Connor E, Kritz-Silverstein DK et al (2000) Hysterectomy, oophorectomy, and endogenous sex hormone levels in older women: the Rancho Bernado Study. J Clin Endocrinol Metab 85:645–651
119. Couzinet B, Meduri G, Lecce MG et al (2001) The postmenopausal ovary is not a major androgen-producing gland. J Clin Endocrinol Metab 86:5060–5066
120. Jabara S, Christenson LK, Wang CY et al (2003) Stromal cells of the human postmenopausal ovary display a distinctive biochemical and molecular phenotype. J Clin Endocrinol Metab 88:484–492
121. Sherwin BB (2002) Randomized clinical trials of combined estrogen-androgen preparations: effects on sexual functioning. Fertil Steril 77(suppl 4):S49–S54
122. Rivera CM, Grossardt BR, Rhodes DJ et al (2009) Increased cardiovascular mortality after early bilateral oophorectomy. Menopause 16:15–23
123. Atsma F, Bartelink ML, Grobbee DE et al (2006) Postmenopausal status and early menopause as independent risk factors for cardiovascular disease: a meta-analysis. Menopause 13:265–279
124. Parker WH, Broder MS, Chang E et al (2009) Ovarian conservation at the time of hysterectomy and long-term health outcomes in the Nurses' Health Study. Obstet Gynecol 113:1027–1037

Chapter 10
Clinical Implications of Prolonged Hypothalamic Amenorrhea

Tammy L. Loucks and Sarah L. Berga

Case Scenario

History – A 26-year-old woman presents to the office with concerns about irregular menstrual periods. The patient reports normal developmental milestones, including menarche at age 13, and regular monthly periods until age 19. Her periods became irregular during college. The physician who saw her attributed the irregular cycles to the stress of college and prescribed oral contraceptive pills (OCPs) to regulate her cycles. The patient did not like the side effects from the OCPs, and so she stopped taking the pill after about 6 months. She reports no more than two episodes of very light vaginal bleeding per year in the past 3 years. She reports regular exercise and that she follows a heart-healthy diet. However, she often skips meals or grabs a piece of fruit for lunch because she is too busy and forgets to eat. She is concerned that her amenorrhea may be impacting her long-term health and in particular her bones. Her mother (age 58) was recently diagnosed with osteopenia and the patient has had two stress fractures in the last 4 years.

The patient reports that she regularly exercises to relieve stress. She began running in college while in an honors program with double major in political science and French literature. She is now enrolled in a JD program and is considering criminal law. She has friends, dates, is on good terms with family, and has no reports of abuse. She reports feeling overwhelmed and that she often says no to social functions because she has too much work and not enough time. She has always been at the top of her class and has always gotten nearly straight A's.

On physical examination, the patient is 5′8″ tall and 130 pounds (BMI 21.7 kg/m^2) and is a nonsmoker. She is Tanner stage 5 for escutcheon and breasts, has a normal gynecoid habitus, and is not hirsute. Her sense of smell is intact. There is no acanthosis nigricans, no abdominal striae, and no areas of hyper- or hypopigmentation. The patient's visual fields are normal to confrontation. There are no focal lateralizing neurological findings. She sustained a minor concussion 6 months ago while playing

S.L. Berga (✉)
Department of Gynecology and Obstetrics, Emory University,
1639 Pierce Drive, Suite 4208-WMB, Atlanta, GA 30322, USA
e-mail: sberga@emory.edu

N.F. Santoro and G. Neal-Perry (eds.), *Amenorrhea: A Case-Based, Clinical Guide*, Contemporary Endocrinology, DOI 10.1007/978-1-60327-864-5_10,

volleyball and an MRI obtained during her ER consult was normal. However, the amenorrhea began before the head injury. You suspect that the patient has functional hypothalamic amenorrhea (FHA).

Baseline Biochemical Evaluation

	Systeme International d'Unites (SI)	Conventional (CI)
Urine βhCG	Negative	
LH	1.2 IU/L (0.8–26)	1.2 mIU (0.8–26)
FSH	1.5 IU/L (1.4–9.6)	1.5 mIU/L (1.4–9.6)
E_2	80.8 pmol/L (70–220)	22 pg/mL (20–60)
P_4	0.8 nmol/L (6–64)	0.25 ng/mL (2–20)
Prl	5 μg/L (2–15)	5 ng/mL (2–15)
TSH	2.3 mU/L (0.5–5)	2.3 μU/mL (0.5–5)
T4	70.8 nmol/L (64–154)	5.5 μg/dL (5–12)
Androstenedione	3.8 nmol/L (3.5–7)	1.10 ng/mL (1–2)
Total testosterone	1.0 nmol/L (<3.5)	0.29 ng/mL (<1 ng/mL)

You offer the patient an opportunity to participate in a study of talk therapy and stress management for women with hypothalamic amenorrhea. The patient consents to participate and is enrolled in the 20 week program. Eight months later, the patient returns and reports that she has had regular menstrual bleeding pattern for 3 of the past 4 months. Her weight has not changed, and she continues to run 10–12 miles each week. With the help of nutrition counseling, she eats more regularly and no longer skips breakfast and plans a break in her day to eat lunch. She also had an opportunity to do a volunteer rotation with a nonprofit human rights foundation and feels less overwhelmed than before. The law school she attends has an excellent international human rights program, and she has changed her focus to this domain of law. She reports that she is now spending more time with friends and enjoys a busy social life and that she has also recently started a new relationship. Her last menstrual cycle was about 23 days ago, and the interval between cycles has been about 30 days.

Followup Biochemical Evaluation

	Systeme International d'Unites (SI)	Conventional (CI)
Urine βhCG	Negative	–
LH	3.0 IU/L (0.8–26)	3 mIU/L (0.8–26)
FSH	4.0 IU/L (1.4–9.6)	4 mIU/L (1.4–9.6)
E_2	367.1 pmol/L (70–220)	100 pg/mL (20–60)
P_4	40.0 nmol/L (6–64)	12.6 ng/mL (2–20)
Prl	8 μg/L (2–15)	8 ng/mL (2–15)
TSH	4.0 mU/L (0.5–5)	4 μU/mL (0.5–5)
T4	96.5 nmol/L (64–154)	7.5 μg/dL (5–12)
Androstenedione	4.4 nmol/L (3.5–7.0 nmol/L)	1.25 ng/dL (1–2)
Total testosterone	0.9 nmol/L (<3.5 nmol/L)	0.26 ng/mL (<1 ng/mL)

You inform the patient that her biochemical evaluation indicates ovulation. You recommend a follow-up in 3 months or sooner should she decide that she needs a reliable form of hormonal contraception.

Overview

Secondary amenorrhea, or the cessation of menses unrelated to pregnancy in a previously eumenorrheic woman, may be the only overt indication of reproductive compromise. Frequently, amenorrhea has as its cause unrecognized metabolic and/or psychogenic stress. Reproductive "alignment" occurs when physiological responses elicited by the external milieu modulate reproductive processes. If the internal or external milieu is stressful, the biological systems mediating reproductive alignment act to halt or compromise gametogenesis or fertilization and effect relative reproductive quiescence until the stress ameliorates. Determinants and mediators of reproductive alignment are many and because factors interact, the independent impact of any one factor may be minimal and difficult to discern [1]. Indeed, a constellation of factors determines whether reproduction is favored or impaired. Stress-induced reproductive compromise is a diagnosis of exclusion. There are many organic, as opposed to functional, conditions that manifest as anovulation or amenorrhea. Congenital and anatomic causes, such as vaginal agenesis or other Muellerian abnormalities, must be excluded. Idiopathic hypothalamic hypogonadism due to Kallman's syndrome is difficult to exclude unless there is anosmia. A careful evaluation is mandated to exclude organic brain, hypothalamic, pituitary, thyroidal, adrenal, or ovarian etiologies. Common organic etiologies include pituitary adenomas, ovarian failure, polycystic ovary syndrome (PCOS), and hypothyroidism. However, the most common cause of hypothalamic hypogonadism with amenorrhea is likely stress. This is important to recognize because stress-induced anovulation is theoretically reversible with appropriate intervention.

Stress may be the underlying cause in the majority of cases of secondary amenorrhea, yet it remains one of the most underappreciated causes of infertility in both women and in men. A clinically recognizable presentation of stress-induced hypothalamic hypogonadism in women is FHA. FHA affects roughly 5% of women of reproductive age but less severe forms of hypothalamic hypogonadism are far more common and occult (i.e., luteal insufficiency with eumenorrhea) and often only recognized clinically when fertility is desired [2]. Women with FHA typically have both subclinical metabolic compromise and psychogenic stress that interacts synergistically to compromise reproductive function. Neuroendocrine concomitants of FHA include activation of the hypothalamic–pituitary–adrenal (HPA) axis with resultant increased cortisol secretion and suppression of the hypothalamic–pituitary–thyroidal (HPT) axis with relatively decreased thyroxine release in the face of normal levels of thyroid stimulating hormone (TSH). Psychosocial correlates of FHA include unrealistic expectations of self and others, poor problem-solving skills, and cognitive distortions related to food and body image that do not meet criteria for an eating disorder. Women with FHA rarely meet criteria for depression or a bonafide syndromal psychiatric disorder. However, they typically report a higher need for social approval which generally reflects an external locus of control. Having an external locus of control heightens psychosocial stressors. Additionally, women with FHA report high degrees of perfectionistism, which may manifest behaviorally as excessive exercise, high achievement or good grades, and/or rigid dietary habits with imbalanced nutrient content or insufficient energy intake relative to expenditure [3–5].

Epidemiological data looking at long-term health of women with FHA are limited in part because most women are not given a concrete diagnosis before initiating treatment with oral contraceptives to regulate menstrual cycles or undergoing fertility procedures when pregnancy is desired. Because women with FHA do not display the same degree of undernutrition as women with anorexia nervosa and they do not meet criteria for depression, it is difficult to gauge the acute and chronic health risks of having untreated FHA by extrapolation from other similar conditions [6]. However, there is evidence to suggest direct negative health effects, including increased risk for osteoporosis, neurodegenerative diseases, and cardiovascular disease (CVD) in women with FHA. In addition, women with FHA who become pregnant are at increased risk for poorer pregnancy outcomes, including intrauterine growth restriction, preterm labor and low birth weight, and possibly congenital birth defects. Taken together, these observations support the notion that unresolved and untreated FHA and even less clinically obvious forms of hypothalamic hypogonadism may heighten acute and chronic health risk to the individual and through epigenetic mechanisms during gestation to future generations.

The conventional therapeutic options offered to women with FHA are oral contraceptives when fertility is not desired and ovulation induction or assisted reproductive interventions when fertility is sought. The rationale for these interventions is based on the view that FHA represents an isolated compromise of reproductive function and that only the reproductive manifestations need to be treated. Herein, we present evidence that challenges this perspective. We highlight the nonreproductive health consequences of stress-induced reproductive compromise in women and discuss nonpharmacological approaches, particularly cognitive behavior therapy (CBT), to ameliorate stress, restore fertility, and improve overall health.

Neuroendocrinology of FHA

Functional hypothalamic hypogonadism is present in about 35% of women seeking clinical evaluation of secondary amenorrhea [7]. The proximate cause of FHA is reduced in central GnRH drive. When sufficient in duration and magnitude, reduced GnRH drive results in anovulation and amenorrhea. Because decrements in central GnRH–LH/FSH drive exist on a continuum and vary from day to day [8], it follows that the associated ovarian compromise exists as a spectrum and manifests as amenorrhea, polymenorrhea, oligomenorrhea, or luteal insufficiency with preserved menstrual interval. The more occult forms of hypothalamic hypogonadism

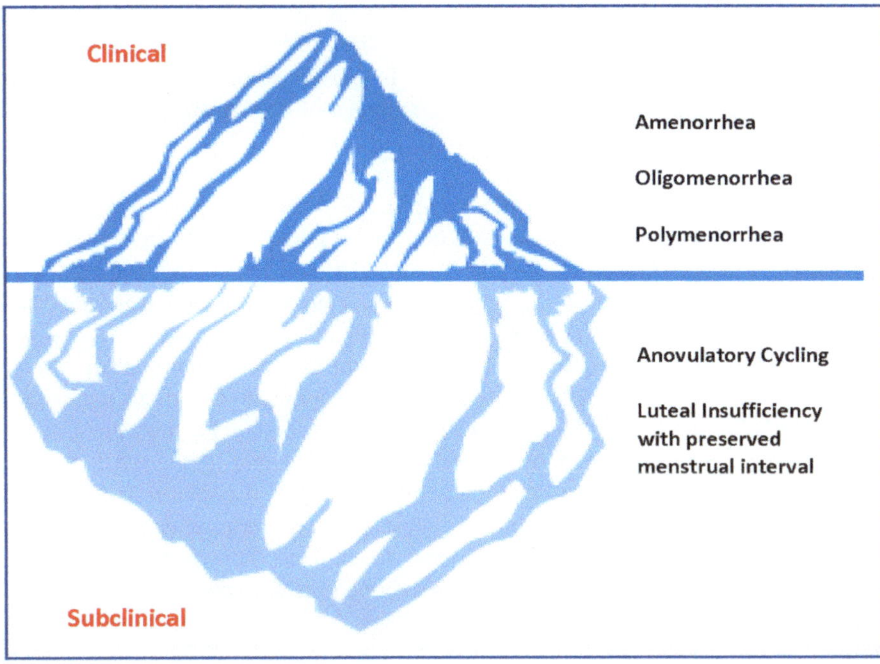

Fig. 10.1 Representation of the spectrum of presentation of functional hypothalamic hypogonadism. Adapted from Berga and Loucks [9]

are estimated to be much more common [2] and likely come to clinical attention when fertility is compromised, see Fig. 10.1 [9].

The purpose of the hypothalamus is to generate an "endocrine action plan" to preserve the organism in the face of challenge. Acutely, stress elicits homeostatic responses designed to restore hormonal equilibrium. When stressed chronically, the resultant adaptive hormonal alterations preserve the individual by conserving metabolic expenditure by limiting reproductive function and by dampening basal metabolic rate. Chronic adaptive responses are termed "allostatic." Women with stress-induced anovulation or FHA show what might be termed neuroendocrine allostasis. Specifically, there is reduced GnRH drive in the face of reduced ovarian secretion of estradiol and progesterone, feedback resistance to the inhibition of corticotrophin-releasing hormone (CRH) release despite increased cortisol in both the circulation and cerebrospinal fluid [10], and lack of a rise in TSH levels despite a decline in thyronine and thyroxine levels. Using a monkey model of stress-induced reproductive compromise, we recently found enhanced sensitivity to the feedback suppression of the pituitary to estradiol [11].

The primary mediators of the stress response are the hypothalamic CRH and the locus coruleus-noradrenergic (LC-NE) neuronal networks and their respective effector systems, the pituitary–adrenal axis, and the autonomic pathways [12]. These systems are linked in a positive feedback loop so that activation of one system activates the other. There are innumerable animal studies demonstrating that the activation of the HPA axis using a variety of stress paradigms induces reproductive compromise. However, only a few studies have been performed to elucidate the mechanisms mediating the disruption of GnRH drive. The evidence that exists supports that hypothalamic GnRH secretion is influenced by both central and peripheral factors and putative regulators include CRH, β-endorphin, dopamine, vasopressin, neuropeptide Y, γ-aminobutyric acid (GABA), and serotonin. For a more extensive review of the neuroendocrine pathways regulating GnRH drive, please refer to Berga and Loucks [13] and Berga and Yen [14].

Evidence supporting the concept that stress impairs ovarian function in women is derived from the consistent demonstration that women with hypogonadotropic hypogonadism not due to defined organic conditions have higher cortisol levels than eumenorrheic, ovulatory women [15–17]. Increased cortisol levels are evident in both the systemic [15, 18] and central [10] compartments. Further, the association between increased cortisol and functional hypothalamic hypogonadism holds in women with athletic amenorrhea [19, 20]. In their study, Loucks et al. found that eumenorrheic athletes had lower luteal progesterone secretion, fewer LH pulses in a day, and higher cortisol levels compared to eumenorrheic sedentary women. Furthermore, anovulatory amenorrheic athletes had the fewest LH pulses in a day and the highest cortisol levels despite comparable levels of exertion and fitness.

In addition to the activation of the HPA axis, women with FHA also display changes in the thyroidal axis. Specifically, women with FHA present with decrements in thyronine and thyroxine, yet TSH levels are preserved [15, 18, 21]. This presentation suggests an altered hypothalamic set point akin to what is seen in hospitalized patients who develop what is referred to as "sick euthyroid syndrome." [15] As was the case of HPA activation, athletic women who have reproductive compromise display hypothalamic hypothyroidism [22]. To summarize, the hypothalamic response to chronic stress causes metabolic mobilization, activation of the HPA axis, and hypothalamic hypothyroidism so as to reduce energy expenditure by lowering basal metabolic rate and reducing the energy spent on reproductive function.

Behavioral Correlates of FHA

Explicating the behaviors and psychosocial factors that promote and sustain the neuroendocrine allostasis of functional hypothalamic hypogonadism has been one of our primary research interests for more than two decades. We have characterized the psychosocial correlates of women with FHA using a wide variety of standardized psychometric inventories and have found that certain characteristics, including mild depressive symptoms, unrealistic expectations of self and others, maladaptive concepts centering on body image, drive for thinness, perfectionism, and need for social approval are more prevalent in women with FHA compared to ovulatory eumenorrheic women and women with other forms of anovulation [3–5].

Two contrasting schools of thought exist regarding the pathogenesis of FHA and the reduction in GnRH/LH drive. One school attributes the disruption of GnRH primarily to psychosocial stress and maladaptive cognitions engendering behaviors, such as undereating and overexercising, that alone or in combination induce mild chronic or intermittent energy deficiency [23]. The other school posits that FHA is primarily caused by volitional energy restriction or expenditure [24]. When subjected prospectively to the combination of running and weight loss, many, but not all women, developed transient anovulation [25]. Cameron et al. showed in monkeys that developed anovulation in response to running that caloric supplementation restored ovulatory function [26]. In unselected eumenorrheic women, GnRH/LH drive was resistant to the acute nutritional challenge of a 72 h fast [27] suggesting that acute caloric restriction alone was not a potent stressor. However, in a study that applied graded energy reductions in eumenorrheic women for a longer duration of 5 days, Loucks and Thuma observed a 40% decline in LH pulse frequency with a 75% reduction in energy availability. These same women displayed a compensatory increase in cortisol secretion and, at the highest level of energy restriction, the cortisol levels increased 30% [28]. Although the increase in cortisol levels observed in this group were comparable to that seen in women with FHA, the level of energy restriction in the experimental paradigm was far greater than that reported by women with FHA. What differs between the subjects in these studies and women with FHA is the psychological compartment. Thus, FHA is more likely to develop when there is both a psychosocial component and an energy deficiency [29]. To look at interactions, we employed a monkey model in which we applied an isolated energy challenge of exercising with mild calorie restriction, an isolated psychosocial challenge of moving to a new milieu, and then we combined both the metabolic and psychosocial challenges. We found that neither metabolic nor psychosocial challenge alone potently compromised menstrual cyclicity, whereas the combination elicited a marked impairment in most [1].

Another factor that differs between research subjects given an energy restriction and women with FHA is that women with FHA "voluntarily" restrict food and calorie intake. The restricted or irregular nutritional intake common in FHA likely indicates a disturbance in appetite and resistance to appetite signals. Ghrelin is a potent orexigenic signal secreted by the cells lining the gastric fundus. Ghrelin administration caused a negative energy balance that decreased GnRH/LH drive and increased cortisol in female rhesus monkeys. Vulliemoz and colleagues used this paradigm to assess the effects of CRH blockade on the effects of energetic challenge caused by ghrelin administration. Astressin B, a CRH receptor antagonist, blocked the reduction of GnRH/LH pulsatility and increased cortisol secretion when coadministered with ghrelin [30]. Interestingly, women with anorexia nervosa have elevated ghrelin levels elicited by chronic energy deprivation, yet they eat less when given ghrelin exogenously [31], indicating "appetite allostasis" or resistance to appetite signals. These results highlight the link between HPA activation and reproductive dysfunction and reinforce the concept that a combination of stressors more potently activates the HPA axis with concomitant neuroendocrine, including reproductive, consequences. These results invalidate the false dichotomy fostered by the question whether reproductive compromise is due to energy deficit vs. psychogenic challenge because in real life these types of stressors travel together [29].

The clinical significance of finding synergism between metabolic/energetic imbalance and psychosocial challenge is that recovery from FHA requires amelioration of energetic imbalance, but not necessarily weight gain, as well as psychosocial support and cognitive restructuring. Further, if FHA is an allostatic state attributable to psychophysiological and behavioral responses to stress that synergistically activate central neuroregulatory networks to concomitantly alter metabolism and suppress the central reproductive axis (GnRH/LH drive), then the neuroendocrine concomitants should reverse when the interaction between energy insufficiency and psychosocial challenge is interrupted. Given that sustained decrements in estradiol, increased cortisol, and subclinical hypothyroidism are likely to negatively impact long-term health for the individual and, through epigenetic mechanisms, fetal development if fertility is induced via reproductive technologies, we sought to determine if FHA could be reversed.

Potential Health Implications of FHA

Increased HPA axis activity is triggered by a variety of different stressors such as restraint or isolation stress, energy depletion, surgery, and psychosocial stress [32, 33]. When stress is defined as the anticipation of an adverse or dangerous situation that exceeds individual coping capacities [34], the ability to delay reproduction until conditions are more favorable makes sense. A decrease in GnRH drive results in a corresponding reduction of pituitary secretion of the gonadotropins LH and FSH and thus reduces the signals for follicle development and ovulation. Correspondingly, follicles make less estradiol and progesterone, which reduces endometrial stimulation and results in amenorrhea. When the HPA axis is chronically activated and results in FHA, the associated estrogen deficiency carries negative health consequences for nonreproductive tissues and heightens the risk for osteoporosis, CVD, and psychiatric syndromes, Table 10.1.

Certainly, bone accretion is compromised in FHA [6], and bone accretion is not readily restored by oral contraceptive use in this context [35–38]. The lack of effectiveness is likely a consequence of chronic or intermittent catabolism and/or

Table 10.1 Putative health consequences associated with functional hypothalamic hypogonadism

Systemic consequences	Reproductive consequences
Osteoporosis	Infertility
Psychiatric syndromes	Preterm labor
Neurodegenerative conditions	Intrauterine growth restriction
Cognitive impairment	Compromised fetal neurodevelopment
Cardiovascular disease (CVD)	Compromised parenting

hypercortisolism blocking the positive effect of sex steroids upon bone accretion. This topic is being addressed in greater detail in another section of this text, but suffice it to say that bone accretion is only possible when an individual is in an anabolic state and sex steroids alone will not reverse catabolism.

We recently found that CSF cortisol concentrations are significantly elevated in women with FHA [10], and this observation raises concern of heightened risk for neurodegenerative disease and dementia [39] as well as other potential health burdens [40, 41]. Further, premenopausal hypogonadism alone, independent of cause, has been linked to an increased late-life risk of depression, Parkinson disease, and dementia [42, 43]. In women with functional hypothalamic hypogonadism who conceive, hypothyroxinemia carries a risk of poor fetal neurodevelopment [44, 45]. Further, maternal stress [46–48] and even brief undernutrition [49] increases the risk of preterm delivery and intrauterine growth restriction. For comprehensive reviews, please refer to Ditzen et al. [50]. What is less often appreciated is the impact of chronic hypoestrogenism coupled with increased cortisol on the cardiovascular system in women with FHA.

CVD is the leading cause of death in women in the USA and more women die from CVD than men. There are two forms of reproductive compromise that increase the risk of CVD, PCOS, and FHA. PCOS is a complex chronic condition associated with oligomenorrhea, hyperandrogenism, and metabolic syndrome, including dyslipidemia and insulin resistance. Women with PCOS display increased risk factors for CVD that are evident at younger age as compared to women with normal menstrual history [51], and these risk factors appear to be associated with the endocrine milieu rather than the appearance of polycystic ovaries on ultrasound evaluation [52]. Conversely, while women with FHA do not have the metabolic syndrome phenotype, they have chronic stress, undernutrition, and hypoestrogenism. Kaplan et al. have demonstrated that monkeys with mild subclinical ovarian compromise related to social subordination have an increased risk of CVD [2, 53]. The monkey model raises concern that women with longstanding FHA may be at increased risk for premature or accelerated CVD.

Indeed, the Women's Ischemia Syndrome Evaluation (WISE) study found a significant association between premenopausal angiographic coronary artery disease (CAD) and hypothalamic hypogonadism [54]. On further analysis, it was found that premenopausal women with both hypothalamic hypogonadism and diabetes had more extensive angiographic CAD than those with either diabetes or hypothalamic hypogonadism alone [55]. Low levels of gonadotropins in this study population argue against underlying PCOS as a contributor to the observed effect. Endothelial function has also been shown to be compromised in women with exercise amenorrhea [56]. O'Donnell et al. recently showed that women athletes with chronic hypoestrogenemia displayed impaired peripheral vascular function that was combined with lower resting blood pressures and heart rate and reduced ischemic responses to occlusion challenge compared to ovulatory exercising and ovulatory sedentary women [57]. These observations substantiate the importance of cyclic ovarian function as an indicator of overall health and wellbeing. When the internal and external environments are sufficiently stressful so as to disrupt systems mediating reproductive alignment, acute and chronic health risks accrue to the individual and future generations. Approaches that address the whole patient, identify and ameliorate stress, and promote balance are warranted as these will likely have the greatest impact on overall health.

Treatment Considerations

As depicted in Fig. 10.1, most functional hypothalamic hypogonadism in women is subclinical and may only come to clinical attention when there is unexplained infertility or when the menstrual interval is markedly short, long, very irregular, or absent. Similarly, luteal insufficiency due to decreased GnRH/LH drive may only be detected when infertility results. Even then, it is difficult using standard office techniques to document intermittent anovulation or luteal insufficiency. It is thus reasonable to say that the more clinically evident the ovarian compromise, the greater the hypothalamic challenge and the more profound the associated HPA, HPT derangements, and sex steroid deprivation. The diagnosis of FHA can be made only by the exclusion of all other organic forms of secondary anovulation, including PCOS, premature ovarian failure, hyperprolactinemia, organic adrenal and thyroidal dysfunction, autoimmune enteropathies, and psychiatric causes.

As mentioned previously, FHA is more than an isolated disruption in central GnRH/LH drive. There is direct evidence of HPA activation in the systemic [15, 18] and central compartments [10] and allostatic adjustments in the thyroidal axis, specifically normal TSH levels despite significantly lower T3 and T4 levels [15, 18, 21]. In women who were in the process of spontaneously recovering from FHA, cortisol levels were comparable to eumenorrheic ovulatory women, but LH pulsatility was not fully restored, and TSH levels were markedly elevated in the face of persistent reductions in T3 and T4 levels [18, 21]. We recently compared metabolic variables in women who did and those who did not recover from FHA after a course of CBT [58]. Taken together, these findings suggest that the thyroidal axis remains restrained by an as yet uncharacterized factor(s) after HPA and HPO recovery or recovers more slowly than the HPA and HPO axes.

The conventional therapy for women with FHA is oral contraceptives when fertility is not desired and ovulation induction or assisted reproduction when it is. These approaches address the symptoms of amenorrhea and infertility but do not address the underlying allostatic adjustments of the adrenal and thyroidal axes. Thus, women with FHA treated with hormone replacement remain at increased risk for bone loss and cardiovascular effects related to chronic activation of the HPA, hypothalamic hypothryroidism and hypoestrogenism [6, 35, 36, 59].

Alternatively, if a woman with functional hypothalamic hypogonadism is seeking to become pregnant, ovulation induction can be accomplished technically with exogenous administration of pulsatile GnRH therapy [60, 61] or exogenous administration of gonadotropins. The obvious advantage of exogenous GnRH therapy is that it diminishes the risk of ovarian hyperstimulation and multiple gestations associated with gonadotropins; however, it is no longer available. Clominphene citrate may not be an effective strategy because it has a hypothalamic site of action, and the hypothalamus is not normoresponsive to estrogen feedback [11]. There also is some concern that ovulation induction may place women with FHA at risk for premature labor and intrauterine growth retardation [62]. The parenting skills of women with FHA may be impaired because they are already overwhelmed and stressed prior to pregnancy and delivery and thus their children may be at risk for poor psychosocial development [63]. Further, children born to mothers with clinically occult autoimmune hypothyroidism had a mean full-scale intelligence quotient that was 7 points lower than the control population [44]. The women with clinically occult hypothyroidism had a 30% reduction in thyroxine, which is roughly what is observed in women with FHA. These findings are explained by the fact that maternal thyroxine is the only source of fetal thyroxine in the first trimester and the predominant fetal source in the second and third trimesters. Appropriate thyroxine is required for fetal neurogenesis and even small decrements may induce neurodevelopmental deficits. Increased maternal cortisol may also have independent effects upon fetal neurodevelopment and organogenesis. Recent evidence showed that severe stress such as that associated with the unexpected death of a child increased the risk of congenital anomalies of the cranial neural crest eightfold [47]. Further, stress and its endocrine concomitants have been implicated as a cause of preterm delivery. It is not known if the endocrine concomitants associated with FHA pose a similar risk, but this is clearly a potential hazard if ovulation induction is undertaken before amelioration of the allostatic changes in the adrenal and thyroidal axes.

Although psychopharmacologic approaches have not been well studied, they probably could be used on an interim basis in special circumstances. The study of Judd suggested that a short course of alprazolam might be effective in reducing HPA activation and permitting hypothalamic–pituitary–ovarian recovery [64]. However, this approach would not be the best for a woman hoping to conceive because of the risk of fetal exposure to benzodiazepines. The optimal intervention is to interdict the stress process so that the hypothalamus recovers and gonadal function resumes. An integral goal of the treatment plan for women with functional hypothalamic hypogonadism is to help them identify and ameliorate the sources of psychogenic and metabolic stress and to provide emotional support while coping mechanisms other than nutrient restriction or exercising are learned. Nonpharmacologic interventions, such as stress management, relaxation training, or psychoeducation, empower individuals by fostering self-care and competency. In this regard, nonpharmacologic therapies have the potential to produce long-term benefits upon psychological, and thereby, physical health. Behavioral therapies acknowledge the wisdom of the body and recognize that FHA represents an endocrine adaptation that can be reversed with appropriate psychogenic and behavioral modifications.

Given these considerations, we recently studied whether CBT aimed at ameliorating problematic attitudes and behaviors would permit reproductive recovery in normal weight women with FHA [65]. Women with FHA were randomized to observation vs. CBT. CBT focused on attitudes rather than behaviors. The program consisted of 16 individual sessions over 20 weeks. Participants met with a trained master's level clinician, a research dietitian, and a reproductive endocrinologist. The sessions occurred in three overlapping stages intended to (1) define healthy eating and exercise patterns; (2) identify stress-enhancing behaviors and guide the participant in developing strategies and problem solving skills to reduce stress; and (3) reinforce strategies and plans for resolving stress and avoiding relapse once CBT concluded [65]. Women in both the observation and CBT groups were followed for the return of menses for up to 8 weeks following the intervention. Regardless of menstrual pattern, estradiol and progesterone levels were monitored at weekly intervals for 4 weeks before and after observation vs. CBT. About 88% of those who underwent CBT had evidence of ovulation, whereas only 25% of those who were observed did. Figure 10.2 shows sex steroid secretion in a woman treated with CBT who showed ovarian recovery contrasted with those in a woman randomized to observation who did not have the recovery of ovarian function.

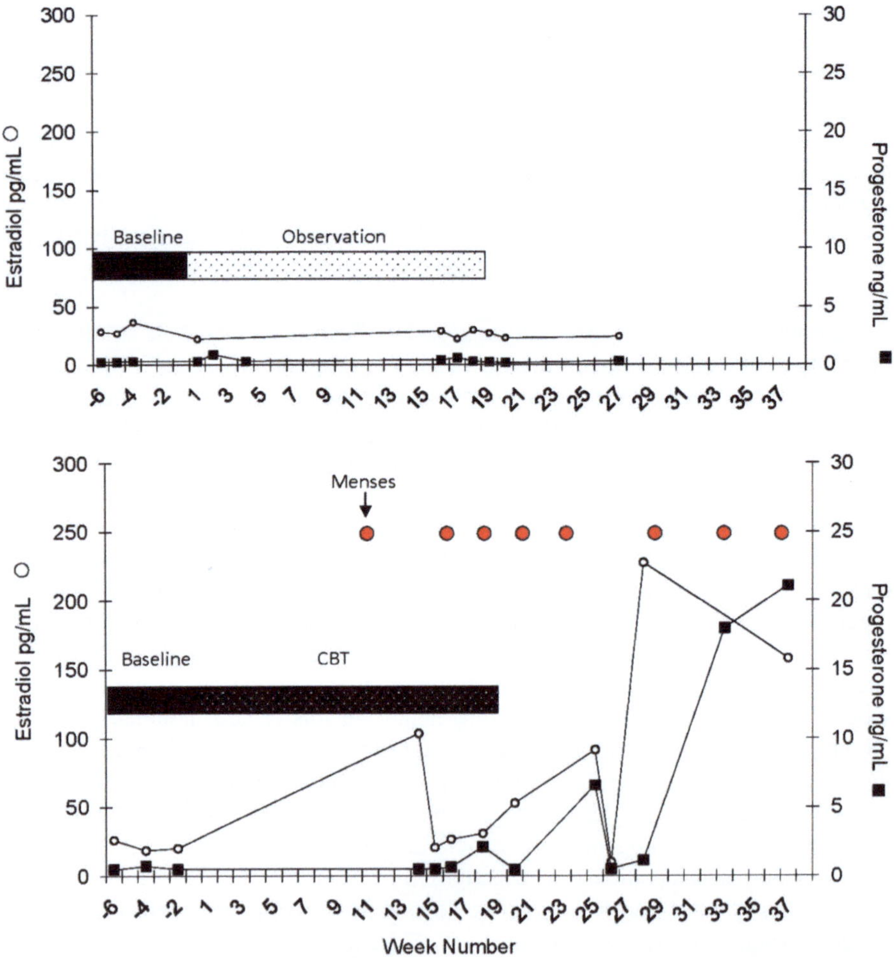

Fig. 10.2 Serum levels of ovarian hormones (estradiol *open circle*) and (progesterone *filled square*) and episodes of vaginal bleeding (*red filled circle*) in a woman with functional hypothalamic amenorrhea (FHA) who was observed and did not recover (*top*) compared to a woman with FHA who was treated with cognitive behavior therapy (CBT) and recovered (*lower*). Adapted from Berga et al. (2003) [65]

Interestingly, when it occurred, ovarian recovery was not associated with significant weight gain. This does not mean that subjects did not alter food intake or energy expenditure, however. Once stress and undernutrition are reduced, the thyroidal axis may increase basal metabolic rate, allowing greater food intake without weight gain.

Persistent HPA activation, which elevates CSF cortisol more than circulating cortisol levels, [10] carries long-term health risks for the woman and, should she conceive, for the fetus [46, 48]. Increased cortisol is one of the factors that suppresses the thyroidal axis. As the mother is the sole source of thyroxine for the fetus during the first and the predominant source during the second and third trimester, the clinician should consider that assisted reproduction presents an unrecognized fetal risk because persistent hypothalamic hypothyroidism may compromise fetal neurodevelopment [44, 45]. Further, psychosocial stress [46–48] and even brief undernutrition [49] increases the risk of preterm delivery and intrauterine growth restriction. In contrast, CBT offers a focused therapeutic option that avoids medical risks and costs associated with ovulation induction and assisted reproduction while at least partially reversing neuroendocrine allostasis. Since the effect of CBT accrues with time while that of pharmacologic interventions does not, CBT should be a mainstay of intervention for stress-related infertility and FHA even if it is not the only therapy the patient receives.

Conclusion

While stress is generally categorized as psychogenic or metabolic, strictly speaking, these are not separable entities. Further, the impact of chronic stress is not limited to the reproductive axis. Adjustments in other systems, specifically HPA and HPT axes occur concomitantly. The health burden of chronic stress puts individuals at increased risk for osteoporosis, CVD, and mental health impairments such as mood disorders, migraines, and insomnia. Thus, when evaluating the patient with hypothalamic amenorrhea, consideration must be given to both long-term and short-term consequences. Behavioral treatments are directed toward amelioration of the underlying stress, are effective, and will likely have a greater positive impact on overall health than pharmacologic approaches.

References

1. Williams NI, Berga SL, Cameron JL (2007) Synergism between psychosocial and metabolic stressors: impact on reproductive function in cynomolgus monkeys. Am J Physiol Endocrinol Metab 293(1):E270–E276
2. Kaplan JR, Manuck SB (2004) Ovarian dysfunction, stress, and disease: a primate continuum. ILAR J 45(2):89–115
3. Giles DE, Berga SL (1993) Cognitive and psychiatric correlates of functional hypothalamic amenorrhea: a controlled comparison. Fertil Steril 60(3):486–492

4. Marcus MD, Loucks TL, Berga SL (2001) Psychological correlates of functional hypothalamic amenorrhea. Fertil Steril 76(2):310–316
5. Berga SL, Girton LG (1989) The psychoneuroendocrinology of functional hypothalamic amenorrhea. Psychiatr Clin North Am 12(1):105–116
6. Grinspoon S, Miller K, Coyle C et al (1999) Severity of osteopenia in estrogen-deficient women with anorexia nervosa and hypothalamic amenorrhea. J Clin Endocrinol Metab 84(6):2049–2055
7. Reindollar RH, Novak M, Tho SP, McDonough PG (1986) Adult-onset amenorrhea: a study of 262 patients. Am J Obstet Gynecol 155(3):531–543
8. Reame NE, Sauder SE, Case GD, Kelch RP, Marshall JC (1985) Pulsatile gonadotropin secretion in women with hypothalamic amenorrhea: evidence that reduced frequency of gonadotropin-releasing hormone secretion is the mechanism of persistent anovulation. J Clin Endocrinol Metab 61(5):851–858
9. Berga SL, Loucks TL (2009) Stress and reproductive function. Female Patient 34:13–16
10. Brundu B, Loucks TL, Adler LJ, Cameron JL, Berga SL (2006) Increased cortisol in the cerebrospinal fluid of women with functional hypothalamic amenorrhea. J Clin Endocrinol Metab 91(4):1561–1565
11. Michopoulos V, Berga SL, Kaplan JR, Wilson ME (2009) Social subordination and polymorphisms in the gene encoding the serotonin transporter enhance estradiol inhibition of luteinizing hormone secretion in female rhesus monkeys. Biol Reprod 81(6):1154–1163
12. Chrousos GP, Gold PW (1992) The concepts of stress and stress system disorders. Overview of physical and behavioral homeostasis. JAMA 267(9):1244–1252
13. Berga SL, Loucks TL (2007) Stress-induced anovulation. In: Fink G (ed) Encyclopedia of stress, vol 3, 2nd edn. Oxford Academic Press, Kidlington, pp 615–631
14. Berga SL, Yen SSC (2004) Reproductive failure due to central nervous system-hypothalamic-pituitary dysfunction, Chap. 18, vol 5. Elsevier Saunders, Philadelphia, PA
15. Berga SL, Mortola JF, Girton L et al (1989) Neuroendocrine aberrations in women with functional hypothalamic amenorrhea. J Clin Endocrinol Metab 68(2):301–308
16. Biller BM, Federoff HJ, Koenig JI, Klibanski A (1990) Abnormal cortisol secretion and responses to corticotropin-releasing hormone in women with hypothalamic amenorrhea. J Clin Endocrinol Metab 70(2):311–317
17. Suh BY, Liu JH, Berga SL, Quigley ME, Laughlin GA, Yen SS (1988) Hypercortisolism in patients with functional hypothalamic-amenorrhea. J Clin Endocrinol Metab 66(4):733–739
18. Berga SL, Daniels TL, Giles DE (1997) Women with functional hypothalamic amenorrhea but not other forms of anovulation display amplified cortisol concentrations. Fertil Steril 67(6):1024–1030
19. De Souza MJ, Miller BE, Loucks AB et al (1998) High frequency of luteal phase deficiency and anovulation in recreational women runners: blunted elevation in follicle-stimulating hormone observed during luteal-follicular transition. J Clin Endocrinol Metab 83(12):4220–4232
20. Loucks AB, Mortola JF, Girton L, Yen SS (1989) Alterations in the hypothalamic-pituitary-ovarian and the hypothalamic-pituitary-adrenal axes in athletic women. J Clin Endocrinol Metab 68(2):402–411
21. Daniels TL, Cameron JL, Marcus MD, Berga SL (1997) Recovery from functional hypothalamic amenorrhea (FHA) involves resolution of hypothalamic hypothyroidism. Paper presented at the 79th annual meeting of the endocrine society, Minneapolis, MN, 11 June 1997
22. Loucks AB, Laughlin GA, Mortola JF, Girton L, Nelson JC, Yen SS (1992) Hypothalamic-pituitary-thyroidal function in eumenorrheic and amenorrheic athletes. J Clin Endocrinol Metab 75(2):514–518
23. Berga SL (1997) Behaviorally induced reproductive compromise in women and men. Semin Reprod Endocrinol 15(1):47–53
24. Redman LM, Loucks AB (2005) Menstrual disorders in athletes. Sports Med 35(9):747–755
25. Bullen BA, Skrinar GS, Beitins IZ, von Mering G, Turnbull BA, McArthur JW (1985) Induction of menstrual disorders by strenuous exercise in untrained women. N Engl J Med 312(21):1349–1353

26. Cameron JL, Nosbisch C, Helmreich D, Parfitt DB (1990) Reversal of exercise-induced amenorrhea in female cynomolgus monkeys (*Macasa fascicularis*) by increasing food intake. Paper presented at the 72nd annual meeting of the endocrine society, Atlanta, GA, 1990
27. Berga SL, Loucks TL, Cameron JL (2001) Endocrine and chronobiological effects of fasting in women. Fertil Steril 75(5):926–932
28. Loucks AB, Thuma JR (2003) Luteinizing hormone pulsatility is disrupted at a threshold of energy availability in regularly menstruating women. J Clin Endocrinol Metab 88(1):297–311
29. Berga SL (2008) Stress and reproduction: a tale of false dichotomy? Endocrinology 149(3): 867–868
30. Vulliemoz NR, Xiao E, Xia-Zhang L, Rivier J, Ferin M (2008) Astressin B, a nonselective corticotropin-releasing hormone receptor antagonist, prevents the inhibitory effect of ghrelin on luteinizing hormone pulse frequency in the ovariectomized rhesus monkey. Endocrinology 149(3):869–874
31. Miljic D, Pekic S, Djurovic M et al (2006) Ghrelin has partial or no effect on appetite, growth hormone, prolactin, and cortisol release in patients with anorexia nervosa. J Clin Endocrinol Metab 91(4):1491–1495
32. Dickerson SS, Kemeny ME (2004) Acute stressors and cortisol responses: a theoretical integration and synthesis of laboratory research. Psychol Bull 130(3):355–391
33. Sapolsky RM, Romero LM, Munck AU (2000) How do glucocorticoids influence stress responses? Integrating permissive, suppressive, stimulatory, and preparative actions. Endocr Rev 21(1):55–89
34. Lazarus RS, Folkman S (1984) Stress, appraisal, and coping. Springer, New York
35. Golden NH, Lanzkowsky L, Schebendach J, Palestro CJ, Jacobson MS, Shenker IR (2002) The effect of estrogen-progestin treatment on bone mineral density in anorexia nervosa. J Pediatr Adolesc Gynecol 15(3):135–143
36. Klibanski A, Biller BM, Schoenfeld DA, Herzog DB, Saxe VC (1995) The effects of estrogen administration on trabecular bone loss in young women with anorexia nervosa. J Clin Endocrinol Metab 80(3):898–904
37. Munoz MT, Morande G, Garcia-Centenera JA, Hervas F, Pozo J, Argente J (2002) The effects of estrogen administration on bone mineral density in adolescents with anorexia nervosa. Eur J Endocrinol 146(1):45–50
38. Warren MP, Miller KK, Olson WH, Grinspoon SK, Friedman AJ (2005) Effects of an oral contraceptive (norgestimate/ethinyl estradiol) on bone mineral density in women with hypothalamic amenorrhea and osteopenia: an open-label extension of a double-blind, placebo-controlled study. Contraception 72(3):206–211
39. Sapolsky RM (2000) Glucocorticoids and hippocampal atrophy in neuropsychiatric disorders. Arch Gen Psychiatry 57(10):925–935
40. McEwen BS (1998) Protective and damaging effects of stress mediators. N Engl J Med 338(3):171–179
41. McEwen BS (2002) Sex, stress and the hippocampus: allostasis, allostatic load and the aging process. Neurobiol Aging 23(5):921–939
42. Rocca WA, Bower JH, Maraganore DM et al (2007) Increased risk of cognitive impairment or dementia in women who underwent oophorectomy before menopause. Neurology 69(11): 1074–1083
43. Rocca WA, Bower JH, Maraganore DM et al (2008) Increased risk of parkinsonism in women who underwent oophorectomy before menopause. Neurology 70(3):200–209
44. Haddow JE, Palomaki GE, Allan WC et al (1999) Maternal thyroid deficiency during pregnancy and subsequent neuropsychological development of the child. N Engl J Med 341(8):549–555
45. Morreale de Escobar G, Obregon MJ, Escobar del Rey F (2000) Is neuropsychological development related to maternal hypothyroidism or to maternal hypothyroxinemia? J Clin Endocrinol Metab 85(11):3975–3987
46. Challis J, Sloboda D, Matthews S et al (2000) Fetal hypothalamic-pituitary adrenal (HPA) development and activation as a determinant of the timing of birth, and of postnatal disease. Endocr Res 26(4):489–504

47. Hansen D, Lou HC, Olsen J (2000) Serious life events and congenital malformations: a national study with complete follow-up. Lancet 9233:875–880
48. Wadhwa PD, Sandman CA, Garite TJ (2001) The neurobiology of stress in human pregnancy: implications for prematurity and development of the fetal central nervous system. Prog Brain Res 133:131–142
49. McMillen IC, Schwartz J, Coulter CL, Edwards LJ (2004) Early embryonic environment, the fetal pituitary-adrenal axis and the timing of parturition. Endocr Res 30(4):845–850
50. Ditzen B, Loucks TL, Berga SL (2009) Role of stress in infertility. In: Dog TL, Maizes V (eds) Weil integrative medicine library: women's health. Oxford University Press, New York
51. Talbott E, Clerici A, Berga SL et al (1998) Adverse lipid and coronary heart disease risk profiles in young women with polycystic ovary syndrome: results of a case-control study. J Clin Epidemiol 51(5):415–422
52. Loucks TL, Talbott EO, McHugh KP, Keelan M, Berga SL, Guzick DS (2000) Do polycystic-appearing ovaries affect the risk of cardiovascular disease among women with polycystic ovary syndrome? Fertil Steril 74(3):547–552
53. Kaplan JR, Manuck SB, Anthony MS, Clarkson TB (2002) Premenopausal social status and hormone exposure predict postmenopausal atherosclerosis in female monkeys. Obstet Gynecol 99(3):381–388
54. Bairey Merz CN, Johnson BD, Sharaf BL et al (2003) Hypoestrogenemia of hypothalamic origin and coronary artery disease in premenopausal women: a report from the NHLBI-sponsored WISE study. J Am Coll Cardiol 41(3):413–419
55. Ahmed B, Bairey Merz CN, Johnson BD et al (2008) Diabetes mellitus, hypothalamic hypoestrogenemia, and coronary artery disease in premenopausal women (from the National Heart, Lung, and Blood Institute sponsored WISE study). Am J Cardiol 102(2):150–154
56. Rickenlund A, Eriksson MJ, Schenck-Gustafsson K, Hirschberg AL (2005) Amenorrhea in female athletes is associated with endothelial dysfunction and unfavorable lipid profile. J Clin Endocrinol Metab 90(3):1354–1359
57. O'Donnell E, Harvey PJ, Goodman JM, De Souza MJ (2007) Long-term estrogen deficiency lowers regional blood flow, resting systolic blood pressure, and heart rate in exercising premenopausal women. Am J Physiol Endocrinol Metab 292(5):E1401–E1409
58. Mancini F, Basanta-Henry P, Corominal A, Loucks TL, Berga SL (2006) Do metabolic variables gate reproductive recovery in functional hypothalamic amenorrhea? Paper presented at the 88th annual meeting of the endocrine society, Boston, MA, 25 June 2006
59. Genazzani AD, Gamba O, Petraglia F (1998) Estrogen replacement therapy modulates spontaneous GH secretion but does not affect GH-RH-induced GH response and low T3 syndrome in women with hypothalamic amenorrhea associated to weight-loss. J Endocrinol Invest 21(6):353–357
60. Hurley DM, Brian R, Outch K et al (1984) Induction of ovulation and fertility in amenorrheic women by pulsatile low-dose gonadotropin-releasing hormone. N Engl J Med 310(17): 1069–1074
61. Miller DS, Reid RR, Cetel NS, Rebar RW, Yen SS (1983) Pulsatile administration of low-dose gonadotropin-releasing hormone. Ovulation and pregnancy in women with hypothalamic amenorrhea. JAMA 250(21):2937–2941
62. van der Spuy ZM, Steer PJ, McCusker M, Steele SJ, Jacobs HS (1988) Outcome of pregnancy in underweight women after spontaneous and induced ovulation. Br Med J (Clin Res Ed) 296(6627):962–965
63. Pike KM, Rodin J (1991) Mothers, daughters, and disordered eating. J Abnorm Psychol 100(2):198–204
64. Judd SJ, Wong J, Saloniklis S et al (1995) The effect of alprazolam on serum cortisol and luteinizing hormone pulsatility in normal women and in women with stress-related anovulation. J Clin Endocrinol Metab 80(3):818–823
65. Berga SL, Marcus MD, Loucks TL, Hlastala S, Ringham R, Krohn MA (2003) Recovery of ovarian activity in women with functional hypothalamic amenorrhea who were treated with cognitive behavior therapy. Fertil Steril 80(4):976–981

Chapter 11
Long-Term Implications of Oophorectomy at the Time of Hysterectomy for Benign Disease

Donna Shoupe and Jonathan S. Berek

Introduction

The National Center for Health Statistics report that in 2004, of the 617,000 hysterectomies performed in the USA, 73% also involved the surgical removal of the ovaries. In the United States, by age 60, about 1/3 of women undergo a hysterectomy [1, 2]. Over the past decade, an average of 622,000 hysterectomies per year have been performed, and it is now estimated that there are 22 million women in the USA who have undergone this procedure [2]. According to the CDC, 52% of all hysterectomies are performed in women aged 44 years of age or younger. Of over 3 million hysterectomies performed between 1994 and 1999 in the USA, slightly over 10% were done for a primary diagnosis of cancer (Table 11.1). It is important to recognize the long-term implications of hysterectomy with and without oophorectomy and to counsel patients accordingly.

Arguments for and Against Oophorectomy

One of the main arguments in the USA for bilateral oophorectomy at the time of hysterectomy for benign disease is to prevent the later development of ovarian cancer. While the overall lifetime risk of ovarian cancer is 1.4% among the U.S. women, the risk varies depending on the presence of risk factors. For white women with three or more term pregnancies and 4 or more years of oral contraceptive use, the risk of ovarian cancer by age 65 is only 0.3% compared to 1.6% among nulliparous women with no prior oral contraceptive use [3]. Other arguments for

J.S. Berek (✉)
Department of Obstetrics & Gynecology, Stanford University Hospital and Clinics,
300 Pasteur Drive Room HH333, Stanford, CA 94305-5317, USA
e-mail: Jberek@stanford.edu

N.F. Santoro and G. Neal-Perry (eds.), *Amenorrhea: A Case-Based, Clinical Guide*,
Contemporary Endocrinology, DOI 10.1007/978-1-60327-864-5_11,

Table 11.1 Estimated hysterectomy rates by age group and primary discharge diagnosis in the United States 1994–1999

Age	Cancer	Hyperplasia	Endometriosis	Leiomyoma	Prolapse	Other
15–29	13,193		53,663	12,312	17,173	165,120
30–34	20,318	3,533	106,575	69,836	47,816	87,806
35–39	29,246	8,026	156,330	222,206	77,818	103,526
40–44	36,906	13,792	143,718	399,277	80,342	69,542
45–54	64,802	44,990	136,060	553,641	126,851	72,132
>55	192,596	49,990	34,488	103,805	241,165	59,024
Total	360,197	121,651	630,834	1,361,786	593,619	457,150

Adapted from ref. [98]

oophorectomy include decreasing the risk of subsequent ovarian pathology or adnexal pain that might require additional surgery. The reoperation rate in hysterectomized women for adnexal pathology is reported to be between 0.895 and 5.5% [4–6].

The chief argument against routine oophorectomy is that premenopausal oophorectomy leads to an abrupt decline in circulating estrogens and androgens, often leading to severe menopausal symptoms, including hot flashes, sleep disturbance, mood alteration, vaginal dryness, and sexual problems. Most importantly, oophorectomy has been associated with higher risks of coronary heart disease (CHD), hip fracture, Parkinsonism, dementia, cognitive impairment, visual declines, depression, and anxiety [7, 8]. There is growing concern that the benefit of reducing a woman's risk of ovarian cancer is outweighed by an increased risk of these serious diseases [9–11]

Long-Term Risks of Hysterectomy

The average age at menopause in women who have had an extrafascial hysterectomy and preservation of the ovaries is 3.7 years earlier than in women who have an intact uterus [12]. This is thought to be due to a decreased blood supply to the ovaries after hysterectomy. Multiple studies have also documented lower androgen levels [13–15] and higher rates of bone loss in older hysterectomized women compared to nonhysterectomized women [16, 17]. A limited number of women report long-term adverse effects on sexual function after hysterectomy, including vaginal shortening or symptoms related to a loss of support to the bladder and bowel. However, improved sexual satisfaction and relief of bladder problems and improvements of bowel function are more commonly reported, especially in women with pain, bleeding problems or bowel or urinary problems prior to surgery. The loss of reproductive function may have emotional implications for a limited number of women.

Long-Term Risks of Oophorectomy in Premenopausal Women

Hot Flashes, Mood, and Quality of Life

Following bilateral oophorectomy in a premenopausal woman, the sudden loss of estrogen often triggers severe menopausal symptoms such as hot flashes, mood changes, headaches, reduced well-being, and sleep disturbances [18–21]. Within a few years, other common problems associated with estrogen deficiency include vaginal dryness, painful intercourse, loss of sex drive, bladder dysfunction, poor sleep quality, and symptoms of depression also emerge [22–25]. The severity of these symptoms and other estrogen deficiency-related problems are increased in oophorectomized women compared to naturally menopausal women, occur at an earlier age, and are usually more difficult to treat with hormonal therapy [21]. It is reported that more than 90% of premenopausal women will have vasomotor symptoms following oophorectomy [26].

Urogenital Atrophy

The loss of estrogen support for the bladder and vagina results in changes in lubrication, pH, normal bacterial flora, and tissue structure. Short-term symptoms associated with estrogen deficiency include decreased vaginal lubrication, itching, dryness, burning, and discharge. Long-term estrogen and possibly also androgen deficiencies lead to thinning of the vaginal epithelium and shrinkage of the tissues. Over time, these changes may result in fissures, ecchymoses, ulcerations, painful intercourse, pruritis, chronic inflammation, and vaginal stenosis. Changes in the urethral and bladder epithelium may cause a sensation of bladder pressure, urethral discomfort, dysuria, incontinence, urinary frequency, and recurrent urinary tract infections.

Oophorectomy, a predisposing factor leading to urogenital atrophy [26, 27] that increased the incidence of urogential atrophy is reported in surgically menopausal women compared to naturally menopausal women [26–28]. This may be related to the low levels of androgens in oophorectomized women, as higher levels of androgens are reported to be protective [28].

Sexual Function

Oophorectomy in premenopausal women is often associated with a negative impact on sexual function. There is strong evidence that sexual desire and motivation in women are highly dependent on androgens [29, 30]. Additionally, androgens appear to impact on sexual sensation and orgasmic response. Studies report that following prophylactic oophorectomy, women with a high risk of hereditary ovarian cancer have significantly lower menopause-specific quality of life scores. In one study, 42–53% of the participants reported that their satisfaction with sexual functioning was moderately to extremely compromised [31]. In a similar study done in 846 high-risk women undergoing prophylactic oophorectomy, participants reported significant postoperative declines in sexual functioning and other endocrine problems [32].

Studies in normal risk women report no decline in sexual function following hysterectomy alone, but dramatic reductions following hysterectomy with oophorectomy. These declines in sexual function were reversed following estrogen and androgen therapy [22].

Central Nervous Effects: Cognitive Thought, Memory, Depression, Parkinson's Disease

Premenopausal oophorectomy is reported to have significant effects on CNS function and is associated with declines in cognitive thought, memory, energy level, mood, and feelings of wellbeing [22, 25, 33–40]. Estrogen has been shown to be neuroprotective in animals and cell culture, [35] suppressing inflammation, reducing oxidative stress, improving synapse formation, upregulating neurotrophic factors, facilitating regeneration of vascular endothelium, [41] protecting dopaminergic neurons, reducing oxidative stress, and upregulating neurotrophic factors. Estrogen may act as an antioxidant, and appears to increase choline acetyltransferase activity and reduce deposition of amyloid [35, 42].

The Mayo Clinic Cohort Study followed women living in Minnesota who underwent either unilateral ($n=1{,}252$) or bilateral oophorectomy ($n=1{,}075$) for 25–30 years. These women were age matched to women ($n=2{,}368$) who had not undergone oophorectomy. The results of this study reported that women who underwent either unilateral or bilateral oophorectomy prior to menopause and did not take hormone therapy had an increased risk of parkinsonism (HR 1.68; 95% CI 1.06–2.67), cognitive impairment or dementia (HR = 1.46; 95% CI 1.13–1.90), and anxiety (HR = 2.29; 95% CI 1.13–3.95) or depression (HR = 1.54 95% CI 1.04–2.26). The risk of each of these conditions increased with younger age at oophorectomy. The authors proposed that ovarian hormones have a neuroprotective effect [10, 36, 37].

Osteoporosis and Hip Fracture

Both androgens and estrogens play important roles in normal bone metabolism as estrogens and androgens inhibit bone resorption and androgens stimulate bone formation [43]. Following oophorectomy in premenopausal women, increased bone turnover, and overall bone loss begins unless adequate hormone therapy is promptly started. Oophorectomy is considered an important risk factor for the development of osteoporosis and hip fracture [44]. After bilateral oophorectomy, women have significantly lower levels of androgens and estrogens compared to those who are naturally menopausal [14, 45–47]. Low levels of these hormones have been linked to lower bone density and increased the risk of hip fracture and vertebral fractures [14, 16, 48–52]. Unfortunately, hip and vertebral fractures are associated with increased morbidity and mortality [53, 54].

Quality of Life: Lens Opacities, Body Mass

Increases in macular degeneration and lens opacities are linked with early menopause [55, 56]. Oophorectomy adversely affects skin, body composition, and central adiposity [57–61].

Cardiovascular Disease

Multiple observational studies report that women with surgical menopause have an increased risk of cardiovascular morbidity and mortality compared to women with natural menopause [7, 8, 62–70]. Data from the Nurses' Health Study (NHS) reported that oophorectomy between ages 40 and 44 doubled the risk of myocardial infarction (RR 2.2 95% CI 1.2, 4.2) compared to that of women with intact ovaries [7, 71]. Even after age 50, oophorectomy increases the risk of developing a first MI compared to controls (RR 1.4, 95% CI 1.0–2.0) A published metaanalysis of observational studies found that oophorectomy doubled the risk of cardiovascular disease (RR 2.62 95% CI 2.05, 3.35) [8].

Other studies support the increased risk of cardiovascular disease following oophorectomy. Data from the Women's Health Initiative (WHI) showed that hysterectomy with oophorectomy was an independent predictor of increased Framingham risk of myocardial infarction or coronary death [67]. Oophorectomy has been shown to increase serum lipids [72, 73], reduce carotid artery blood flow, [74] and have adverse effects on other atherosclerotic risk factors [75–77]. Women having earlier menopause, as a result of bilateral oophorectomy, have more subclinical atherosclerosis compared to age-matched women who had natural menopause [78].

In a substudy of WHI placebo-controlled trial of conjugated estrogens, the authors aimed to determine the associations between coronary artery calcium (CAC) and hysterectomy, oophorectomy, and hormone therapy. CAC was measured by computed tomography in participants 1.3 years after the trial was stopped. Participants included 1,064 women with previous hysterectomy, aged 50–59 years at baseline. The mean trial period was 7.4 years. Imaging was performed at a mean of 1.3 years after the trial was stopped. The mean age was 55.1 years at randomization and 64.8 years at CAC measurement. There was a significant interaction between bilateral oophorectomy and prerandomization HT use for the presence of any CAC ($p=0.05$). When multivariable analyses were restricted to women who reported no previous HT use, those with bilateral oophorectomy had an odds ratio of 2.0 (95% CI: 1.2–3.4) for any CAC compared with women with no history of oophorectomy, whereas among women with unilateral or partial oophorectomy, the odds of any CAC was 1.7 (95% CI: 1.0–2.8). Among women with bilateral oophorectomy, HT use within 5 years of oophorectomy was associated with a lower rate of CAC. The authors concluded that factors related to oophorectomy and the lack of estrogen treatment may be related to CHD [79].

Long-Term Risks of Oophorectomy in Postmenopausal Women

Hormone Production in the Postmenopausal Ovary

During the reproductive years, ovarian follicles secrete relatively large amounts of estrogens and androgens. During the menopausal transition, there is a loss of follicular activity and a resultant drop of estrogen, progesterone, and androgens. It is believed that the postmenopausal ovarian stromal tissues continue to produce substantial amounts of androgens and remain an important source of androgens for the remainder of a woman's lifetime [45–47, 80–82]. The peripheral conversion of these androgens to estrogens also provides low levels of circulating estrogens. Postmenopausal women with intact ovaries have significantly higher levels of plasma testosterone, androstenedione, and estrogens than oophorectomized women [45–47, 80] (Table 11.2). The benefits of postmenopausal ovarian androgens on bone and their derivatives and the consequences of their removal are well documented [45–48, 50–52].

In a cross-sectional study in 684 postmenopausal women ages 50–89 in a community-dwelling postmenopausal women, both total and bioavailable testosterone levels were 40% lower ($p<0.001$) in hysterectomized women with bilateral oophorectomy compared to those in intact women. Women with ovarian conservation and hysterectomy had intermediate levels. Total estradiol levels tended to be

Table 11.2 Steroid hormone levels in natural vs. surgical menopause

	Mean steroid levels in women (pg/mL)		
	Reproductive age (luteal phase)	Natural menopause	Surgical menopause
Estradiol	150	10–15	10
Testosterone	400	290	110
Progesterone	12,000–20,000	<100	<100

Adapted from refs. [45–47]

lower ($p=0.095$) in bilaterally oophorectomized women. Interestingly, among intact women, total testosterone levels increased with age ($p=0.015$) peaking in the 70s to premenopausal levels and there on remaining relatively stable. Among intact women, total, but not bioavailable, testosterone levels increased with age ($p=0.015$), reaching premenopausal levels for the 70–79 decade with relatively stable levels thereafter. The authors concluded that the postmenopausal ovary remains a critical source of androgen throughout the lifespan of older women. They suggested that reconsideration of prophylactic oophorectomy and further study of the effects of androgen replacement after oophorectomy are needed [14].

Controversies on Postmenopausal Ovarian Enzyme Activity

Despite a large body of research studies demonstrating substantial production of androgens from postmenopausal ovaries, [45–47, 80–84] controversy remains regarding steroidogenic enzyme expression in the postmenopausal ovary. Investigators have demonstrated gonadotropin binding sites in the postmenopausal ovary, [85, 86] responsiveness to gonadotropins, [87] and decreases in serum androgen levels after postmenopausal women are treated with GnRH agonists [88]. Studies in women with endometrial hyperplasia or cancer, demonstrated by northern analysis that the postmenopausal ovary possesses all the enzymes necessary for androgen synthesis [89]. However, in a well-known study of ovarian steroidogenic enzymes by immunohistochemistry, the authors reported that the postmenopausal ovary lacked aromatase. They also reported that the enzymes necessary for ovarian androgen synthesis were detected very weakly and were scattered in hilar cells [90].

Recently, more sensitive detection methods have been used to determine the steroidogenic enzymes expressed in the human postmenopausal ovary. Real-time RT-PCR detected the presence of steroidogenic acute regulatory protein transcripts, cholesterol side-chain cleavage transcripts, 3β-hydroxysteroid dehydrogenease type II transcripts but undetectable 17α-hydroxylase transcripts [91]. In another study using microarray analysis and real-time RT-PCR, the authors reported that the postmenopausal ovary retained the ability to produce androgens with a unique pattern of steroidogenic enzyme expression [92].

Osteoporosis and Hip Fracture

For many years, oophorectomy prior to age 45 or early menopause has been considered an important risk factor for the development of osteoporosis and hip fracture [50, 93]. Less well appreciated, however, are the studies linking oophorectomy done in older, postmenopausal women to osteoporosis risk. In a 16-year study tracking 340 postmenopausal women, those elderly women undergoing an oophorectomy for benign conditions had 54% more osteoporotic fractures than those with intact ovaries [50]. The authors' findings support the hypothesis that androgens produced by the postmenopausal ovary are important and protect against fracture risk.

In a related study investigating the effect of oophorectomy in postmenopausal women on bone metabolism, investigators measured serum and urinary markers of bone resorption and bone density in 80 menopausal women divided into 4 groups as follows: ≤3 years since natural menopause; ≥3 years since natural menopause; ≤3 years since oophorectomy; ≥3 years since oophorectomy. Lumbar BMD was lowest in the groups ≥3 years since oophorectomy. Serum markers of bone resorption were significantly higher in the early postoophorectomy group compared to all other groups. The authors concluded that women are at the greatest risk of bone resorption during the first few years following oophorectomy and that bone loss following oophorectomy is greater than that seen following natural menopause [51].

Quality of Life

Removal of ovaries in postmenopausal women usually results in the minimal change in estrogen levels and will rarely trigger the onset of hot flashes or other estrogen deficiency symptoms. However, there is generally a substantial effect on circulating androgen levels [46–48], and the impact of this change may not be appreciated for many years. Androgens protect bone and muscle mass and affect the distribution of muscle mass, percent body fat, and skin thickness. A lack of these hormones, over many years, is believed to result in muscle loss, weakness, increased body fat, and skin changes.

Examining the Effect of Oophorectomy on Overall Mortality

Several analyses have been done to look at the overall survival impact of oophorectomy. In one of these, a decision analysis was performed using survival information from previously published observational studies. That analysis found that ovarian conservation maximized the survival for healthy women aged 40–65 (without a family history of ovarian cancer) who have a hysterectomy for benign disease. Women having had a hysterectomy at age 55 or younger with ovarian conservation had a 8.6% survival advantage over women with oophorectomy. There was never a survival benefit for removing ovaries in any age group [9].

A study from the Mayo Clinic found that mortality was not increased overall in women who underwent bilateral oophorectomy compared with referent women. However, mortality was significantly higher in women who had prophylactic bilateral oophorectomy before the age of 45 years and had not received estrogen up to the age of 45 years (HR 1.67, 95% CI 1.16–2.40). Specifically, mortality for neurological or mental disorders was significantly increased [10].

In a third study, NHS cohort database was analyzed, which included 122,700 married registered nurses ages 30–55 years in 1976 when the initial questionnaires were mailed. A total of 29,380 hysterectomized women were included in the analysis; 13,035 (44.4%) had a hysterectomy alone (ovarian conservation) and 16,345 (55.6%) with hysterectomy with bilateral oophorectomy. During the 24 years of follow-up through 2002, nonfatal events and death due to the CHD, stroke, breast cancer, epithelial ovarian cancer, lung cancer, colorectal cancer, hip fracture, pulmonary embolus, and death due to all causes were tabulated. Each outcome analysis was adjusted for multiple-related risk factors. Oophorectomy was associated with an increased risk of CHD for all women (HR 1.17 95% CI 1.02, 1.35) and was greater for women with oophorectomy before age 45 (HR 1.26 95% CI 1.04, 1.54). Breast cancer was less frequent among all women with oophorectomy (HR 0.75 95% CI 0.68, 0.84), and the risk was lower among women having oophorectomy before the age of 45 (HR 0.62 95% CI 0.53, 0.74). Oophorectomy was associated with a very low risk of ovarian cancer (HR 0.04; 95% CI, 0.01–0.09) and a slight reduction in total cancers (HR 0.90 95% CI 0.84, 0.96), but an increased risk of lung cancer (HR 1.26; 95% CI, 1.02–1.56) [11].

Controversies on Hormone Replacement

For most of the studies, the long-term effects of oophorectomy are mitigated in women taking hormone replacement therapy for extended periods of time. In the study mentioned above, for oophorectomized women without hormone therapy, the risks of stroke (HR 1.85 95% CI 1.09, 3.16) and lung cancer (HR 2.09 95% 1.01, 4.33) were significantly higher. For women having oophorectomy before age 50 without hormone therapy, the risk of incident CHD (HR 1.98 95% CI 1.18, 3.32) was higher and the risk of death from all causes was higher (HR 1.40 95% CI 1.01, 1.96) [11].

These data, along with the many studies, supporting the use of hormone replacement in women appear to be at odds with the findings of WHI that reported an absolute excess risk of 8 more strokes per 10,000 person-years attributable to estrogen plus progestin treatment [94]. However, the data above taken from the observational cohort of NHS, represent real life hormone use that typically begins at in early menopause with the onset of hot flashes. In order to better define the risks of starting hormone therapy in early menopause, several subsequent publications of the WHI divided the study group into 10-year age groups based on age or years since menopause. These studies reported that the age of initiation of therapy had a profound effect on the risk of cardiovascular events. One of these studies, reported that for women treated within 10 years since their menopause began, the hazard ratio (HR) for CHD was 0.76 (95% confidence interval (CI), 0.50–1.16). For those treated 10–19 years, the HR was 1.10 (95% CI, 0.84–1.45) and for 20 or more years, the HR was 1.28 (95% CI, 1.03–1.58) (p for trend = 0.02) [95]. In another of these studies, the authors found no increase risk of stroke if estrogen was started between the ages of 50 and 59 [96].

Oophorectomy increased the risk of death from any cause (HR 1.12 95% CI 1.03, 1.21). Analysis of cause-specific mortality found an increased risk of death from CHD (HR 1.28, 95% CI 1.00, 1.64), lung cancer (HR 1.31, 95% CI 1.02, 1.68), and all cancers (HR 1.17, 95% CI 1.04, 1.32) and no overall difference in deaths from stroke, breast cancer, or colorectal cancer. While there was a reduced risk of death from ovarian cancer (HR 0.06; 95% CI, 0.02–0.21), during the 24 years of follow-up only 34 (0.7%) women died from ovarian cancer. *At no age did oophorectomy show an overall survival benefit* [11].

These data together would support the concept that there is an optimum therapeutic window for the initiation of estrogen therapy and that beginning estrogen during this window allows for the most benefit and lowest risk and may indeed offer substantial protection from cardiovascular disease [79, 97].

Conclusions

The purpose of prophylactic surgery is to provide a health benefit to patients. There is growing evidence that oophorectomy in many, if not most, women is associated with more risk than benefit (Table 11.3). Unless well-designed prospective, randomized

Table 11.3 Risks linked to oophorectomy

Body composition changes
Increase in adipose tissue and decreased muscle mass
Fat accumulation in central, abdominal area
Cardiovascular disease
Adverse effects on lipids and other risk factors
Increased rates of myocardial infarction
Accelerated atherosclerosis
Increased mortality
CNS
Short-term memory declines
Dementia
Decreased wellbeing
Parkinson's disease
Len opacities and macular degeneration
Menopausal symptoms
Osteoporosis and fractures
Accelerated bone loss
Increased risk of hip and spinal fracture and associated morbidity and mortality
Sexual dysfunction and loss of desire
Skin changes
Loss of collagen, thinning, wrinkling
Urogenital atrophy
Bladder and vaginal symptoms

studies can demonstrate clearly those women who will benefit, removing the ovaries at the time of hysterectomy should be approached with caution. For women without a genetic mutation or family history of ovarian cancer, current practice suggests that prophylactic oophorectomy is generally not beneficial for women under age 40–45 but recommendations vary greatly for ages 45 and older. It is important that both women and their healthcare providers consider the most reliable evidence regarding the potential risks and benefits of prophylactic oophorectomy in order to make appropriate decisions.

References

1. Wu JM, Wechter ME, Geller EJ et al (2007) Hysterectomy rates in the United States, 2003. Obstet Gynecol 110:1091
2. Hysterectomy. National women's Health Information center (2006-07-01). http://www.4women.gov/faq/hysterestecomy.htm. Accessed 4 Oct 2009
3. Hartge P, Whittemore AS, Itnyre J, McGowan L, Cramer D (1994) Rates and risks of ovarian cancer in subgroups of white women in the United States. The Collaborative Ovarian Cancer Group. Obstet Gynecol 84(5):760–764
4. Dekel A, Efrat Z, Orvieto R, Levy T, Dicker D, Gal R, Ben-Rafael Z (1996) The residual ovary syndrome: a 20 year experience. Eur J Obstet Gynecol Reprod Biol 68(1–2):159–164
5. Holub Z, Jandourek M, Jabor A, Kliment L, Wagnerova M (2000) Does hysterectomy without salpingo-oophorectomy influence the reoperation rate for adnexal pathology? A retrospective study. Clin Exp Obstet Gynecol 27(2):109–112
6. Christ JE, Lotze EC (1975) The residual ovary syndrome. Obstet Gynecol 46(5):551–556
7. Colditz CA, Willett W, Stampfer M, Rosner B, Speizer F, Hennekens C (1987) Menopause and the risk of coronary heart disease in women. N Engl J Med 316:1105–1110
8. Atsma F, Bartelink M, Grobbee D, van der Schouw Y (2006) Postmenopausal status and early menopause as independent risk factors for cardiovascular disease: a meta-analysis. Menopause 13(2):265–279
9. Parker WH, Broder M, Liu Z, Shoupe D, Farquhar C, Berek J (2005) Ovarian conservation at the time of hysterectomy for benign disease. Obstet Gynecol 106:219
10. Rocca W, Grossardt BR, de Andrade M, Jalkasian GD, Melton LJ III (2006) Survival patterns after oophorectomy in premenopausal women: a population based cohort study. Lancet Oncol 7(10):821–828
11. Parker WH, Broder MS, Change E, Feskanich D, Farquhar C, Shoupe D, Berek J, Hankinson S, Mason JE (2009) Ovarian conservation and long-term health outcome in the Nurses' Health Study. Obstet Gynecol 113(5):1027–1037
12. Farquhar CM, Sadler L, Harvey SA, Stewart AW (2005) The association of hysterectomy and menopause: a prospective cohort study. BJOG 112(7):956–962
13. Menon RK, Okonofua FE, Agnew JE et al (1987) Endocrine and metabolic effects of simple hysterectomy. Int J Gynaecol Obstet 25(6):459–463
14. Laughlin GA, Barrett-Connor E, Kritz-Silverstein D, von Muhlen D (2000) Hysterectomy, oophorectomy, and endogenous sex hormone levels in older women: the Rancho Bernardo study. J Clin Endocrinol Metab 85(2):645–651
15. Nahas E, Pontes A, Traiman P, NahasNeto J, Dalben I, DeLuca L (2003) Inhibin B and ovarian function after total abdominal hysterectomy in women of reproductive age. Gynecol Endocrinol 17:125–131
16. Hreshchyshyn MM, Hopkins A, Zylstra S, Anbar M (1988) Effects of natural menopause, hysterectomy, and oophorectomy on lumbar spine and femoral neck bone densities. Obstet Gynecol 72(4):631–638

17. Watson NR, Studd JW, Garnett T, Savvas M, Milligan P (1995) Bone loss after hysterectomy with ovarian conservation. Obstet Gynecol 86(1):72–77
18. Nieman LK (2003) Management of surgically hypogonadal patients unable to take hormone replacement. Endocrinol Metab 32:325–336
19. Thompson B, Hart SA, Durno D (1973) Menopausal age and symptomatology in a general practice. J Biosoc Sci 5:71–82
20. Madalinska JB, van Beurden M, Bleiker EM et al (2006) The impact of hormone replacement therapy on menopausal symptoms in younger high-risk women after prophylactic salpingo-oophorectomy. J Clin Oncol 24(22):3519–3521
21. Gallicchia L, Whiteman MK, Tomic D, Miller KP, Lanagerberg P, Flaws JA (2006) Type of menopause, pattern of hormone use, and hot flashes. Fertil Steril 95(5):1432–1440
22. Melville JL, Katon W, Delaney K, Newton K (2005) Urinary incontinence in US women: a population based study. Arch Intern Med 165(5):537–542
23. Roos NP (1984) Hysterectomies in one Canadian province: a new look at risks and benefits. Am J Public Health 74:39–46
24. Sherwin BB, Gelfan MM (1978) The role of androgens in the maintenance of sexual functioning in oophorectomized women. Psychosom Med 49:397–409
25. Nathorst-Boos J, von Schoultz B, Carlstrom K (1993) Elective ovarian removal and estrogen replacement therapy-effects on sexual life, psychological well-being and androgen status. J Psychosom Obstet Gynaecol 14(4):283–293
26. Hansen KA (2007) Female reproductive biology. In: O'Leary P, Tabuenca A, Capote LR (eds) The physiologic basis of surgery. Lippincott Williams and Wilkins, Hagerstown, MD, pp 314–315
27. Bachman GA, Nevadunsky NS (2000) Diagnosis and treatment of atrophic vaginitis. Am Fam Physician 61:3090–3096
28. Lieblum S, Bachmann G, Kemmann E, Colburn D, Swartzman L (1983) Vaginal atrophy in the postmenopausal woman. The importance of sexual activity and hormones. JAMA 249: 2195–2198
29. Schifren JL, Braustein GD, Simon JA, Casson PR, Buster JE, Redmond GP, Burki RE, Ginsburg ES, Rosen RC, Leiblum SR, Caramelli KE, Mazer NA (2000) Transdermal testosterone treatment in women with impaired sexual function after oophorectomy. N Engl J Med 343(10):682–688
30. Shifren JL, Braunstein GD, Simon JA, Casson PR, Buster JE, Redmone GP, Burki RE, Gkinsburg ES, Rosen RC, Leiblum SR, Carameli KE, Mazer NA (2001) Transdermal testosterone treatment in women with impaired sexual function after oophorectomy. Obstet Gynecol Surv 56(2):95–96
31. Elit I, Esplen MJ, Butler K, Narod S (2001) Quality of life and psychosexual adjustment after prophylactic oophorectomy for a family history of ovarian cancer. Fam Cancer 1(3–4):149–156
32. Madalinska JB, Hollenstein J, Bleiker E, van Beurden M, Valdimarsdottir HB, Massuger LF, Gaarenstroom KN, Mouritis JM, Verheijen RH et al (2005) Quality of life effects of prophylactic salpingo-oophorectomy versus gnecolgic screening among women at increased risk of hereditary ovarian cancer. J Clin Oncol 23(29):2690–2698
33. Sherwin BB (1988) Affective changes with estrogen and androgen replacement in surgically menopausal women. J Affect Disord 14(2):177–178
34. Farrag AK, Khedr EM, Abdel-Aleem H, Rageh TA (2002) Effect of surgical menopause on cognitive functions. Dement Geriatr Cogn Disord 13(3):193–198
35. Nilsen J, Chen S, Irwin RW, Iwamoto S, Brinton RD (2006) Estrogen protects neuronal cells form amyloid beta-induced apoptosis via regulation of mitochondrial proteins and function. BMC Neurosci 3:7–74
36. Rocca WA, Bower JH, Maraganore DM, Ahiskog JE, Grossartdt BR, DeAndrade M, Melton LH (2007) Increased risk of cognitive impairment or dementia in women who underwent oophorectomy before menopause. Neurology 69(11):1074–1083
37. Rocca W, Grossardt BR, Maraganore DM (2008) The long-term effects of oophorectomy on cognitive and motor aging are age dependent. Neurodegener Dis 5:257–260

38. Halbreich U, Lumley LA, Palter S et al (1995) Possible acceleration of age effects on cognition following menopause. J Psychiatr Res 29:153–163
39. Dennerstein L, Guthrie JF, Clark M, Lehert P, Henderson VW (2004) A population-based study of depressed mood in middle aged Australian-born women. Menopause 11:563–568
40. McKinlay JB, McKinlay SM, Brambilla DJ (1987) The relative contribution of endocrine changes and social circumstances to depression in middle aged women. J Health Soc Behav 28(4):345–363
41. Billon A, Lehoux S, Shang Leen LL et al (2008) The estrogen effects on endothelial repair. Am J Pathol 172:830–838
42. Behl C, Skutella T, Lezoualc'H F, Post A, Widmann M, Newton CJ, Holsboer F (1997) Neuroprotection against oxidative stress by estrogens: structure-activity relationship. Mol Pharmacol 51:535–541
43. Raisz RK, Wilta B, Artis A, Bowen A, Schwartz S, Trahiotis M, Shoukri K, Smith J (1996) Comparison of the effects of estrogen alone and estrogen plus androgen on biochemical markers of bone formation and resorption in postmenopausal women. J Clin Endocrinol Metab 81(1):37–43
44. National Osteoporosis Foundation (1998) Physician guide to prevention and treatment of osteoporosis. Excerpta Medica, Belle Mead, NJ
45. Vermeulen A (1976) The hormonal activity of the postmenopausal ovary. J Clin Endocrinol Metab 42:247–253
46. Fogle R, Stanczyk F, Zhang X, Paulson R (2007) Ovarian androgen production and the postmenopausal ovary. J Clin Endocrinol Metab 92:3040–3043
47. Davidson SL, Bell R, Donath S, Montalto JF, Davis SR (2005) Androgen levels in adult females: changes with age, menopause, and oophorectomy. J Clin Endocrinol Metab 90(7):3847–3853
48. Davidson BJ, Ross RK, Paganini-Hill A, Hammond GD, Siiteri PK, Judd HL (1982) Total and free estrogens and androgens in postmenopausal women with hip fractures. J Clin Endocrinol Metab 54(1):115–120
49. Longcope C, Baker RS, Hui SL, Johnston CC Jr (1984) Androgen and estrogen dynamics in women with vertebral crush fractures. Maturitas 6(4):309–318
50. Kreiger N, Kelsey J, Holford TR, O'Connor T (1982) An epidemiologic study of hip fracture in postmenopausal women. Am J Epidemiol 116(1):141–148
51. Ohtaa H, Makitab K, Komukaib S, Nozawab S (2002) Bone resorption versus estrogen loss following oophorectomy and menopause. Maturitas 43(1):27–33
52. Johansson C, Mellstrom D, Milsom I (1993) Reproductive factors as predictors of bone density and fracture in women at the age of 70. Maturitas 17(1):39–50
53. Keene G, Parker M, Pryor G (1993) Mortality and morbidity after hip fractures. BJM 13:1248–1250
54. Center J, Nguyen T, Schneider D, Sambrook P, Eisman J (1999) Mortality after all major types of osteoporotic fracture in men and women: an observational study. Lancet 353:878–882
55. Vingerling JR, Dielemans I, Witteman CM et al (1994) Macular degeneration and early menopause: a case-control study. Br Med J 310:1570
56. Worzala K, Hiller R, Sperduto RD, Mutalik K, Murabito JM, Moskowitz M, D'Agostino RB, Wilson PWF (2001) Postmenopausal estrogen use, type of menopause, and lens opacities. The Framingham Studies. Arch Intern Med 161:1448–1454
57. Floter A, Nathorst-Boos J, Carlstrom K, Ohlsson C, Ringertz H, Schoultz B (2005) Effects of combined estrogen/testosterone therapy on bone and body composition in oophorectomized women. Gynecol Endocrinol 20(3):155–160
58. Brincat M, Moniz CJ, Studd JW, Darby A, Magos A, Emburey G, Versi E (1985) Long-term effects of the menopause and sex hormones on skin thickness. Br J Obstet Gynaecol 92(3):256–259
59. Brincat M, Kabalan S, Studd JW, Moniz CF, de Trafford J, Montgomery J (1987) A study of the decrease in skin collagen content, skin thickness, and bone mass in the postmenopausal woman. Obstet Gynecol 70(6):840–849

60. Donato GB, Fuchs SC, Oppermann K, Bastos C, Spritzer PM (2006) Association between menopause status and central adiposity measured at different cutoffs of waist circumference and waist-to-hip ratio. Menopause 13(2):280–285
61. Haarbo J, Marslew U, Gotfredsen A, Christiansen C (1991) Postmenopausal hormone replacement prevents central distribution of body fat after menopause. Metabolism 40(12): 1322–1326
62. Falkeborn M, Schairer C, Naessen T, Persson I (2000) Risk of myocardial infarction after oophorectomy and hysterectomy. J Clin Epidemiol 53:832–837
63. Rosenberg L, Hennekens CH, Rosner B, Belanger C, Rothman KJ, Speizer FE (1981) Early menopause and the risk of myocardial infarction. Am J Obstet Gynecol 139:47–51
64. Kanel WB, Hjortland MC, McNamara PM, Gordon T (1976) Menopause and risk of cardiovascular disease. The Framingham Study. Ann Intern Med 85:447–452
65. Matthews KA, Meilahn E, Kuller LH, Kelsey SF, Caggiula AW, Wing RR (1989) Menopause and risk factors for coronary heart disease. N Engl J Med 321(10):641–652
66. Wuerst J, Dry T, Edwards J (1953) The degree of coronary atherosclerosis in bilaterally oophorectomized women. Circulation 7:891–899
67. Hsia J, Barad D, Margolis K, Rodabough R, McGovern P, Limacher M et al (2003) Usefulness of prior hysterectomy as an independent risk predictor of Framingham risk score. Am J Cardiol 92:264–269
68. Robinson RW, Higano N, Cohen WD (1959) Increased incidence of coronary heart disease in women castrated prior to the menopause. Arch Intern Med 104:908–913
69. Van der Schouw Y, van der Fraaf Y, Steyerberg E, Elijkemans M, Banga J (1996) Age at menopause as a risk factor for cardiovascular mortality. Lancet 347:714–718
70. Lokkegaard E, Jovanovic Z, Heitmann BL, Keidling N, Ottesen B, Pedersen AT (2006) The association between early menopause and risk of ischemic heart disease: influence of hormone therapy. Maturitas 53(2):226–233
71. Hu FB, Grodstein F, Hennekens CH, Colditz GA, Hohnson M, Manson JE, Rosner B, Stampfer MJ (1999) Age at natural menopause and risk of cardiovascular disease. Arch Intern Med 159:1061–1066
72. Cheung LP, Pang MW, Lam CW, Tomlinson B, Chung TK, Haines CJ (1998) Acute effects of a surgical menopause on serum concentrations of lipoprotein(a). Climacteric 1(1):33–41
73. Suda Y, Makita KI, Takamatsu K, Horiguchi F, Nozawa S (1998) Influence of bilateral oophorectomy upon lipid metabolism. Maturitas 29:147–154
74. Mihmanli V, Mihmanli I, Kantarci F, Aydin T, Yilmaz MH, Ogut G (2002) Carotid pulsatility indices in surgical menopause. Arch Gynecol Obstet 266(2):96–100
75. Mollica G (1993) Influence of spontaneous and surgical menopause on atherogenic metabolic risk. Maturitas 17(3):181–190
76. Schulman JH, Aranda P, Roij L, Veronesi M, Aranda FJ, Martin R (2006) Surgical menopause increases salt sensitivity for blood pressure. Hypertension 47(6):1168–1174
77. DeLeo V, La Marca A, Agricol E, Morgante G, Mondillo S, Setacci C (2002) Resting ECG is modified after oophorectomy and regresses with estrogen replacement therapy in premenopausal women. Maturitas 31(1):43–47
78. Mack WJ, Slater CC, Xiang M, Shoupe D, Lobo RA, Hodis HN (2004) Elevated subclinical atherosclerosis associated with oophorectomy is related to time since menopause rather than type of menopause. Fertil Steril 82(2):391–397
79. Allison MA, Manson JE, Langer RD, Carr JJ, Rossouw JE, Pettinger MB, Phillips L, Cochrane BB, Eaton CB, Greenland P, Hendrix S, Hsia J, Hunt JR, Jackson RD, Johnson KC, Kuller LH, Robinson J; Women's Health Initiative and Women's Health Initiative Coronary Artery calcium study investigators (2008) Oophorectomy, hormone therapy, and subclinical coronary artery disease in women with hysterectomy: The Women's Health Initiative Coronary Artery Calcium Study. Menopause 15:639–647
80. Longcope C, Baker S (1993) Androgen and estrogen dynamics: relationship with age, weight, and menopausal status. J Clin Endocrinol Metab 76:601–210

81. Meldrum DR, Davidson BJ, Tatryn IV, Judd HL (1981) Changes in circulating steroids with aging in postmenopausal women. Obstet Gynecol 57:624–628
82. Longcope C, Johnston CC Jr (1990) Androgen and estrogen dynamics: stability over a two year interval in perimenopausal women. J Steroid Biochem 35(1):91–95
83. Adashi EY (1994) The climacteric ovary as a functional gonadotropin-driven androgen-producing gland. Fertil Steril 62:20–27
84. Ushiroyama T, Sugimoto O (1995) Endocrine function of the peri- and postmenopausal ovary. Horm Res 44:64–68
85. Puluso JJ, Steger RW, Jaszezak S, Hafez ES (1976) Gonadotropin binding sites in human postmenopausal ovaries. Fertil Steril 27:789–795
86. Nakano R, Shima K, Yamoto M, Kobayashi M, Nishimori K, Hiraoka J (1989) Binding sites for gonadotropins in human postmenopausal ovaries. Obstet Gynecol 73:196–200
87. Dennefors BL, Janson PO, Hamberger L, Knutsson F (1982) Hilus cells from human postmenopausal ovaries: gonadotrophin sensitivity, steroid and cyclic AMP production. Acta Obstet Gynecol Scand 61:413–416
88. Dowsett M, Cantwell B, Lal A, Jeffcoate SL, Harris AL (1988) Suppression of postmenopausal ovarian steroidogenesis with the luteinizing hormone-releasing hormone agonist goserelin. J Clin Endocrinol Metab 66:672–677
89. Nagamani M, Urban RJ (2003) Expression of messenger ribonucleic acid encoding steroidogenic enzymes in postmenopausal ovaries. J Soc Gynecol Invest 10:37–40
90. Couzinet B, Meduri G, Leece MG, Young J, Brailly S, Loosfelt H, Milgrom E, Schaison G (2001) The postmenopausal ovary is not a major androgen-producing gland. J Clin Endocrinol Metab 86:5060–5066
91. Jabara S, Christenson LK, Wang CY, McAllister JM, Javitt NB, Dunaif A, Strauss JF III (2003) Stromal cells of the human postmenopausal ovary display a distinctive biochemical and molecular phenotype. J Clin Endocrinol Metab 88:484–492
92. Havelock JC, Rainey WE, Bradshaw KD, Carr BR (2006) The post-menopausal ovary displays a unique pattern of steroidogenic enzyme expression. Hum Reprod 21(1):309–317
93. Melton J, Khosla S, Malkasian G, Achenbach S, Oberg A, Riggs L (2003) Fracture risk after bilateral oophorectomy in elderly women. J Bone Miner Res 18:900–905
94. Writing Group for the WHI Investigators (2002) Risks and benefits of estrogen plus progestin in healthy postmenopausal women. Principal results from the Women's Health Initiative Randomized Controlled Trial. JAMA 288:321–333
95. Rossouw JE, Prentice RL, Manson JE, Wu L, Barad D, Barnabei VM, Ko M, LaCroix AZ, Margolis KL, Stefanick ML (2007) Postmenopausal hormone therapy and risk of cardiovascular disease by age and years since menopause. JAMA 297(13):1465–1477
96. Hsia J, Langer RD, Manson JE, Kuller L, Johnson KC, Hendrix SL, Pettinger M, Heckbert SR, Greep N, Crawford S, Eaton CB, Kostis JB, Caralis P, Prentice R (2006) Conjugated equine estrogens and coronary heart disease: the Women's Health Initiative. Arch Intern Med 166:357–365
97. Manson JE, Allison MA, Rossouw JE, Carr JJ, Langer RD, Hsia J, Kuller LH, Cochrane BB, Hunt JR, Ludlam SE, Pettinger MB, Gass M, Margolis KL, Nathan L, Ockene JK, Prentice RL, Robbins J, Stefanick ML; for the WHI and WHI-CACS Investigators (2007) Estrogen therapy and coronary-artery calcification. N Engl J Med 356(25):2591–2602
98. Keshavarz H, Hillis SD, Kieke BA, Marchbanks PA (2002) Hysterectomy surveillance – United States, 1994–1999. MMWR Surveill Summ 51(SS05):1–8

Chapter 12
Ethnicity and Amenorrhea

Benjamin M. Lannon and Kim L. Thornton

Discussion preceding this chapter has addressed various physiological and pathophysiological states that affect the menstrual cycle. This chapter focuses on the role of race and/or ethnicity on menstrual physiology. Our discussion about the impact of race and ethnicity on amenorrhea focuses on two factors: (1) the physiologic variations in the menstrual cycle among different racial and ethnic groups and (2) variations in cultural attitudes and beliefs about the cessation of menses. While these cultural differences may not always impose specific diagnostic or management dilemmas, awareness may be essential to the goal of providing comprehensive care to our diverse patient population.

Ethnic Variations in Menstrual Physiology

Menarche

Failure to recognize interracial variations in the onset of puberty can have a profound effect on subsequent evaluation and management.

An analysis of the National Health and Nutrition Examination Survey (NHANES) 1999–2004, showed a significant decrease in age at menarche in women born in 1920's compared to 1980's across Mexican Americans, non-Hispanic Whites, and African Americans [1]. While these data were based on retrospective self-reported age at menarche, the trends are real.

While there may be an overall reduced age for menarche, the generational differences in pubertal onset are not the same across all racial and ethnic groups. Results from the Pediatric Research in Office Settings (PROS) network study in 1997 suggested that

B.M. Lannon (✉)
Division of Reproductive Endocrinology and Infertility, Department of Obstetrics and Gynecology and Reproductive Biology, Beth Israel Deaconess Medical Center, Harvard Medical School, Boston, MA 02215, USA

N.F. Santoro and G. Neal-Perry (eds.), *Amenorrhea: A Case-Based, Clinical Guide*, Contemporary Endocrinology, DOI 10.1007/978-1-60327-864-5_12,

black girls in particular had a mean age of menarche more than 6 months earlier than white girls (12.16 vs. 12.88 years) [2]. A subsequent analysis of the data revealed that increases in body mass index (BMI) may have accounted for the earlier onset of puberty in white girls [3]. Unlike white girls, BMI alone did not completely explain the earlier onset of the pubertal transition observed in black girls, leading the authors to speculate that genetic factors such as leptin levels and environmental factors such as nutrition may contribute to interracial differences in pubertal development [3].

Controversy exists regarding the validity of these findings, and the mechanisms underlying racial and ethnic variations in pubertal/menarcheal onset [3]. Nonetheless, these data can clearly impact the evaluation and referral of young girls from different racial and ethnic groups for presumed abnormal pubertal development.

Menstruation

In addition to differences in the timing of menarche, there are also variations in specific menstrual patterns among various racial and ethnic groups. As we discuss later in this chapter, these differences can influence perceived attitudes about menstruation and menstrual cyclicity and management approaches offered to and selected by women from different racial and ethnic groups.

A study by Harlow and colleagues investigated the effect of ethnicity and/or race on the duration, amount, and length of postmenarcheal bleeding [4, 5]. They enrolled 125 African American and 123 European American girls between 12 and 14 years old living in North Carolina in a 2-year study of postmenarcheal bleeding patterns. The participants kept menstrual calendars and records of weight, exercise, and stress. Although they were twice as likely to have an episode of heavy bleeding, African American girls reported a half day shorter mean duration of bleeding [4]. Although mean cycle length was similar in both groups, European American girls had an increased cycle length variability and an increased probability of having a cycle length more than 45 days [5]. These studies were limited by sample size and applicability of results to other age groups. Nonetheless, they suggest that an association between race and variations in the pattern of menstrual cycle length exists. Understanding these variations may help physicians counsel patients and their families about normal and abnormal menstruation patterns and management options.

The role of genetics and the exact biological mechanism giving rise to apparent ethnic and/or racial differences in menstrual duration and flow and menstrual cycle length are unknown. Additional studies are needed to characterize menstrual cycle phenotypes with hormonal profiles and their relation to ovulatory function as a function of ethnicity and/or race.

Ovulation/Anovulation

Even after menarche, variations in ovulatory function and hormonal profiles among various racial and ethnic groups continue to exist. It is important to recognize that these differences may alter the risk of developing other hormonally responsive conditions such as fibroids, breast cancer, and endometrial neoplasia.

Haiman et al. investigated the effect of race and/or ethnicity on the rates of anovulation in groups of students in greater Los Angeles area [6]. They found a trend for a greater frequency of anovulation in white women vs. African American and Latina women. In addition, they noted differences in hormone profiles between the groups with higher follicular phase estradiol (E2) and luteal phase E2 and progesterone levels in African American compared to all other women. Likewise, Latina women had elevated follicular phase E2 and luteal phase E2 and progesterone compared to white women [6]. These differences may account for increased rates of fibroids and invasive breast cancer and breast cancer mortality in African American women [7].

Understanding the role of race and ethnicity in hormonal and menstrual cycle variations may provide a means to assess the risk for future morbidities. For example, Rieder et al., determined markers of insulin resistance and hyperandrogenemia in an unselected group of Caribbean Hispanic and African American women aged 12–21 [8]. The women were grouped according to menstrual regularity and physical exam characteristics. They found that waist circumference, free androgen index, and sex hormone binding globulin (SHBG) levels correlated best with ovulatory and menstrual dysfunction and a hyperandrogenic phenotype. Identification of these young women who are at risk of developing adult polycystic ovarian syndrome (PCOS) may afford an opportunity for intervention and subsequent minimization of the metabolic disruption that frequently plague women with PCOS [8].

Ovarian Insufficiency

Abnormal cessation of ovarian function has also been shown to vary by ethnic group. While many aspects of primary ovarian insufficiency, also known as premature ovarian failure (POF), remain uncertain, there appear to be differences in the prevalence and risk factors among ethnic and racial groups. In a study by Luborsky and colleagues, a part of the Study of Women Across the Nation (SWAN), women aged 40–55 were interviewed at seven sites in the US as part of a multiethnic longitudinal study [9]. The investigators defined POF as spontaneous cessation of menses less than 40 years old with uncertain etiology. In this population, the highest reported rate of POF was in Black and Hispanic women (1.4%) followed by Caucasian (1%) and then Chinese (0.5%) and Japanese (0.14%). Similar trends were observed for women reporting early menopause (age 40–45) as well [9].

A multivariate subgroup analysis of factors associated with POF in African American and Caucasian women suggested the use of female hormones (other than oral contraceptives) was predictive of POF risk. Additionally, in Caucasian women, osteoporosis, severe disability and smoking were significantly associated with POF. While in African American women, higher BMI but not osteoporosis was associated with POF [9].

Although this study was limited by retrospective self-reporting and a cross-sectional design, it still provides some insight into how risk factors for POF vary across ethnic groups as well as information about the overall prevalence of POF in each group.

Menopausal Transition

One of the most studied areas of ethnic variations in amenorrhea is the change during the menopausal transition. As described above, there are differences in hormonal profiles in postmenarchal girls across various racial and ethnic groups. This finding is consistent in women making the menopausal transition and is reflected in studies that evaluate the role of the pituitary, adrenal, and ovarian axes.

Several analyses of the SWAN data have reported racial and ethnic differences in hormone levels in pre- and perimenopausal women. Dehydroepiandrosterone (DHEAS), testosterone (T), and E2 levels in serum collected from 3,029 women in five racial and ethnic groups aged 42–54 for over 2 years suggested DHEAS levels were highest in Chinese and Japanese women and lowest among African American and Hispanics [10]. These differences persisted even after adjusting for age, smoking, and BMI with a multivariate analysis. In some women DHEAS levels exhibited transient elevations, with the greatest increases in Chinese, Hispanic and Japanese women and less for African American and Caucasians. Racial and ethnic changes in T and E2 correlated with changes in DHEAS [10].

A second report from the SWAN study looked at a sub-cohort of 848 women of whom daily urinary hormone levels were measured during the peri-menopausal transition. They found that Chinese- and Japanese American women had lower urinary estrogen conjugates. Other variables including FSH, LH, and progesterone metabolites were not significantly different amongst various racial and ethnic groups when adjusted for BMI [11].

The third analysis of the SWAN data by Randolph et al., looked at changes in E2 and FSH across the early menopausal transition. They found similarities in age-related E2 reductions and FSH increases across racial and ethnic groups studied. They also found that in Caucasians, FSH levels were lower than African American women, and similar to Chinese and Japanese women. However, Chinese and Japanese women had lower E2 levels, while the African American women were comparable to Caucasians. These findings suggest that ethnic variations in hypothalamic-pituitary-ovarian communication and/or response [12].

The varied relationship between hormone profiles with age across ethnic groups was also supported by data from a 4-year cohort study from the University of Pennsylvania [13]. This study tracked E2, FSH, DHEAS, and T levels in 436 women, equally divided between African American and Caucasian women and found African American women demonstrated an age-related decrease of E2 and DHEAS as compared to Caucasians. Moreover, African American women had decreased E2 and increased DHEAS with increasing BMI [13].

One of the most important concerns raised from all of this data is to what extent do differences in hormone profiles influence racial differences in the rates of hormone sensitive breast cancer. This question was addressed in a subgroup analysis form the Nurse Health Study II. This retrospective study included 116,671 nurses aged 25–42. In a follow up 8–10 years from the initial survey, over 19,000 women submitted a menstrual cycle timed blood sample. A subgroup of women was selected to submit samples over several years. Ultimately, 111 Caucasian women were included and matched with African American and Asian American women. E2, P, prolactin, SHBG, insulin-like growth factor-1 (IGF-1), and insulin-like growth factor binding protein-3 (IGFBP-3) were assayed and analyzed across racial and ethnic groups. African American women had higher levels of E2 and IGF-1 and lower levels of SHBG and IGFBP-3 as compared to Caucasian women. Asian Americans had higher E2 and IGF-1 and lower SHBG as compared to Caucasians. There were no differences in P or prolactin across the groups [14].

Variations in Cultural Beliefs and Attitudes Toward Normal and Abnormal Menstrual Cycles

Equally important to the biological differences, are the cultural beliefs and attitudes that can impact the evaluation and subsequent treatment recommendations. A woman's perception of what is normal and abnormal menstrual function is dictated by a number of factors. These beliefs can modestly affect her decision to seek treatment as well as her choice of management.

Menstrual Symptoms

While a number of anthropologic studies have investigated cultural attitudes toward menses, few have focused on symptom reporting. One such study from England looked at women's self-assessment of menses across three racial groups. A total of 153 women (48 Afro-Caribbean, 73 Caucasian, and 32 Asian) between the ages of 18 and 48 were enrolled in the study and administered standardized questionnaires about mood, behavior, and menstrual symptoms over a monthly cycle [15]. While intermenstrual symptoms were similar, Caucasian women reported significantly more premenstrual and menstrual related symptoms compared to the other groups. Symptoms reported were primarily attributed to psychological mood, body symptoms and pain categories, rather than mental performance or social behavior [15]. The authors propose that sociocultural mechanism account for racial differences; Caucasian women perceive menstrual bleeding as an aversive event, thereby leading to increased vigilance and more complaints. While these theories are difficult to substantiate, it is hard to deny that there are differences in the way different racial groups report menstrual physiology and symptoms. It remains to be seen whether menstrual cycle and symptom difference across racial groups reflect physiologic or sociologic divergence. Nonetheless, it is important for the physician to recognize perceived or physiological differences in the menstrual cycle and symptoms can ultimately affect a woman's decision to seek treatment, the type of treatment that she seeks, and whether she is compliant with treatment.

Contraceptive-Induced Amenorrhea

For women seeking treatment for menstrual cycle dysfunction, contraceptive methods are among the most commonly offered. One potential and possibly unintended consequence of treatment is amenorrhea. For some women, this may be a desired effect, while others prefer to maintain monthly menstrual bleeds. Edelman and colleagues assessed whether there were ethnic variations in women's attitudes toward contraceptive-induced amenorrhea [16]. This study surveyed 292 women with mean age of 27 years in Atlanta, Georgia and Portland, Oregon. They found that 69% of participants welcomed amenorrhea and 58% preferred to have menses every 3 months. However, significantly fewer black women would consider using birth control to induce amenorrhea vs. white women (29 vs. 49%) [16]. The study was limited by the sample size as well as several possible confounders that included education level, geographic location, and prior use of contraception. As a result, the author's interpretation of their data was limited with regard to the relationship between race and attitude toward amenorrhea. Nonetheless, in light of possible existence of differences in cultural beliefs about menses, race and ethnicity should be seriously considered and cultural attitudes discussed with the patient prior to crafting management plans for menstrual cycle regulation.

Racial Differences in Hysterectomy

Another commonly offered treatment modality for menstrual dysfunction is hysterectomy. Whether racial differences in the decision to seek definitive treatment exist is an area of active investigation. However, race and/or ethnicity may affect counseling received by patients regarding management options for menstrual dysfunction. These differences may reflect underlying disparities in access to healthcare between groups or disparities in physician attitudes rather than differences in racial and/or ethnic physiology or cultural attitudes.

Hysterectomy is the most frequently performed surgery on women in the US. Epidemiological data has suggested that over the past decade, while overall hysterectomy rates have declined, there was an increase in its use for treatment of leiomyoma. For women aged 40–44, there is a significant difference in the hysterectomy rate among African American women [17]. Some have speculated that increased rates of fibroids in African American women explain increased hysterectomy rates, however definitive studies are needed.

Using SWAN data, Powell et al., investigated racial/ethnic differences in hysterectomy for benign conditions [17]. After adjusting for adjusted for age, education, fibroids, BMI, marital status, smoking, geography, and country of education, Powell et al., found that race and ethnicity was associated with past hysterectomy. Increased odds in African American (1.66) and Hispanic (1.64) women, and decreased odds in Asian American (0.44) women compared to Caucasians were specifically noted. The authors contend that the highest rates of hysterectomy occurred in disadvantaged African American and Hispanic groups. More importantly, because the differences could not be explained by other factors, the authors conclude that this could reflect health disparity resulting in the overuse of hysterectomy in this groups [17].

Interestingly, a recent analysis of the Coronary Artery Risk Development in Young Adults (CARDIA) Women's Study addressed the potential issue of health disparity as well [18]. This cohort study included 1,863 black and white women in the US from 2000 to 2002, 15 years after the baseline study. Again black women were more likely (3.5 times) to undergo hysterectomy than white women. This association was observed after the adjustment for age, educational status, perceived barriers to medical care, BMI, PCOS, tubal ligation, age at menarche, depressive symptoms and geographic location [18]. Further analysis of a subset of women in whom fibroids were directly visualized by ultrasound revealed only a minimal reduction in the difference between the two groups, implying that fibroids alone did not explain the racial differences in hysterectomy. They speculate that while biologic factors may contribute to these racial disparities, there may be nonclinical modifiers such as education about alternative treatments, cultural beliefs, communication issues, or other psychosocial factors.

Menopause

Just as ethnicity and race appears to modify how some women experience menstruation, attitudes about menopause and the climacteric are also effected by ethnicity and race. A subgroup of the SWAN dataset analyzed attitudes toward menopause in over 12,000 women aged 40–55 years. They were surveyed by telephone using standardized questionnaires to assess whether they had positive or negative attitudes about menopause [19]. The five racial and ethnic groups included were African American, White, Chinese American, Japanese American, and Hispanic. All of the groups tended to report a positive attitude toward menopause, while slightly more positive in African American and less so in Chinese- and Japanese Americans. Group attitudes did not vary significantly across the stages of menopause [19].

Another SWAN report studied symptom reporting across the groups [20]. They used factor analysis to identify two consistent factors affecting menopausal women; vasomotor symptoms (hot flashes and night sweats) and psychosomatic symptoms. In a regression analysis, controlling for age, education, health, and economic strain, they found that Caucasian women reported more psychosomatic symptoms than all other groups, while African American women reported more vasomotor symptoms [20]. This suggests that race and ethnicity may differentially affect the way menopause and the climacteric manifests and thus counseling and treatment may need to be tailored accordingly.

Summary

In this chapter, we have discussed ethnic differences in amenorrhea, the menstrual cycle and the menopause. These range from biologic variations in hormone profiles and endocrine function, to complex cultural and psychosocial interactions. While the majority of these studies may be limited by sample size, retrospective review, or reporting biases, the overall theme is the same and suggests that the physical and psychological experience of amenorrhea varies across different racial and ethnic groups and that this could negatively impact the effectiveness of a "one size fits all" approach to counseling, treatment, and healthcare policy.

References

1. McDowell MA, Brody DJ, Hughes JP (2007) Has age at menarche changed? Results from the National Health and Nutrition Examination Survey (NHANES) 1999–2004. J Adolesc Health 40(3):227–231
2. Herman-Giddens ME, Slora EJ, Wasserman RC et al (1997) Secondary sexual characteristics and menses in young girls seen in office practice: a study from the Pediatric Research in Office Settings network. Pediatrics 99(4):505–512
3. Kaplowitz PB, Slora EJ, Wasserman RC, Pedlow SE, Herman-Giddens ME (2001) Earlier onset of puberty in girls: relation to increased body mass index and race. Pediatrics 108(2):347–353
4. Harlow SD, Campbell B (1996) Ethnic differences in the duration and amount of menstrual bleeding during the postmenarcheal period. Am J Epidemiol 144(10):980–988
5. Harlow SD, Campbell B, Lin X, Raz J (1997) Ethnic differences in the length of the menstrual cycle during the postmenarcheal period. Am J Epidemiol 146(7):572–580
6. Haiman CA, Pike MC, Bernstein L et al (2002) Ethnic differences in ovulatory function in nulliparous women. Br J Cancer 86(3):367–371
7. Chlebowski RT, Chen Z, Anderson GL et al (2005) Ethnicity and breast cancer: factors influencing differences in incidence and outcome. J Natl Cancer Inst 97(6):439–448
8. Rieder J, Santoro N, Cohen HW, Marantz P, Coupey SM (2008) Body shape and size and insulin resistance as early clinical predictors of hyperandrogenic anovulation in ethnic minority adolescent girls. J Adolesc Health 43(2):115–124
9. Luborsky JL, Meyer P, Sowers MF, Gold EB, Santoro N (2003) Premature menopause in a multi-ethnic population study of the menopause transition. Hum Reprod 18(1):199–206
10. Lasley BL, Santoro N, Randolf JF et al (2002) The relationship of circulating dehydroepiandrosterone, testosterone, and estradiol to stages of the menopausal transition and ethnicity. J Clin Endocrinol Metab 87(8):3760–3767
11. Santoro N, Lasley B, McConnell D et al (2004) Body size and ethnicity are associated with menstrual cycle alterations in women in the early menopausal transition: the Study of Women's Health across the Nation (SWAN) Daily Hormone Study. J Clin Endocrinol Metab 89(6):2622–2631
12. Randolph JF Jr, Sowers M, Bondarenko IV, Harlow SD, Luborsky JL, Little RJ (2004) Change in estradiol and follicle-stimulating hormone across the early menopausal transition: effects of ethnicity and age. J Clin Endocrinol Metab 89(4):1555–1561
13. Manson JM, Sammel MD, Freeman EW, Grisso JA (2001) Racial differences in sex hormone levels in women approaching the transition to menopause. Fertil Steril 75(2):297–304
14. Pinheiro SP, Holmes MD, Pollak MN, Barbieri RL, Hankinson SE (2005) Racial differences in premenopausal endogenous hormones. Cancer Epidemiol Biomarkers Prev 14(9):2147–2153

15. van den Akker OB, Eves FF, Service S, Lennon B (1995) Menstrual cycle symptom reporting in three British ethnic groups. Soc Sci Med 40(10):1417–1423
16. Edelman A, Lew R, Cwiak C, Nichols M, Jensen J (2007) Acceptability of contraceptive-induced amenorrhea in a racially diverse group of US women. Contraception 75(6):450–453
17. Powell LH, Meyer P, Weiss G et al (2005) Ethnic differences in past hysterectomy for benign conditions. Womens Health Issues 15(4):179–186
18. Bower JK, Schreiner PJ, Sternfeld B, Lewis CE (2009) Black-White differences in hysterectomy prevalence: the CARDIA study. Am J Public Health 99(2):300–307
19. Sommer B, Avis N, Meyer P et al (1999) Attitudes toward menopause and aging across ethnic/racial groups. Psychosom Med 61(6):868–875
20. Avis NE, Stellato R, Crawford S et al (2001) Is there a menopausal syndrome? Menopausal status and symptoms across racial/ethnic groups. Soc Sci Med 52(3):345–356

Index

H

I

K

L

M

MIX
Papier aus verantwortungsvollen Quellen
Paper from responsible sources
FSC® C105338

If you have any concerns about our products,
you can contact us on
ProductSafety@springernature.com

In case Publisher is established outside the EU,
the EU authorized representative is:
Springer Nature Customer Service Center GmbH
Europaplatz 3, 69115 Heidelberg, Germany

Printed by Libri Plureos GmbH
in Hamburg, Germany